An Atlas of

HUMAN GAMETES AND CONCEPTUSES

An Illustrated Reference for Assisted Reproductive Technology

THE ENCYCLOPEDIA OF VISUAL MEDICINE SERIES

An Atlas of HUMAN GAMETES AND CONCEPTUSES

An Illustrated Reference for Assisted Reproductive Technology

Lucinda L. Veeck, MLT, hDSc

Assistant Professor of Embryology and Director, Embryology Laboratories
The Center for Reproductive Medicine and Infertility
Cornell University Medical College, New York Hospital, New York

Foreword by

Zev Rosenwaks, MD

Revlon Distinguished Professor of Reproductive Medicine in Obstetrics and Gynecology
Professor, Obstetrics and Gynecology
Cornell University Medical College, New York

The Parthenon Publishing Group

International Publishers in Medicine, Science & Technology

NEW YORK LONDON

Library of Congress Cataloging-in-Publication Data
Veeck, Lucinda L.
An atlas of human gametes and conceptuses : an illustrated reference for assisted reproductive technology / Lucinda L. Veeck ; foreword by Zev Rosenwaks.
p. cm. -- (The Encyclopedia of visual medicine series)
Includes bibliographical references and index.
ISBN 1-85070-016-8
1. Fertilization in vitro, Human--Atlases. I. Title. II. Series
[DNLM: 1. Germ Cells--ultrastructure atlases. 2. Germ Cells--growth & development atlases. 3. Blastocyst--ultrastructure atlases. 4. Fertilization in Vitro atlases. WQ 17 V417a 1998]
RG135.V438 1998
618.1'78059--dc21
DNLM/DLC
for Library of Congress 98-26503
CIP

British Library Cataloguing in Publication Data
An atlas of human gametes and conceptuses : an illustrated reference for assisted reproductive technology. – (The encyclopedia of visual medicine series)
1. Gametes 2. Conception 3. Reproductive technology 4. Fertilization in vitro, Human
I. Veeck, Lucinda L.
612.6'4
ISBN 1-85070-016-8

Published in the USA by
The Parthenon Publishing Group Inc.
One Blue Hill Plaza
PO Box 1564, Pearl River
New York 10965, USA

Published in the UK and Europe by
The Parthenon Publishing Group Limited
Casterton Hall, Carnforth
Lancs. LA6 2LA, UK

Printed and bound in Spain
by T.G. Hostench, S.A.

Contents

This work is dedicated to the many couples who suffer from infertility and who bravely seek to overcome it.

Foreword

A prerequisite to the practice of the assisted reproductive technologies, particularly *in vitro* fertilization (IVF), is a thorough understanding of normal gametogenesis and early embryological events. This discipline, more than any other, requires great expertise in the microscopic anatomy of human gametes and preembryos as well as a thorough grounding in the basic physiology of early reproductive processes.

Lucinda Veeck has played a major role in advancing this dynamic discipline with her two previous landmark volumes comprising the *Atlas of the Human Oocyte and Early Conceptus*. In these classic treatises, she meticulously described and catalogued, for the first time, the microanatomy of human oocytes, fertilization, and the critical events in the development of the early human conceptus following IVF. These comprehensive atlases have served as essential reference resources for students, physicians, and laboratory personnel for both learning and practicing the art of human IVF. These seminal contributions were grounded in the belief that a thorough knowledge of, and the ability to recognize, both normal and abnormal maturational processes in human gametes and preembryos are fundamental to the practice of sound laboratory technique and clinical success.

This latest of Lucinda Veeck's outstanding works elegantly depicts a remarkable collection of previously unpublished photographs and graphics obtained with the author's usual meticulous manner. This volume beautifully demonstrates the normal and abnormal morphology of human oocytes, spermatozoa, and preembryos cultured during the course of IVF treatment. Indeed, many of the abnormalities depicted in this exhaustive work have hitherto never been described. This work has been further expanded to include the many remarkable new developments that have taken place in the IVF laboratory. Not only is intracytoplasmic sperm injection described by its pioneers, but other procedures, such as assisted hatching and fragment removal, are also exquisitely illustrated. These magnificent descriptions of micromanipulation techniques pioneered in our unit are complemented by a chapter on preimplantation genetic diagnosis, an exciting new application in IVF technology.

An Atlas of Human Gametes and Conceptuses is a dynamic authoritative work on the microanatomy of normal and abnormal human gametes, fertilization, and human preembryos. It superbly captures the early events of human development and will serve as a most significant and indispensable reference resource to all those involved in the study of human reproduction.

Zev Rosenwaks, MD
Cornell University Medical College, New York

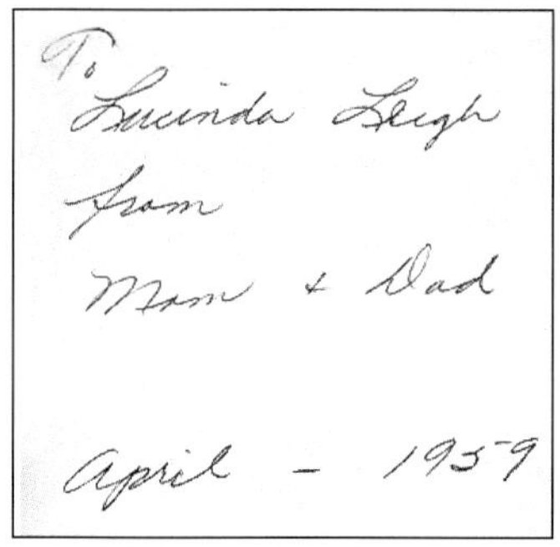

"Until recently, nobody had ever seen a human embryo from the very start. The smallest that had been seen was eleven days old and not larger than, well, just a speck. But today, in this age of wonders, an American scientist made an experiment that broke the record for seeing the earliest beginning of human life. He brought a newly discharged ovum and a new sperm together just at the proper moment (high fertility), put them tenderly in a test tube in his laboratory and was rewarded with the first known, first observed, spark of human existence — the spark that starts the little you or me, the human embryo. This tiny baby lived but a few days, yet it served to show how each of us and the great world about us made their first beginnings."

From *Being Born* by Frances Bruce Strain,
Appleton–Century–Crofts, New York, 1954

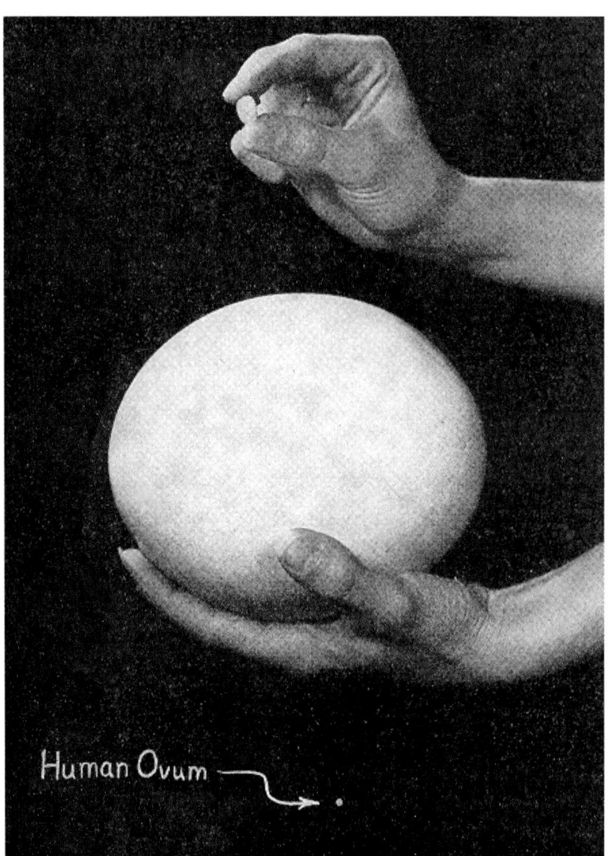

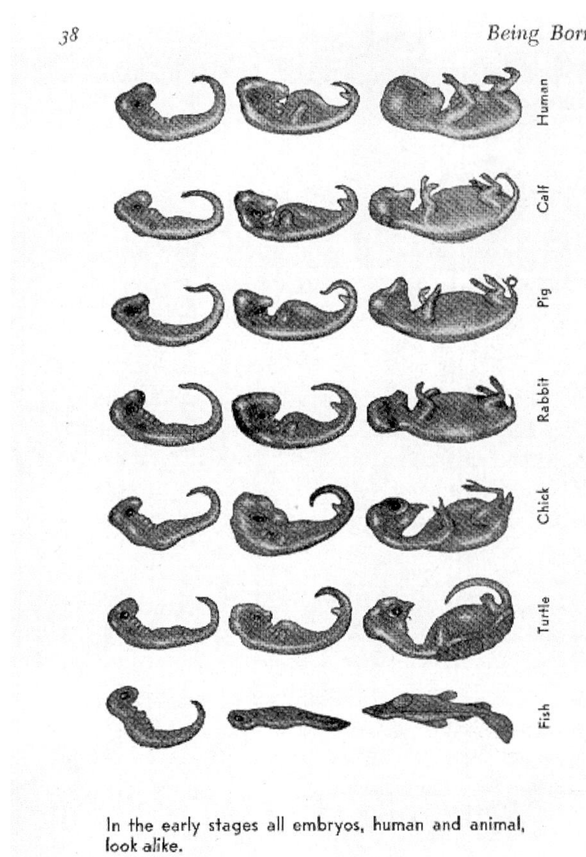
38 *Being Born*

In the early stages all embryos, human and animal, look alike.

Preface

Perhaps my first interest in embryology began with the book, *Being Born,* in 1959. Meant as an educational tool to enlighten an 8-year-old girl in the intimacies of reproduction, it took the edge off having to explain these things in the first-person by proper parents of the 1950s. Having just reread it, I am amazed at how very well it was written and how much valuable information it imparts. From this book, at a very young age, I became familiar with the basic anatomy of male and female reproductive tracts, came to the conclusion that marriage was not a requirement for mating, and learned that the gestational period of the elephant was 600 days. When a confounding question arose during puberty, I always looked for reference in this book; it was gentle and tactful, yet informative. It set the stage for a life-long interest in genetics and reproduction.

Twenty years later, when I joined Eastern Virginia Medical School in January of 1979, I was 28 years old, fresh from taking the National Board Examinations, and excited about the future. Who could not be excited about the changing events in infertility treatment? The first birth after *in vitro* fertilization (IVF) had recently been reported from the United Kingdom. There was soon to be a surprisingly large local and national debate over our intention to establish the first clinic offering IVF technology in the United States. The newspapers and local community were excited; so were we.

Since then, the scientific advances have been most extraordinary. We have matured in our laboratory methods, from collecting and culturing a single oocyte from the natural cycle to treating intractable male infertility with microsurgical techniques, storing healthy preembryos through cryopreservation, and diagnosing inherited gene defects before implantation.

My first laboratory at the Norfolk General Hospital was located on a labor and delivery floor, and was no larger in size than a generous walk-in closet. A single incubator served as home for oocytes collected from those first brave patients embracing the new and controversial technology of IVF. I recall feeling the pain of those couples as they walked past the nursery viewing area and gazed at the newborn infants on their way to the operating room for an arduous laparoscopic oocyte retrieval. I also remember the anguish I felt when an oocyte was not successfully collected or failed to become fertilized *in vitro*. I felt then, and still do, a deep and personal guilt when events do not go as well as anticipated.

On the other hand, the joy associated with successfully treating a difficult infertility problem cannot be overstated. The entire team relishes these happy moments, probably to an extent that passes unrecognized by patients over the telephone or during follow-up consultation. These successes keep us going despite the long hours and often stressful workload. These successes motivate us to continue our attempts to overcome the next stubborn obstacle to the natural desire that we as humans possess for forming a family unit.

Today, I am fortunate to be moving into new laboratories within New York Hospital in Manhattan. Five separate areas define spaces for andrology and cryopreservation, oocyte and preembryo culture, micromanipulation, preimplantation genetic diagnosis, and endometrial cell coculture. Research facilities are located at three separate locations. No fewer than 20 incubators now serve our work, and the range of complex and modern equipment is impressive. Such a long road we have traveled since 1979!

All along the way, we have been in a partnership with our patients in the quest to combat childlessness. Working together, the majority of couples will achieve their goal, especially so if treatment commences before the female partner enters her fourth decade of life. Nevertheless, it is a difficult and emotionally vexing process. For this reason, I dedicate this work to our patients, to those who have been successful and, most particularly, to those who are still trying.

Lucinda L. Veeck
New York

Acknowledgements

Sincere appreciation is extended to the physicians, scientists, nurses, technicians, and support staff of the Center for Reproductive Medicine and Infertility of Cornell University Medical College / New York Hospital for their support of this work, and to Laurel Halsey, who helped with the references and editing.

Special acknowledgement is given to those who contributed photographic material or text:

Dr Robert Bargalló, Dr Simón Marina, Silvia Menéndez, MS, Dr Maureen Moomjy, Dr Gianpiero Palermo, Dr Zev Rosenwaks, Dr Kangpu Xu, Zhen Ye, and Nikica Zaninovic.

The author also wishes to thank Drs Berrin Ergun and Takumi Takeuchi for assisting Dr Palermo in preparing the manuscript for Chapter 10 on assisted fertilization by intracytoplasmic sperm injection.

All figures, except for the electronmicrographs in Chapter 3 and the fluorescence microscopy in Chapters 8, 11 and 12, were photographed using a Nikon Diaphot microscope equipped with a Sony CatsEye camera.

Finally, Parthenon Publishing is responsible for the excellent format and layout of the photographs selected for inclusion in this atlas.

Section I A Review of Human Gametes and Conceptuses

1 Gamete maturation

Sexual differentiation and germ cells

Gonadal sex is determined by testis-determining factor (TDF), which is coded on the short arm of the Y chromosome. TDF directs testicular differentiation. In the XY embryo, Leydig cells produce testosterone to stimulate the development of male genital ducts and, eventually, male genitalia. Müllerian inhibiting factor (MIF), produced by testicular Sertoli cells, further inhibits the development of female ducts. Alternatively, in the absence of TDF and MIF, and in the presence of two X chromosomes, ovaries develop.

The primordia that give rise to the gonads are identical in both sexes. During the early undifferentiated stage, the embryo possesses the potential to develop into either a phenotypic male or phenotypic female. Although genetic sex is established at fertilization by the participation of either an X-bearing or Y-bearing spermatozoon, the embryonic gonad does not attain sexual characteristics until around week 7, and fetal genitalia do not acquire masculine or feminine characteristics until week 12.

Primordial germ cells form during week 4 of gestation and migrate into developing embryonic gonads, where they differentiate into definitive germ cells called *oogonia* or *(pre)spermatogonia.*

The spermatozoon

Spermatogenesis comprises several stages: *mitotic division of spermatogonia; meiotic divisions of spermatocytes;* and *transformation of round spermatids into spermatozoa (spermiogenesis).* Over his lifetime, a man may produce as many as two trillion or more spermatozoa. All of these are descended from only 1000–2000 diploid spermatogonia, which were generated through mitosis in the fetal testis. An *early type A, intermediate stage* and a *late type B* generation of spermatogonia can be clearly distinguished by microscopy. Type A spermatogonia are classified into four increasingly differentiated subtypes (A1–A4), which are continuously generated from undifferentiated type A throughout adult life.

Type A spermatogonia pass through the intermediate stage to become type B. These undergo mitotic divisions to form diploid primary spermatocytes. After a lengthy prophase, the first meiotic division results in two haploid secondary spermatocytes. The second meiotic division gives rise to four haploid round spermatids. Further maturation involving growth of the tail and loss of cytoplasm then occurs as round spermatids are transformed into spermatozoa, which possess both motility and fertilizing potential.

As genetic sex is determined by whether a spermatozoon contributes an X or a Y chromosome to the embryo, it is reasonable to expect the primary sex ratio of conceptuses at fertilization to be 1.00 (100 males per 100 females). However, in reality, more female than male embryos are lost in early pregnancy, as the actual secondary sex ratio observed at birth is approximately 1.05 (105 males per 100 females).

The oocyte

Once ovarian differentiation has taken place, the female germ cells are called *oogonia*. These cells divide mitotically over several months before the process of meiosis is initiated. The enormous increase in the number of oogonia produced by mitotic divisions results in each female beginning her life with over half a million germ cells. Shortly after the last mitotic division of the oogonium, the cell enters an interphase, when DNA is replicated in preparation for meiosis I.

In the human ovary, the transformation of oogonia into oocytes begins from month 3 or 4 of gestation; by the time of birth, all germ cells are oocytes and the meiotic process is arrested (first meiotic arrest). The oocyte, with a prominent nucleus or germinal vesicle, rests in the diplotene stage (also called the *dictyate stage*), which persists through infancy until just before ovulation.

Meiotic events

Meiosis is termed *cell reduction* because it reduces the number of chromosomes in the gamete to a haploid number (n; 23 chromosomes). When a mature oocyte with a haploid number of chromosomes unites with a mature spermatozoon of haploid number, a diploid zygote (2n; 46 chromosomes) is formed.

Meiosis also creates new gene combinations by mixing the parent chromosomes; for example, each oogonium and spermatogonium possesses a pair of number 1 chromosomes, one from each parent. During meiosis I, replicated homologs exchange genetic material between them so that gametes inherit chromosomes that are derived from, but not identical to, the homologous pair from the parents. This genetic exchange is responsible for the variation in phenotype found in all sexually reproducing organisms.

Meiosis is a complex and important process. It provides the means for maintaining a constant number of chromosomes from generation to generation and spawns genetic diversity through mixing maternal and paternal chromosomes **and** genes.

Meiosis has two stages, meiosis I and meiosis II (Figure 1.1). During meiosis I, the homologs separate whereas, during meiosis II, the chromatids separate. The result of this is four cells (four spermatids which mature into spermatozoa in the male; one oocyte plus two or three polar bodies in the female), each with a haploid set of chromosomes (Figure 1.2).

Unlike meiosis in the male, meiosis in the female results in only one viable gamete containing the bulk of cytoplasm and several smaller polar bodies. Thus, the majority of the cytoplasmic components of the oocyte are conserved for use during future early embryogenesis. Theoretically, three polar bodies should be formed as a result of meiotic divisions in the oocyte: one during meiosis I, and two during meiosis II. However, in reality, first polar bodies rarely divide during meiosis II.

Meiosis I has a complex prophase, which is divided into five substages: leptotene; zygotene; pachytene; diplotene; and diakinesis. Meiosis II has only a brief prophase as there has been no replication of DNA and no genetic material is exchanged. Both stages of meiosis have metaphase, anaphase, and telophase components.

Meiosis I

Prophase I

(1) **Leptotene** Nuclear chromatin begins to condense; both ends of the chromosomes are attached to the nuclear envelope.

(2) **Zygotene** Homologous chromosomes align side-by-side and attach to one another (point-by-point pairing), thus allowing homologous loci to come into contact or to *synapse*. A definite structural material, termed the *synaptinemal complex*, holds chromosomes close and is the likely site for the exchange of genetic material. This exchange is

called *crossing-over* or *recombination*. Each set of synapsed homologs is called a *bivalent* as the two chromosomes do not yet appear differentiated into chromatids. Zygotene ends when all homologs have been paired.

(3) **Pachytene** Bivalents become shorter and thicker. At this stage, the bivalent, because of its four closely opposed chromatids, is termed a *tetrad*. *Crossing-over* (the exchange of genetic material between non-sister chromatids of paired homologous chromosomes) occurs.

(4) **Diplotene** Tetrads come apart except at one or more certain points called *chiasmata* where crossing-over has occurred. Chromosomes take on a cross-like appearance. At this point, in females, meiosis is halted before diakinesis. Many thousands of oocytes remain in this stage (also called the *dictyate stage* or *dictyotene stage*) until just before ovulation or degeneration, and perhaps for more than 50 years. In the oocyte, this stage is marked by the morphological appearance of a germinal vesicle.

(5) **Diakinesis** The primary oocyte or primary spermatocyte (Figure 1.3 and Table 1.1) begins a period of dramatic growth under stimulation. The nucleolus dissipates and the nuclear envelope disappears.

Metaphase I

A spindle is formed and the chromosomes line up on the equatorial plate. In females, the spindle is off-center and, by its position, determines which of the daughter cells will inherit most of the cytoplasm. Those chromosomes of rearranged maternal and paternal origin line up randomly toward the poles, and whole chromosomes sort independently to daughter cells. In this manner, maternal and paternal chromosomes are mixed and can theoretically result in more than 8 000 000 chromosomally different gametes (2^{23}). In the oocyte, this stage is marked by the absence of the germinal vesicle before first polar-body extrusion.

Table 1.1 Comparison of meiosis duration in females compared with males

Oogonium	Formed in fetal life (month 2 or 3 of gestation)	**Spermatogonium**	Formed in fetal life / throughout adult life
OOGENESIS begins during embryogenesis		**SPERMATOGENESIS begins at puberty**	
Primary oocyte	Formed in fetal life; remains in meiosis I until ovulation 12–50 years after formation	**Primary spermatocyte**	~16 days
Secondary oocyte	Formed after puberty; usually viable for < 1 day until fertilization occurs	**Secondary spermatocyte**	~16 days
Pronuclear oocyte	Approximately 12 h (requires fertilization)	**Spermatid**	~16 days
Zygote		**Mature sperm**	
Total time	**12–50 years**	**Total time**	**~48 days**

Anaphase I

Whole chromosomes, with centromeres intact, move to opposite ends of the cells.

Telophase I

Cell division occurs and daughter cells are formed. In the male, two *secondary spermatocytes* are formed; in the female, one *secondary oocyte* and one *polar body* are formed, and are connected by a cytoplasmic bridge. The nuclear envelope reforms and the chromosomes remain attached to it until meiosis II.

Meiosis II

Prophase II

There is no replication of DNA in interphase and, therefore, no synapsis. The chromosomes condense and begin to move towards the equator of the cell.

Metaphase II

The nuclear envelope again disappears and the spindle reforms. The 23 chromosomes, each with two chromatids, line up on the equatorial or metaphase plate. Spindle fibers attach to the centromeres. Although only a haploid set of double-stranded chromosomes is present, there is still a diploid amount of DNA because the strands have not yet separated. Secondary oocytes arrest at this stage until sperm penetration or environmental activation triggers the resumption of meiosis II (Figure 1.4); secondary spermatocytes continue into anaphase without arrest.

Anaphase II

Chromatids split at the centromeres and move to opposite ends of the cell. This occurs in oocytes only after an activating factor has stimulated the resumption of meiosis (sperm penetration, chemical exposure or environmental / electrical trauma).

Telophase II

Cell division occurs. In males, four round spermatids (1 n) are produced from the original single spermatogonium and undergo maturation in the male reproductive tract before they participate in unassisted fertilization events; in females, the activated (presumably fertilized) oocyte continues to retain the bulk of the cytoplasm and a second polar body inherits a smaller amount. Unlike meiosis in the male wherein four viable spermatozoa are likely to represent the endpoint of meiotic and biochemical maturation, in the female, only the oocyte itself is viable; polar bodies degenerate over time.

Suggested reading

Austin CR. *The Mammalian Egg*. Oxford: Blackwell Scientific Publications, 1961:21

Baker TG. Oogenesis and ovulation. In: Austin CR, Short RV, eds. *Germ Cells and Fertilization, Book 1, 2nd edn*. Cambridge: Cambridge University Press, 1982:17

Beatty RA. The genetics of the mammalian gamete. *Biol Rev* 1970;45:73

Byskov AG. Primordial germ cells and regulation of meiosis. In: Austin CR, Short RV, eds. *Germ Cells and Fertilization, Book 1, 2nd edn*. Cambridge: Cambridge University Press, 1982:1

Fowler RE, Edwards RG. The genetics of early human development. *Prog Med Genet* 1973;9:49

Grootegoed JA. The testis: Spermatogenesis. In: Hillier SG, Kitchener HC, Neilson JP, eds. *Scientific Essentials of Reproductive Medicine*. London: W.B. Saunders, 1996:172

Lindner HR, Bar-Ami S, Tsafriri A. Control of the resumption of meiosis in mammals. In: Serra GB, ed. *The Ovary*. New York: Raven Press, 1983:83

2 The human oocyte

General structure

In most species, there are only two types of gametes, each of which is radically different from the other. Except for motor neurons with their remarkably long axons, the oocyte is among the largest cells of the human organism. In contrast, spermatozoa and red blood cells are two of the smallest.

The diameter of the mature human oocyte is approximately 110–115 μm and bounded by a plasma membrane called the *oolemma*. Surrounding the oocyte / oolemma is a glycoprotein envelope called the *zona pellucida*, a structure approximately 15–20 μm wide (becoming slightly thinner after fertilization) that protects the oocyte during transport and fertilization. Between the oolemma and the zona pellucida is the fluid-filled *perivitelline space*. The use of this term persists despite its inaccuracy when describing the oocytes of humans or most other mammals; it acknowledges the word *vitellus*, traditionally used to describe the yolky substance of a hen's egg, which contains abundant nutrient reserves. The cytoplasm of the mammalian oocyte is usually referred to as the *ooplasm*, a more appropriate term for describing the living portion of the human gamete. The main organelles of the ooplasm are the mitochondria, the endoplasmic reticulum, and the Golgi system.

When fully capable of undergoing a normal fertilization process, the secondary oocyte is briefly arrested in its course of maturation at metaphase II (MII) of meiosis. Nuclear maturation is usually closely attended by a general maturation of the cytoplasm and is characterized by an increase in the number of organelles scattered throughout the ooplasm. The presence of a first polar body indicates that nuclear maturation has reached this stage.

With the added breadth of the zona pellucida and perivitelline space, the entire structure of the preovulatory oocyte and its shell ultimately spans a diameter of 150 μm (Figure 2.1).

An oocyte incubated with spermatozoa before reaching M II may incorporate a spermatozoon into its ooplasm and yet fail to initiate events leading to sperm decondensation; such an oocyte ultimately lacks a functional male pronucleus[1]. One study, involving examination of 518 non-fertilized oocytes, demonstrated that 22% had, in fact, been penetrated by sperm, but without oocyte activation or pronuclear formation[2]. Many of these oocytes may have been immature at the time they were combined with spermatozoa.

In addition to the requirement of nuclear maturation, it is believed that a brief lapse of time is necessary after extrusion of the first polar body to allow the oocyte to gain full cytoplasmic competence. An oocyte that is meiotically mature, but slightly under- or overdeveloped with regard to its cytoplasm, may be more apt to display one, three or more pronuclei. With immature cytoplasm, the cortical granule numbers and response may be inadequate; with post-mature cytoplasm, cortical granule release may be inhibited due to the inward migration of the granules towards the interior of the cell. In either instance, there is evidence that the zona reaction also often functions poorly when sperm / oocyte interaction is not appropriately timed with regard to oocyte nuclear and cytoplasmic maturity[3].

Oocytes collected for *in vitro* fertilization (IVF) are generally surrounded by several layers of cells which define the *cumulus oophorus*. Cells of the cumulus are instrumental, *via* gap junctions, in nurturing the oocyte during growth and possibly in passing inhibiting factors, such as adenosine 3′:5′-cyclic phosphate (cAMP), necessary for deterring the resumption of meiosis[4]. The innermost layer of cells is called the *corona* or *coronal layer*. This layer expands and presents a radiant pattern as oocytes mature in response to exogenous human chorionic gonadotropin (hCG) or a midcycle surge of luteinizing hormone (LH). Near ovulation, as they loosen and expand, cumulus cells are observed to retract from the zona pellucida of the oocyte, presumably cutting off the previously important cellular / oocyte communication. It has been proposed that oocytes not associated with proliferative cellular changes near ovulation have limited potential for implantation despite fertilization and apparently normal development *in vitro*[5].

In most mammalian species studied *in vivo*, the oocyte arrives at the site of fertilization in the ampulla of the Fallopian tube still surrounded by the cumulus mass. The cumulus may play a role in assisting transport of the oocyte into the Fallopian tube through fimbrial cilia / cumulus cell contact. It has also been proposed that the radially arranged cells of the cumulus after oocyte maturation may help to guide spermatozoa towards the oocyte just before fertilization; however, there is no hard evidence for this speculation. Breakdown of the cumulus mass is brought about by dissolution of its mucoid hyaluronic acid matrix by enzymes released by the spermatozoa.

Follicular *membrana granulosa cells* dissociated from cumulus cells are found in follicular aspirates collected for *in vitro* fertilization (IVF). The number of cells collected varies from follicle to follicle according to the extent of negative pressure exerted during suction, the size of the needle, and the overall maturity of the follicle. As with cumulus cells, the correlation between morphological aspects of free granulosa cells and oocyte nuclear maturity is not exact, but apparently mature cells (large well-dispersed cells) are generally collected along with mature oocytes, and apparently immature cells (smaller tightly packed cells) with immature oocytes. Follicular membrana granulosa cells may be assessed at the time of oocyte harvest to aid in the evaluation of follicular maturity. These cells are often subsequently used during studies *in vitro* to examine metabolic activity or steroid synthesis.

The oocyte observed while its chromosomes are at metaphase I (M I) of maturation lacks a first polar body and requires time in culture before attaining full meiotic competence[6]. More than 98% of these oocytes complete their journey towards M II and first polar-body extrusion (Figure 2.2).

Oocytes with chromosomes at prophase I (P I) of maturation exhibit a nucleus or germinal vesicle. More than 80% of these continue through M I to M II if isolated and incubated in an appropriate medium for 24 h (Figure 2.3).

Assessment of maturity

By tradition, evaluation of oocyte maturity has been based upon the expansion and radiance of the cumulus / corona complex which surrounds the harvested oocyte[7,8]. At this assessment, oocytes are rapidly categorized as 'mature' (which correlates to M II of maturation), when they possess an expanded and luteinized cumulus matrix and a radiant or *sunburst* corona radiata (Figure 2.4). A less-expanded cumulus / corona complex denotes an intermediate stage of maturity (which correlates to M I of maturation), and the absence of an expanded cumulus is generally associated with immaturity (which correlates to P I of maturation). Although this type of analysis usually closely approximates the true nuclear status of the oocyte, it is too often imprecise and may lead to subsequent laboratory errors in the handling of gametes.

Indeed, nuclear maturation of the oocyte and cellular maturation of the cumulus are frequently disparate[8–12]. When disparity occurs, immature oocytes may be inseminated prematurely and fail to produce a favorable outcome. In addition to fertilization failure, other detrimental side-effects accompany combining sperm and eggs at suboptimal times; ovulation-induction protocols may not be suitably appraised and male factor issues become difficult to interpret when based on poor fertilization results.

Because of these pitfalls, techniques have been developed to assess more accurately the meiotic status of the oocyte. A systematic approach, which can be used to produce a *maturation score*, grades the size of the follicle, expansion of the cumulus mass, radiance of the corona cells, size / cohesiveness of associated membrana granulosa cells, and shape / color of the oocyte itself, if visible within the mass of surrounding cellular investments (Figures 2.5 and 2.6). Alternatively, frank visualization of the oocyte and its germinal vesicle or first polar body can be attempted by spreading out the cumulus mass or by removing it altogether with the aid of enzymes.

If clearly visible or denuded of cells, oocytes are classified according to the presence or absence of first polar bodies / germinal vesicles and are inseminated or injected as follows:

Metaphase II (M II) First polar body present, no germinal vesicle; inseminated or injected 3–5 h after collection;

Metaphase I (M I) No first polar body, no germinal vesicle; inseminated or injected 1–5 h after extrusion of the first polar body;

Prophase I (P I) Germinal vesicle present; inseminated or injected 26–29 h after collection.

Our experience has been that oocytes collected at more advanced stages of maturation *in vivo* demonstrate the greatest ability to form two pronuclei after insemination[6,13,14]. Fertilization rates drop only slightly during the 5–15 h of culture required by oocytes before extruding the first polar body, but fertilization is markedly reduced when more than 15 h pass before the maturational process is completed. The reason for this is probably related to sperm functionality as well as oocyte maturity as processed sperm may be >24 h old before being placed with an early M I or P I oocyte. Under these conditions, the precise cause of the lower incidence of fertilization of very immature oocytes is difficult to interpret[6].

Approximately 20–30% of oocytes collected for IVF are meiotically immature at the time of harvest from the ovary. This is undoubtedly due to the stimulation of multiple follicles during clinical ovulation induction, some of which are large and well vascularized, but others small, having been recruited late. If all oocytes are placed with sperm at the same time, then slightly more than 20–30% will fail to become fertilized normally. Thus, it follows logically that, when oocytes are placed with sperm only when they have reached full maturity, far better fertilization results are attained.

The incidence of abnormal fertilization (one pronucleus, three or more pronuclei) does not differ between M II oocytes and M I or P I oocytes that have matured in culture before insemination or injection[6,13,14]. Pregnancy potential after the transfer of preembryos developed from M II and M I oocytes is similar regardless of whether 0 h or 20 h has been required for maturation before insemination or injection[15]. Only preembryos developing from P I oocytes demonstrate a significantly reduced potential for implantation and live birth, although such births are certainly within the realm of possibility[6,16–19].

Metaphase II oocyte

The M II oocyte is often termed *mature, ripened*, or *preovulatory*, vague descriptions that fail to specify the exact meiotic status of the gamete. This oocyte is at a resting stage of meiosis II after extrusion of the first polar body and direct passage to M II.

Chromosomes are divided between the oocyte and the polar body (23 chromosomes, 46 chromatids, 2 n DNA in each), with those in the oocyte attached to spindle microtubules[1].

For a while after its formation, the first polar body remains connected to the oocyte by the meiotic spindle, forming a cytoplasmic bridge. Chromosomes within the first polar body may either remain clumped together, undergo a second meiotic division, or scatter within the cytoplasm; usually, a nucleus is not formed[1,20]. The first polar body contains cortical granules because of its extrusion before sperm penetration and cortical-granule release; in the oocyte, one to three layers of cortical granules are present at the periphery.

Under the microscope, the oocyte is characterized by a round, even shape and displays an ooplasm of a light color and homogeneous granularity (Figures 2.7–2.12). It is usually associated with an expanded luteinized cumulus and a sunburst corona radiata. Membrana granulosa cells harvested along with the M II oocyte are loosely aggregated and display features of maturity[6,8,11,19].

Metaphase I oocyte

The M I oocyte is considered nearly mature or intermediate in maturation (Figure 2.13). The oocyte has completed prophase of meiosis I; the germinal vesicle and its nucleolus have faded and disappeared. During this stage, a spindle forms, and recombined maternal and paternal chromosomes line up randomly towards the poles. Later, at telophase, whole chromosomes sort independently to either oocyte or first polar body.

An M I oocyte requires 1–24 h in culture before reaching full maturity. Those requiring < 15 h are considered late in maturity whereas those needing > 15 h are defined as early[6,8,11–14].

Under the microscope, the M I oocyte is characterized by the absence of both the germinal vesicle and first polar body. A late M I oocyte is round and even in form, with a homogeneously granular and light-colored ooplasm (Figures 2.14 and 2.15). Early M I oocytes may display minor central granularity (Figures 2.16 and 2.17). Mature-appearing (luteinized) cumulus cells are usually associated with late stages.

Because first polar-body extrusion can occur at any time after harvest, it is necessary to examine the oocyte at regular intervals to determine the correct timing for insemination. If sperm are placed with the oocyte before nuclear and cytoplasmic maturation are complete, they generally fail to decondense within the ooplasm, or abnormal fertilization occurs. If insemination is delayed too long, aging *in vitro* may follow, with similar undesirable consequences[1,6].

Prophase I oocyte

The P I oocyte is often termed *immature* or *unripened*. It possesses a tetraploid amount of DNA due to the presence of 46 double-stranded chromosomes. This oocyte begins to mature in response to gonadotropin surges and reduction of follicular maturation-inhibiting factors. The germinal vesicle, which has persisted throughout earlier growth phases, begins its progression to germinal-vesicle breakdown (GVBD), and the oocyte enlarges (Figure 2.18). Most P I oocytes collected for IVF have been stimulated to resume meiosis, are in the final stages of the first meiotic prophase, and have already reached full size. If a spermatozoon penetrates this immature oocyte, it will fail to promote activation, as the oocyte is not meiotically mature and its chromosomes will undergo premature condensation[21].

GVBD may occur within minutes or require up to several hours after harvest; the length of time necessary appears to depend on how far maturational events have progressed within the follicle before collection. More than 80% succeed in passing through M I of maturation to ultimately reach M II[6].

The germinal vesicle, or nucleus, of the human oocyte is spherical and contains a large refractile exocentric nucleolus (Figures 2.19–2.21). Upon closer examination, a second smaller nucleolus may be detected. The germinal vesicle is centrally located within the ooplasm of young PI oocytes and in those exhibiting developmental arrest (Figure 2.22). It migrates to a more cortical position in healthy oocytes before GVBD. The dissolution of the germinal vesicle marks the first practical microscopic indication that meiosis has resumed. As the oocyte matures, defenses against polyspermy are established in the form of cortical granule accumulation and alignment at the oocyte periphery. These granules are sparse and discontinuous in immature oocytes[1].

On microscopy, the PI oocyte is characterized by its distinct germinal vesicle and refractile nucleolus. An irregular shape, a darkened center, and granular ooplasm are almost always displayed (Figures 2.23 and 2.24). Attached cumulus cells are usually compact and multilayered, but may be proliferative. Free follicular membrana granulosa cells within the immature follicle are usually small and found in compact masses. PI oocytes with mature characteristics of the cumulus (expanded appearance and a very radiant corona) generally fail to undergo GVBD[11,12].

References

1. Sathananthan AH, Trounson AO, Wood C. *Atlas of Fine Structure of Human Sperm Penetration, Eggs, and Embryos Cultured in Vitro.* New York: Praeger, 1986:2(penetration of immature oocytes); 4(chromosomes and spindle microtubules);10(cortical granules);42,126 (oocyte aging);90(polar body nucleus)

2. Van Blerkom J, Davis PW, Merriam J. A retrospective analysis of unfertilized and presumed parthenogenetically activated human oocytes demonstrates a high frequency of sperm penetration. *Hum Reprod* 1994;9:2381

3. Edwards RG. *Conception in the Human Female.* New York: Academic Press, 1980:634

4. Dekel N, Beers WH. Development of the rat oocyte in vitro: Inhibition and induction of maturation in the presence or absence of the cumulus oophorus. *Dev Biol* 1980;75:247

5. Gregory L, Booth AD, Wells C, Walker SM. A study of the cumulus-corona cell complex in in-vitro fertilization and embryo transfer; a prognostic indicator of the failure of implantation. *Hum Reprod* 1994;9: 1308

6. Veeck LL. Oocyte assessment and biological performance. *Ann NY Acad Sci* 1988;541:259

7. Veeck LL. Extracorporeal maturation, Norfolk, Virginia. *Ann NY Acad Sci* 1985;442:357

8. Veeck LL. The morphologic estimation of mature oocytes and their preparation for insemination. In: Jones HW Jr, Jones GS, Hodgen GD, Rosenwaks Z, eds. *In Vitro Fertilization – Norfolk.* Baltimore: Williams & Wilkins, 1986:81

9. Hammitt DG, Syrop CH, Van Voorhis BJ, *et al.* Maturational asynchrony between oocyte cumulus–coronal morphology and nuclear maturity in gonadotropin-releasing hormone agonist stimulations. *Fertil Steril* 1993;59:375

10. Laufer N, Tarlatzis BC, DeCherney AH, *et al.* Asynchrony between human cumulus-corona cell complex and oocyte maturation after human menopausal gonadotropin treatment for in vitro fertilization. *Fertil Steril* 1984;42:366

11. Veeck LL. *Atlas of the Human Oocyte and Early Conceptus, Vol I.* Baltimore: Williams & Wilkins, 1986:7,127(mature granulosa);57,68(oocyte classification);74(disparity between cumulus and nucleus)

12. Veeck LL. *Atlas of the Human Oocyte and Early Conceptus, Vol II.* Baltimore: Williams & Wilkins, 1991:3,13,27(membrana granulosa);13(oocyte classification);27(disparity between cumulus and nucleus)

13. Veeck LL. Pregnancy rate and pregnancy outcome associated with laboratory evaluation of spermatozoa, oocytes, and preembryos. In: Mashiach S, Ben-Rafael Z, Laufer N, Schenker JG, eds. *Advances in Assisted Reproductive Technologies.* New York: Plenum Press, 1990:745

14. Veeck LL. The morphological assessment of human oocytes and early concepti. In: Keel BA, Webster BW, eds. *Handbook of the Laboratory Diagnosis and Treatment of Infertility.* Boca Raton: CRC Press, 1990:353

15. Coetzee K, Windt ML. Fertilization and pregnancy using metaphase I oocytes in an intracytoplasmic sperm injection program. *J Assist Reprod Genet* 1996;13:768

16. Barnes FL, Crombie A, Gardner DK, *et al.* Blastocyst development and birth after in-vitro maturation of human primary oocytes, intracytoplasmic sperm injection, and assisted hatching. *Hum Reprod* 1995; 10:3243

17. Cha KY, Koo JJ, Choi DH, *et al.* Pregnancy after in vitro fertilization of human follicular oocytes collected from non-stimulated cycles, their culture in vitro, and their transfer in a donor oocyte program. *Fertil Steril* 1991;55:109

18. Liu J, Katz E, Garcia JE, *et al.* Successful in vitro maturation of human oocytes not exposed to human chorionic gonadotropin during ovulation induction, resulting in pregnancy. *Fertil Steril* 1997;67:566

19. Veeck LL, Wortham JWE, Witmyer J, *et al.* Maturation and fertilization of morphologically immature human oocytes in a program of in vitro fertilization. *Fertil Steril* 1983;39:594

20. Austin CR. *The Mammalian Egg.* Oxford: Blackwell Scientific Publications, 1961:75

21. Plachot M, Crozet N. Fertilization abnormalities in human in vitro fertilization. *Hum Reprod* 1992; 7(Suppl 1):89

3 The human spermatozoon

Silvia Menéndez, MS and Simón Marina, MD

Spermatogenesis

Spermatogenesis is the sequence of events that begins at puberty after the preparatory period of prespermatogenesis in the fetus and infant. The process takes place in the testis, specifically, inside the seminiferous tubules, and leads to the production of functional male gametes. Basically, under the control of the central nervous system, the anterior pituitary gonadotropins follicle-stimulating hormone (FSH) and luteinizing hormone (LH) are the agents that directly affect adult testicular function and spermatogenesis, as has been known for more than 60 years[1].

FSH and LH are synthesized by stimulation of gonadotropin-releasing hormone (GnRH) in the same cells of the pituitary, termed the gonadotrophs. FSH receptors are localized to Sertoli cells whereas LH receptors are localized to Leydig cells in the interstitium. Leydig cells are stimulated by LH and synthesize testosterone, which passes to the lumen of the seminiferous tubules. FSH and testosterone are the main agents responsible for spermatogenesis. Spermatozoa can be considered the secretory product of spermatogenesis.

The histology of the testis depends on the stage of sexual development. The lamina propria surrounds the germinal tissue which, in the fertile adult, contains all germ cells at different maturation stages. The supporting elements of the germinal tissue are the Sertoli cells, which are non-mitotic and fixed in their location. They have a foot on the basal lamina and extend between the germ cells to the lumen of the seminiferous tubules. Sertoli cells have specialized cell junctions (tight junctions). These junctions divide the seminiferous tubule into two compartments, basal and luminal. The basal compartment houses the spermatogonia, and the luminal compartment contains the rest of the spermatogenic cells. Each compartment has its own environment, which is maintained by tight junctions. In the interstitium are found Leydig cells, fibrocytes and blood vessels.

During spermatogenesis, diploid spermatogonia divide by mitosis to replicate and produce cells that enter the spermatogenic process. Three types of spermatogonia can be clearly distinguished[2]: type A dark spermatogonium; type A pale spermatogonium (intermediate); and type B. Type A remain at the basement membrane to maintain the germ cell line. Type B are the immediate precursors of primary spermatocytes. Spermatogonial cell divisions are incomplete as the daughter cells remain interconnected by cytoplasmic bridges that are dissolved only in advanced stages of spermatid development. Because maturing spermatogonia and spermatocytes fail to complete cytokinesis, the progeny of a single spermatogonium develop as a syncytium.

Each primary spermatocyte undergoes meiosis I, forming two haploid secondary spermatocytes (see Chapter 1). Secondary spermatocytes contain half the number of chromosomes, but the total DNA content is equivalent to that of diploid cells, as each chromosome is composed of a pair of daughter chromatids. After a short period of time, meiosis II occurs and the chromatids of each chromosome separate to daughter cells, called spermatids. Each of the two spermatids contains a haploid number of chromosomes and half the DNA content of secondary spermatocytes.

Each spermatid differentiates into a spermatozoon through a process called spermiogenesis, which ends when the male gametes are released from the Sertoli cells to the lumen of the seminiferous tubules (Figure 3.1). The process of spermiogenesis is simply a cellular differentiation without division, which involves the following stages[3]:

(1) Fusion of the proacrosomic granules and subsequent spreading of the early acrosome over the nucleus (Figure 3.2);

(2) Rounding of the nucleus (Figure 3.3). In this stage, the tail begins its development, which continues throughout the entire process of spermiogenesis;

(3) Further development of the acrosomal cap;

(4) Elongation of the nucleus and its movement to an eccentric position, towards the basement membrane of the seminiferous tubule (Figure 3.4);

(5) Progressive nuclear condensation;

(6) Reduction and shedding of cytoplasm, resulting in the residual body; the spermatid at this stage has become more flattened and oval as a result of further nuclear condensation. In this process, mitochondria migrate to the proximal portion of the tail to form the midpiece (Figure 3.5).

Late spermatids progressively lose their contact with Sertoli cells. The release of mature spermatids from the epithelium is called spermiation and the released cell is termed a spermatozoon when it is finally shed into the lumen of the tubule. Spermiation may be altered due to inadequate hormonal support or exposure to chemicals[4]. Cells that are not released normally are phagocytosed by Sertoli cells.

After their release into the lumen of the tubule, spermatozoa are transported through the epididymis to the ejaculatory duct. During their passage through the epididymis, spermatozoa undergo maturation, involving morphological, physiological and metabolic changes. This maturation depends mainly on testicular androgens, but also involves the secretory and absorptive activity of the principal cells (Figure 3.6) in the epididymal epithelium[5]. The presence of lymphocytes in the epididymis may favor an immunological reaction[5] (Figure 3.7).

There is now strong evidence for the existence of genes on the Y chromosome that regulate spermatogenesis. Using DNA probes, reports of submicroscopic chromosomal Yq deletions in azoospermic men have been documented[6].

A review of the literature of somatic chromosome investigations in infertile males has shown that 13.7% of azoospermic males and 4.6% of oligozoospermic males have abnormal karyotypes. Sex chromosome abnormalities predominate in azoospermic men (mostly 47,XXY) whereas Robertsonian and reciprocal translocations are more frequent in oligozoospermic men[7].

Spermatozoon morphology

The evaluation of sperm morphology has greatly changed over the last two decades. The percentage of normal forms considered acceptable for an ejaculate has also been modified (lowered)[8–13]. The following facts may explain these changes:

(1) Every ejaculate contains high percentages of abnormal spermatozoa;

(2) A wide variety of abnormalities is observed even in otherwise normal semen samples;

(3) The incidence of spermatozoa with simultaneous abnormalities of head, midpiece and tail components is high;

(4) It is difficult to clinically evaluate the relationship between sperm morphology and a given sample's fertility potential either *in vivo* (coitus or intrauterine insemination) or *in vitro* (traditional IVF or ICSI).

Different methods may be used to assess sperm morphology. Studying stained smear preparations by light microscopy (LM) is the most useful and common method employed for routine evaluation (Figures 3.8–3.25). However, LM evaluation has two major limitations: only the surface of the spermatozoon is seen; and the magnification cannot be greater than ×2000.

In Figures 3.8–3.25, two staining techniques were employed for LM photography:

(1) **Testsimplet slides**: These are commercial ready-to-use prestained slides. One drop of unwashed sperm was placed on a Testsimplet slide and kept frozen until evaluation. The method is quick and renders results that are comparable to other, more complicated, staining methods[14];

(2) **Papanicolaou staining method**, modified for spermatozoa[12]. Samples for this staining technique were washed once with phosphate buffer before making the smears. The smears were then air-dried and fixed in equal parts of 95% ethanol and ether for 30 min.

Scanning electron microscopy (SEM) gives a three-dimensional image and a higher resolution than does LM but, again, has the limitation that only the sperm surface is observable; intrinsic alterations cannot be seen.

Transmission electron microscopy (TEM), due to its high-power resolution and use of ultrathin sections, has the advantage of detecting anomalies not seen with either LM or SEM, but is not easily applied for routine evaluation.

SEM and TEM samples (Figures 3.26–3.43) were prepared using the following technique[15]. Briefly, samples were fixed in a phosphate-buffered glutaraldehyde-paraformaldehyde solution. Osmium tetroxide was used as the post-fixation agent, Araldite® as the inclusion material and uranyl acetate / lead citrate as contrast. The microscopes used were the Philips 200EM, Philips 301M and Joel 840.

Normal morphology

On light microscopy

As well as the different methods of sample preparation, there are different criteria for the assessment of sperm morphology. The two most frequently used are the World Health Organization (WHO) criteria and Kruger's strict criteria.

WHO criteria A semen sample is considered normal if it presents with ≥30% sperm cells with a normal morphology, defined as follows[12]:

- Length of the head: 4.0–5.5 μm
- Width of the head: 2.5–3.5 μm
- Length-to-width ratio (length : width): 1.5 to 1.75
- Well-defined acrosomal region comprising 40–70% of the head area
- No neck, midpiece or tail defects
- No cytoplasmic droplets more than one-third the size of a normal sperm head.

Kruger's strict criteria For a sample to be considered fertile, ≥14% of the sperm must display normal morphology [16]:

- Length of the head: 4.0–5.5 μm
- Width of the head: 2.5–3.5 μm
- Shape: Smooth oval (acorn-shaped)
- Acrosome: 40–70% of head
- Midpiece: 6–10 μm

- Tail: Approximately 45 μm.

On transmission electron microscopy

The complex structural organization of the human spermatozoon can be seen with electron microscopy[17].

Head The sperm head consists of the nucleus, which houses compact chromatin, and some areas of dispersed chromatin and vacuoles. Its anterior two-thirds are covered by the acrosome. A single membrane, the postnuclear cap, covers its posterior region. The site of overlap of the acrosome and postnuclear cap is called the 'equatorial segment'.

Midpiece A basal plate sits at the site of attachment of the head to the midpiece. The midpiece consists of two centrioles, an axoneme, and a mitochondrial sheath that surrounds the axial filament in a helicoidal pattern. An outer ring of nine coarser fibrils surrounds the central axial core of nine fine fiber microtubule doublets and a central pair of microtubules.

Tail The tail has two differentiated areas: the principal piece or mainpiece; and the endpiece. In the mainpiece, the 9 + 2 system of axonemal microtubules is surrounded by the coarse fibrous sheath, which consists of semicircular strands or ribs. The outer doublets consist of microtubules A and B. Inner and outer dynein arms extend from the A microtubule towards the B microtubule of the adjacent pair. The endpiece has a length of 4–10 μm and a small diameter (< 1 μm) due to the absence of the outer fibers and sheath.

Abnormal morphology

On light microscopy

Identification of the abnormal and slightly abnormal sperm cells shown in Figures 3.8–3.25 was carried out using Kruger's strict criteria, summarized as follows:

Acrosomal defects

- Small acrosome: < 40% of head
- Large acrosome: > 70% of head

Structural defects

- Pyriform: Narrow head at tail junction site
- Tapered: Narrow head (entire)
- Dumb-bell: Narrow head in the middle
- Surface irregularity: Non-oval head
- Vacuolated: More than two vacuoles present
- Flattened head at the tail implantation site
- Round head: Globular shape

Size defects

- Too small
- Too large

Double head

Loose head (decapitated)

Neck / midpiece defect

- Bent neck: Neck and tail form an angle > 90° to the head
- Immature spermatozoa: Cytoplasmic droplet present behind the head, or around the midpiece or tail

Tail defects

- Attachment incorrect: Tail attached at site other than at base of head
- Coiled tail: Curled below the head or encircling the entire cell
- Bent > 90° in relation to the main axis of the head
- Multitailed.

Table 3.1 Sperm abnormalities observed with transmission electron microscopy (TEM)

Site of defect	*Type of defect*
General	Dead (necrozoospermia)
Head	Cephalic cytoplasm; microcephalic; discoidal, isolated, or bi- or polynucleated head
Acrosome	Deformed and / or recoiled; separated from nucleus and / or plasma membrane; with vesicles; reacted; hypoplasic; absent
Nucleus	Deformed; with vacuoles and / or inclusions; subcondensed chromatin
Connecting piece	Axial flexion; absence of centriole microtubules
Midpiece	Mitochondrial sheath partially missing; disorganized, empty or absent mitochondria
Fibrous sheath	Deformed; hypertrophied
Tail	Angulated; coiled
Axoneme	Polyaxoneme; disorganized; with vesicles; outside of fibrous sheath; supernumerary microtubules; loss of peripheral doublets, central pair, peripheral fibers, inner or outer dynein arms, or radial spokes

On transmission electron microscopy

Table 3.1 summarizes the type of abnormalities commonly observed in spermatozoa from infertile men. Among the abnormalities listed, some may be diagnosed, or at least suspected, with the use of LM (necrozoospemia, decapitation, cephalic cytoplasm, acrosomal defect, and bent / coiled tail). A high frequency of concomitant defects of more than one structure is commonly observed[15].

Special acknowledgement

The EM photographs are courtesy of Robert Bargalló, PhD, Servei de Microscopia Electronica, Universitat de Barcelona, Spain.

References

1. Greep RO, Fevold HL. The spermatogenic and secretory function of the gonads of hypophysectomized adult rats treated with pituitary FSH and LH. *Endocrinology* 1937;21:611

2. Clermont Y. Spermatogenesis in man. A study of the spermatogonial population. *Fertil Steril* 1966;17:705

3. Stevens RW. Basic spermatozoon anatomy and physiology for the clinician. In: Acosta AA, Swanson RJ, Ackerman SB, *et al*., eds. *Human Spermatozoa in Assisted Reproduction*. Baltimore: Williams & Wilkins, 1990:1

4. Russell LD. Role in spermiation. In: Russell LD, Griswold MD, eds. *The Sertoli Cell*. Clearwater, Florida: Cache River Press, 1993:269

5. Hafez ESE, Prasad MRN. Functional aspects of the epididymis. In: Hafez ESE, ed. *Human Semen and Fertility Regulation in Man*. St Louis: C.V. Mosby Co, 1976:31

6. Reijo R, Lee TY, Salo P, *et al*. Diverse spermatogenic defects in humans caused by Y chromosome deletions encompassing a novel RNA-binding protein gene. *Nat Genet* 1995;10:383

7. Van Assche E, Bonduelle M, Tournaye H, *et al*. Cytogenetics of infertile men. *Hum Reprod* 1996;11 (Suppl):1

8. Freund M. Standards for the rating of human sperm morphology. A comparative study. *J Fertil* 1966;11:97

9. Eliasson R. Standards for investigation of human semen. *Andrologia* 1970;3:49

10. Freund M, Peterson RN. Semen evaluation and fertility. In: Hafez ESE, ed. *Human Semen and Fertility Regulation in Man*. St. Louis: C.V. Mosby Company, 1976:344

11. World Health Organization. *WHO Laboratory Manual for the Examination of Human Semen and Sperm–Cervical Mucus Interaction*. Cambridge: Cambridge University Press, 1980

12. World Health Organization. *WHO Laboratory Manual for the Examination of Human Semen and Sperm–Cervical Mucus Interaction*. Cambridge: Cambridge University Press, 1992

13. Kruger TF, Menkveld R, Stander FSH, *et al.* Sperm morphology features as a prognostic factor in in vitro fertilization. *Fertil Steril* 1986;46:1118

14. Schirren C, Eckhardt U, Jachczik R, Carstensen CA. Morphological differentiation of human spermatozoa with Testsimplets slides. *Andrologia* 1977;9:191

15. Marina S, Franco J, Fontarnau R, Bargalló R. The value of electron microscopy in the study of sperm morphology. In: Serio M, ed. *Perspectives in Andrology. Serono Symposia Publication.* New York: Raven Press 1989;53:399

16. Kruger TF, Franken DR, Menkveld R. *Strict 1-2-3. A self-teaching program for strict sperm morphology.* Tygerberg-Capetown, South Africa: MQ Medical, 1993

17. Zamboni L. Sperm ultrastructural pathology and infertility. In: Gondos B, Riddick DH, eds. *Pathology of Infertility. Clinical Correlations in the Male and Female.* New York: Thieme Medical Publishers, 1987:353

18. Afzelius BA. Electron microscopy of the sperm tail: Results obtained with a new fixative. *J Biophys Biochem Cytol* 1959;5:269

19. Mann T, Lutwak-Mann C. *Male Reproductive Function and Semen*. Berlin: Springer-Verlag, 1981:258

20. Gagnon C, Sherins RJ, Phillips DW, Bardin CW. Deficiency of protein-carboxyl methylase in spermatozoa of infertile men. *N Engl J Med* 1982;306:821

21. Tournaye H, Liu J, Nagy Z, *et al.* The use of testicular sperm for intracytoplasmic sperm injection in patients with necrozoospermia. *Fertil Steril* 1996; 66:331

22. Lüders G. Ein defekt der Kopf-Schwanz-Ver-knüpfung beim menschlichen spermatozoen. *Andrologia* 1976;8:365

23. LeLannou D. Tératospermie consistant en l'absence de tête spermatique par défaut de connexion tête-col chez l'homme. *J Gynecol Obstet Biol Reprod* 1979; 8:43

24. Baccetti B, Selmi MG, Soldani P. Morphogenesis of "decapitated" spermatozoa in a man. *J Reprod Fertil* 1984;70:395

25. Kjessler B. Chromosomal constitution and male reproductive failure. In: Mancini RE, Martini L, eds. *Male Fertility and Sterility*. London: Academic Press, 1974:231

26. Silvestroni L, Frajese G. Abnormal structure of spermatozoa in infertile oligospermic men. In: Fabbrini A, Steinberger E, eds. *Recent Progress in Andrology*. London: Academic Press, 1978:415

27. Pedersen H, Rebbe H. Fine structure of round-headed human spermatozoa. *J Reprod Fertil* 1974; 37:51

28. Anton-Lamprecht I, Kotzur B, Schopf E. Round-headed human spermatozoa. *Fertil Steril* 1976;27:685

29. Florke-Gerloff S, Topfer-Petersen E, Muller-Esterl W. Biochemical and genetic investigation of round-headed spermatozoa in infertile men, including two brothers and their father. *Andrologia* 1984;16:187

30. Liu J, Nagy Z, Joris H, *et al.* Successful fertilization and establishment of pregnancies after intracyto-

plasmic sperm injection in patients with globozoospermia. *Hum Reprod* 1995;10:626

31. Zamboni L, Zemjanis R, Stefanini M. The fine structure of monkey and human spermatozoa. *Anat Rec* 1971;169:129

32. Feneux D, Serres C, Jouannet P. Sliding spermatozoa: A dyskinesia responsible for human infertility? *Fertil Steril* 1985;44:508

33. Chemes HE. The significance of flagellar pathology in the evaluation of abnormal sperm motility. In: Baccetti B, ed. *Comparative Spermatology 20 Years After. Serono Symposia Publication.* New York: Raven Press, 1991;75:815

34. Fawcett DW, Phillips DM. The fine structure and development of the neck region of the mammalian spermatozoon. *Anat Rec* 1969;165:153

35. Walt H, Campana A, Balerna M. Mosaicism of dynein in spermatozoa and cilia and fibrous sheath aberrations in an infertile man. *Andrologia* 1983;15:295

36. Jonsson MS, McCormick JR, Gillies CG. Kartagener's syndrome with motile spermatozoa. *N Engl J Med* 1982;307:1131

37. Afzelius BA, Eliasson R. Male and female infertility problems in the immotile cilia syndrome. *Eur J Resp Dis* 1983;64(Suppl 127):144

38. Chao J, Turner JAP, Sturgess JM. Genetic heterogeneity of dynein deficiency in cilia from patients with respiratory disease. *Am Rev Respir Dis* 1982;126:302

39. Jouannet P, Escalier D, Serres C. Motility of human sperm without outer dynein arms. *J Submicrosc Cyto* 1983;115:67

4 The sperm-penetrated human oocyte

Process of fertilization

Human fertilization begins when a spermatozoon, with its haploid number of chromosomes, passes through oocyte cellular investments and makes contact with the protective zona pellucida that surrounds the oocyte. This contact induces an acrosomal reaction whereby the spermatozoon releases the contents of its acrosomal vesicle, including enzymes that aid the sperm in digesting its way through the zona to the oocyte plasma membrane. The equatorial segment of the sperm head attaches to the plasma membrane of the oocyte, and sperm incorporation occurs through a process similar to phagocytosis. Only acrosome-reacted sperm are believed to be capable of fusing with the oolemma of the oocyte. Spermatozoon / oolemma fusion is bypassed when performing intracytoplasmic sperm injection (ICSI) to assist the fertilization process (see Chapter 10).

It has been reported that, with insemination *in vitro*, spermatozoa traverse oocyte cellular investments within 3 h and first appear in the oocyte cortex within 4 h. An interesting fact is that oocytes need only be incubated with spermatozoa for 1 h to achieve fertilization outcomes similar to that with controls exposed for 16 h[1].

Fusion of gametes invokes a cascade of events that are initiated by the hydrolysis of phosphatidylinositol biphosphate in the oolemma[2]. Electrical changes occur on the oolemma and intracellular calcium levels rise in the oocyte. Cortical granule exocytosis from the ooplasmic periphery causes a chemical alteration of the zona pellucida which generally renders it impermeable to other sperm. Thus, the oocyte is said to become *activated* by its fusion with the spermatozoon. It completes its second meiotic division: 23 double-stranded chromosomes split at their centromeres, and chromatids separate to the oocyte or a second polar body. In this manner, a haploid number of chromosomes and a haploid amount of DNA are contributed by the oocyte. Activation does not necessarily require the stimulus of a spermatozoon. Oocytes may be activated through mechanical trauma, temperature shock, chemical stimuli, or electrical signals. Oocytes are commonly activated during ICSI procedures simply by piercing the oolemma or aggressively disturbing the ooplasm.

Within a few hours, male and female pronuclei are formed from the sperm and oocyte chromatin. The stage at which pronuclei are visible is termed the *pronuclear stage*, and the specimen is defined as a *prezygote* or *ootid*. Technically, the zygote has not yet formed (see page 106). During pronuclear formation, the zygotic centrosome is assembled; centrosomal proteins and sperm aster microtubules gather around the sperm centriole. Assembly of the zygotic centrosome is a crucial step for subsequent pronuclear apposition and genomic union[3]. Pronuclei come into close contact, eventually lose their apposed pronuclear membranes, and enter into syngamy.

This final event of the fertilization process involves the reorganization and pairing of maternal and paternal chromosomes, and formation of the zygote. As already described in Chapter 1, mixing of maternal and paternal gamete chromosomes during meiosis I results in a mathematical probability of more than 8 000 000 possible chromosome combinations (2^{23}) for each gamete. If each parent has this many possible combinations, then one couple could produce more than 7×10^{13} offspring with different combinations of parental chromosomes. This astronomical number does not take into consideration the additional genetic variability generated by crossing-over events that occur during meiosis I. Without crossing-over, gene combinations on a given chromosome would remain coupled indefinitely. With crossing-over, the theoretical possibility of creating genetically different offspring after fertilization reaches 80^{23}. This is why it is impossible, or nearly so, for any two individuals other than monozygotic twins (or, in this era, clones) to be genetically identical.

There is a brief period after pronuclei breakdown during which the zygote remains single-celled. In humans, the nearly 24-h fertilization process is completed with the initiation of the first (mitotic) cleavage.

Block to polyspermy

One consequence of sperm / oolemma fusion is the exocytosis of cortical granules from the oocyte periphery. This release, occurring within minutes of fusion, is a key component of the oocyte's strategy for preventing polyspermy. The dispersal of cortical granule contents into the perivitelline space is followed by a chemical alteration of the zona pellucida, an event often termed *zona hardening* or the *zona reaction*. Before fusion, the zona exhibits a porous appearance and is composed of a large number of ring-shaped structures called *hoops*, randomly superimposed in several layers. Pore diameter decreases towards the inside of the zona. After fusion, the zona appears to be more compact and its diameter is slightly decreased; the hoops can no longer be distinguished, and the pores are obliterated by an amorphous material emerging from the inner zona[4]. The zona reaction may render the zona pellucida impenetrable by other sperm, or may cause secondary sperm to become entrapped within its altered matrix, unable to pass the highly condensed inner layer of the zona. A slow or incomplete cortical granule exocytosis and zona reaction may represent the most common causes of polyspermic fertilization. Premature or failed cortical granule discharge may be responsible for some instances of failed fertilization after standard insemination.

It has been postulated that human oocytes do not possess a true block to polyspermy at the level of the oolemma[5]. This theory was recently supported by a study that retrospectively examined the polyspermy rate in over 3000 human oocytes subjected to subzonal insemination techniques (SUZI) after 1–20 sperm were placed under their zonae. The authors concluded that all sperm possessing fertilizing ability were indeed capable of fusing with the oocyte cell membrane, indicating the absence of a polyspermy block at this level[6].

However, in another experiment where zona-free human oocytes were exposed to high concentrations of sperm, it appeared that sperm were not able to indiscriminately penetrate oocytes at the expected rates[7]. At 30 min, an average of 1.3 sperm had penetrated the oocytes and, at 60 min, 2.9 had succeeded in penetration. The number of penetrating sperm peaked at 2 h, regardless of sperm concentration. In addition, the sperm demonstrated a reduced ability to bind to membranes of previously fertilized oocytes, with few or none binding to the membranes of four-cell preembryos. The authors concluded that, in fact, the oolemma has a role in preventing polyspermy and that a plasma membrane block may involve permanent changes to sperm binding / fusion ability.

Based on these and other conflicting reports[8], it is only possible to conclude that, at this time, the question of a membrane block in humans remains unresolved.

Usually, 5–10% of oocytes cultured *in vitro* are observed to incorporate more than one spermatozoon, as indicated by the subsequent development of three or more pronuclei. The reported frequency in the literature ranges from as low as 1–2% after insemination of mature oocytes[1,9] to over 30% after insemination of immature oocytes[10].

Some investigators have found a high correlation between triploidy and inseminating sperm concentration. As early as 1986, one such study reported a tripling of polyspermy with increasing sperm concentrations[11]. Others have reported that the incidence of abnormal fertilization is no higher when oocytes are exposed to large numbers of sperm[12,13].

Although it is tempting to correlate polyspermic fertilization to the unnaturally high numbers of spermatozoa used for standard insemination *in vitro*, it has been our observation that this incidence is better correlated to oocyte maturity and viability than to gross numbers of inseminating spermatozoa. Approximately 5% of mature oocytes exhibit three pronuclei after injection of a single sperm during ICSI procedures (they are largely *digynic*), indicating a relatively high occurrence of second polar-body suppression at meiosis II.

Although it is possible that the ICSI procedure itself may be instrumental in causing this effect or that a sperm possessing two nuclei was injected, digynic fertilization has been noted sufficiently often after natural intercourse and insemination *in vitro* to suggest that digyny is not restricted to assisted fertilization techniques. Most late-term triploid fetuses and liveborn triploid children have been shown to have developed from digynic preembryos[14,15]. Moreover, recent studies confirm that digyny is clearly the most common origin of triploidy in humans[16]. These studies indicate that oocyte factors are commonly accountable for triploid fertilization.

Which oocyte factors might this include? Certainly, oocyte aging has been shown to be associated with an increased incidence of spindle defects; retention of chromosomes within the ooplasm after suppression of first or second polar body extrusion may represent one possible mechanism for digyny. Poor culture conditions *in vitro* may be implicated in some cases of spindle damage if oocytes are allowed to chill for long periods[17] or overheat. In addition, mature oocytes may develop from binucleate primary oocytes; an example of a binucleate oocyte displaying two germinal vesicles is shown in Figure 8.11 (see page 163).

Other factors may also be responsible for allowing polyspermic fertilization to occur. Oocytes that are postmature (aged) have been shown to exhibit a centripetal migration of their cortical granules when analyzed under the electron microscope[18,19] which, at best, would trigger a retarded zona reaction and may result in multiple sperm fusion during fertilization. Conversely, oocyte immaturity has been implicated in contributing to polyspermic fertilization, presumably through delayed cortical-granule release[20].

In all probability, polyspermy is the result of different mechanisms, or combinations of different mechanisms, in different oocytes. In some oocytes, immaturity or postmaturity may be implicated, or they may be intrinsically abnormal. In others, minute cracks may be present in the zona pellucida after oocyte harvest procedures, thereby allowing multiple sperm entry. In further oocytes, entry of two sperm may simply be a random event that occurs when two sperm simultaneously make their way through the zona and concurrently fuse with the oolemma; whether the chance of this happening increases in the presence of high numbers of motile spermatozoa remains to be elucidated.

Male and female pronuclei

Male and female pronuclei (Figures 4.1–4.13) are usually formed simultaneously. The male pronucleus forms near the site of sperm entry whereas the female pronucleus originates at the ooplasmic pole of the meiotic spindle[21]. These structures, although small and faint, may be visualized as early as 4 h after ICSI or 5–6 h after insemination. The male pronucleus may be somewhat larger in humans[22], but the difference is difficult, if not impossible, to discern with LM. When a group of investigators attempted to distinguish pronuclear gender by using morphological criteria under LM, they observed sperm tail remnants in only 3 out of 342 pronucleate oocytes. Furthermore, pronuclear diameter and position within the ooplasm failed to yield any informative distinctions between male and female pronuclei[23].

Early in their formation, pronuclei are seen at a distance from each other; later, they migrate together towards the center of the cell. By 15 h after insemination, pronuclei are most often observed lying close to one another; they may present a *figure-8* configuration if viewed in an overlapping position. Although they appear to have touched and fused, TEM has demonstrated that they remain separated by a narrow strip of ooplasm, which may contain mitochondria and elements of smooth endoplasmic reticulum, or be altogether free of organelles[5,18,24]. As male and female pronuclei become closely associated, adjacent areas of each appear to become flattened. At the same time, nucleoli move from random locations within each pronucleus to line up at the regions of juxtaposition. One to nine nucleoli can be observed in each structure, the smaller pronucleus often containing a lower number.

Pronuclei are surrounded by a dense aggregation of cellular organelles which may appear granular or even darkened under LM. The female pronucleus envelope often dismantles and undergoes membrane breakdown slightly ahead of that of the male[25] (Figure 4.14). During the human pronuclear phase, DNA synthesis within male and female pronuclei begins synchronously at around 12 h after sperm / oocyte fusion. Errors of DNA synthesis may be responsible for developmental arrest at the pronuclear stage; it may be that pronuclear membranes require signaling of DNA replication before dismantling. By 20 h postinsemination / injection, male and female pronuclei have both begun to fade (Figures 4.15–4.17). The first cleavage soon follows.

In an elegant study performed by Payne and coworkers[26], oocytes in the process of fertilization were monitored for up to 20 h by time-lapse videocinematography following ICSI. The fertilization patterns in 50 oocytes followed a defined course of events, but varied markedly in timing from one prezygote to another.

The investigators described a circular wave of granulation moving throughout the cytoplasm that lasted for approximately 20–53 min. Granulation occurred in cortical regions of the oocyte and completed two to ten full circular rotations, some clockwise and others counterclockwise. During this active phase, the sperm head decondensed. This was followed by extrusion of the second polar body and central development of the male pronucleus. After polar-body extrusion (mean time from injection was 2.5 h), the granulation wave ceased in all oocytes.

At the same time or immediately after male pronucleus formation, the female pronucleus was seen to form near the site of second-polar-body extrusion, which was not always near the site of first-polar-body extrusion. The female pronucleus was then gradually drawn towards the male pronucleus until the two were in abutment. Finally, both pronuclei increased in size and showed moving nucleoli, some of which coalesced over time.

During the period of pronuclear growth, cytoplasmic organelles were observed to migrate inwardly towards the center of the oocyte, leaving a clear zone at the cortex. Measurement of these specimens confirmed that the female pronucleus was indeed smaller than the male pronucleus (22.4 *vs* 24.1 μm, respectively), and possessed fewer nucleoli (4.2 *vs* 7.0). It was discovered that subsequent preembryo quality, as determined by morphology and developmental rate, was correlated to sequential timing of events and duration of the cytoplasmic granulation wave: good preembryos showed uniform (but not necessarily more rapid) progression and longer granulation waves. Of interest is the fact that, in this series, pronuclei could be identified as early as 3 h postinjection and, by 5 h, over half of the oocytes possessed visible small pronuclear structures. In this fascinating study, the cytoplasmic granulation wave proved to be a novel and unique finding.

In the absence of videocinematography, the embryologist has to rely on the presence and number of pronuclei, assessed during one or two brief examinations, to determine whether or not normal fertilization is ongoing[27]. Practical criteria for sperm penetration in living material include:

(1) Observation of two pronuclei at 10–18 h postinsemination; and

(2) Visualization of two polar bodies in the perivitelline space.

Assessment of these two parameters is rapid and simple. Unfortunately, the identification of pronuclei neither ensures a normal fertilization process nor guarantees paternal and maternal origins for each pronucleus. Evaluating second polar bodies is also potentially misleading because of first-polar-body fragmentation.

Another serious drawback of the use of a single observation to assess pronuclear number arises from the fact that pronuclear counts have been observed to change during the pronuclear period. Most embryologists can recall instances where two pronuclei were visualized in an oocyte at an initial observation, but only one (or three) pronucleus(i) were subsequently seen during a follow-up evaluation or *vice versa*.

Although pronuclear and polar-body determinations are not ideal for assessment of sperm penetration, they do provide the most useful and least time-consuming means of clinical evaluation. Perhaps, in future, all evaluations of fertilized oocytes will be as described by Payne *et al.* Until then, less informative methods will have to suffice.

Chromosomes and fertilization

Fusion between male and female gametes is not always successful even under optimal conditions. When investigating causes of fertilization failure, gamete maturity and *genetic health* emerge as two important factors related to fertilizing potential. In a study carried out to examine fertilization failure in 293 oocytes inseminated *in vitro*, it was discovered that 30% of the oocytes were not fully mature at the time of sperm / oocyte interaction (chromosomes at M I or P I of maturation), and a full 59% were chromosomally abnormal[28]. Similar numbers are often reported in the literature, indicating that a large proportion of human gametes are genetically incapable of generating normal offspring.

Nowadays, gamete immaturity represents less of a problem than it did in the past, during the early days of our attempts to optimize IVF techniques. Certainly, ovarian-stimulation regimes have been refined over the last 20 years so that virtually all patients are now able to produce healthy mature oocytes. There has also been mild success in the clinical application of *in vitro* maturation methods. Healthy babies have been generated from germinal vesicle-bearing immature oocytes collected from stimulated[29,30] and unstimulated[31,32] cycles. Unfortunately, implantation rates are not in the range expected compared with oocytes matured *in vivo*.

Recently, immature spermatozoa have also generated considerable interest. Almost unthinkable two decades ago, it is now possible to use haploid round and elongated spermatids in the clinical treatment of azoospermia[33,34] and healthy children have been conceived[35–38]. It now appears, based on experiments in the mouse, that injecting secondary spermatocytes may prove to be a future treatment modality. Incredibly, normal offspring have been born after such cells had completed meiosis II within oocytes following injection and electroactivation. The extra set of chromosomes was extruded into the perivitelline space as an extra (male) polar body[39].

The fact that many gametes are genetically abnormal probably accounts for much of the failed fertilization observed in our programs. If the numerous reports describing very high percentages of chromosome abnormalities in sperm, eggs, and developing preembryos are to be believed, it becomes a wonder that humans have managed so well to overpopulate the earth. It is well documented that chromosomal abnormalities among first trimester spontaneous abortions occur at a rate of around 60%[40]. It is estimated that more than one-quarter of oocytes[41,42], and up to 10% of spermatozoa[43], that fail fertilization carry a chromosomal aberration. A review of the literature led one investigator to conclude that at least 50% of conceptuses developing after natural conception are chromosomally abnormal[44].

Males with non-mosaic Klinefelter's syndrome (47,XXY) are now capable of fathering children if even one or two mature or maturing sperm cells can be isolated from testicular tissue and used in assisted-fertilization procedures[45]. Whether the very presence of spermatozoa or spermatids in the testicular tissue indicates mosaicism in germ-cell lines must be further investigated. Several cases have thus far been reported to show normal karyotypes of preembryos generated from men who show no evidence of mosaicism in peripheral blood cells. In one report, after performing preimplantation genetic diagnosis on five preembryos from three Klinefelter's patients, all were found to be chromosomally normal[46].

In our own program at Cornell thus far, three clinical pregnancies have been established using testicular spermatozoa from husbands with presumed non-mosaic Klinefelter's syndrome. The results of these pregnancies so far have been one normal baby boy and a set of normal twins (a boy and a girl); the third is currently ongoing[45].

The course and harmony of events that define the fertilization process are indeed fascinating. There continues to be more to learn regarding the complex stages of reproduction from extensive animal research and clinical investigation of human infertility. Perhaps no other branch of science is as interesting as the exploration of this fundamental life-generating process.

References

1. Gianaroli L, Magli MC, Ferraretti AP, *et al.* Reducing the time of sperm–oocyte interaction in human in-vitro fertilization improves the implantation rate. *Hum Reprod* 1996;11:166

2. Alberts B, Bray D, Lewis J, *et al.* Germ cells and fertilization. *Molecular Biology of the Cell, 2nd edn.* New York: Garland Publishing, 1989:877

3. Sutovsky P, Hewitson L, Simerly C, Schatten G. Molecular medical approaches for alleviating infertility and understanding assisted reproductive technologies. *Proc Assoc Am Physicians* 1996;108:432

4. Nikas G, Paraschos T, Psychoyos A, Handyside AH. The zona reaction in human oocytes as seen with scanning electron microscopy. *Hum Reprod* 1994;9: 2135

5. Soupart P, Strong PA. Ultrastructural observations on human oocytes fertilized in vitro. *Fertil Steril* 1974; 25:11

6. Wolf JP, Ducot B, Aymar C, *et al.* Absence of block to polyspermy at the human oolemma. *Fertil Steril* 1997;67:1095

7. Sengoku K, Tamate K, Horikawa M, *et al.* Plasma membrane block to polyspermy in human oocytes and preimplantation embryos. *J Reprod Fertil* 1995; 105:85

8. Van Blerkom J, Davis PW, Merriam J. The developmental ability of human oocytes penetrated at the germinal vesicle stage after insemination in vitro. *Hum Reprod* 1994;9:697

9. Van Blerkom J, Henry GH, Porreco R. Preimplantation human embryonic development from polypronuclear eggs after in vitro fertilization. *Fertil Steril* 1984;41:686

10. Van der Ven HH, Al-Hasani A, Diedrich K, *et al.* Polyspermy in in vitro fertilization of human oocytes: Frequency and possible causes. *Ann NY Acad Sci* 1985;442:88

11. Englert Y, Puissant F, Camus M, *et al.* Factors leading to tripronucleate eggs during human in vitro fertilization. *Hum Reprod* 1986;1:117

12. Diamond MP, Rogers JB, Webster BW, *et al.* Polyspermy: Effect of varying stimulation protocols

and inseminating sperm concentrations. *Fertil Steril* 1985;43:777

13. Veeck LL. Abnormal morphology of the human oocyte and conceptus. *Atlas of the Human Oocyte and Early Conceptus, Vol. 2*. Baltimore: Williams & Wilkins, 1991:218

14. Dietzsch E, Ramsay M, Christianson AL, *et al.* Maternal origin of external haploid set of chromosomes in third trimester triploid fetuses. *Am J Med Genet* 1995;58:360

15. Miny P, Koppers B, Dworniczak B, *et al.* Parental origin of the extra haploid chromosome set in triploidies diagnosed prenatally. *Am J Med Genet* 1995;57:102

16. McFadden DE, Pantzar JT. Placental pathology of triploidy. *Hum Pathol* 1996;27:1018

17. Almeida PA, Bolton VN. The effect of temperature fluctuations on the cytoskeletal organization and chromosomal constitution of the human oocyte. *Zygote* 1995;3:357

18. Sathananthan AH. Ultrastructural morphology of fertilization and early cleavage in the human. In: Trounson A, Wood C, eds. *In Vitro Fertilization and Embryo Transfer*. London: Churchill Livingstone, 1984:131(cortical granules),110 (pronuclei)

19. Sathananthan AH, Trounson AO, Wood C. *Atlas of Fine Structure of Human Sperm Penetration, Eggs, and Embryos Cultured In Vitro*. New York: Praeger, 1986:5

20. Sathananthan AH, Trounson AO. Ultrastructure of cortical granule release and zona interaction in monospermic and polyspermic human ova fertilized in vitro. *Gamete Res* 1982;6:225

21. Wright G, Wiker S, Elsner C, *et al.* Observations on the morphology of pronuclei and nucleoli in human zygotes and implications for cryopreservation. *Hum Reprod* 1990;5:109

22. Edwards RG. *Conception in the Human Female*. New York: Academic Press, 1980:617

23. Wiker S, Malter H, Wright G, Cohen J. Recognition of paternal pronuclei in human zygotes. *J In Vitro Fert Embryo Transf* 1990;7:33

24. Zamboni L. *Fine Morphology of Mammalian Fertilization*. New York: Harper & Row, 1971

25. Sathananthan AH, Trounson AO. The human pronuclear ovum: Fine structure of monospermic and polyspermic fertilization in vitro. *Gamete Res* 1985; 12:385

26. Payne D, Flaherty SP, Barry MF, Matthews CD. Preliminary observations on polar body extrusion and pronuclear formation in human oocytes using time-lapse video cinematography. *Hum Reprod* 1997; 12:532

27. Veeck LL. Penetrated human oocytes (prezygotes) after in vitro fertilization. *Atlas of the Human Oocyte and Early Conceptus, Vol I*. Baltimore: Williams & Wilkins, 1986:142

28. Almeida PA, Bolton VN. Immaturity and chromosomal abnormalities in oocytes that fail to develop pronuclei following insemination in vitro. *Hum Reprod* 1993;8:229

29. Veeck LL, Wortham JWE, Witmyer J, *et al.* Maturation and fertilization of morphologically immature human oocytes in a program of in vitro fertilization. *Fertil Steril* 1983;39:594

30. Nagy ZP, Cecile J, Liu J, *et al.* Pregnancy and birth after intracytoplasmic sperm injection of in vitro matured germinal vesicle stage oocytes: Case report. *Fertil Steril* 1996;65:1047

31. Cha KY, Koo JJ, Ko JJ, *et al.* Pregnancy after in vitro fertilization of human follicular oocytes collected from nonstimulated cycles, their culture in vitro and their transfer in a donor oocyte program. *Fertil Steril* 1991;55:109

32. Barnes FL, Crombie A, Gardner DK, *et al.* Blastocyst development and birth after in vitro maturation of human primary oocytes, intracytoplasmic sperm injection, and assisted hatching. *Hum Reprod* 1995; 10:3243

33. Vanderzwalmen P, Lejeune B, Nijs M, *et al.* Fertilization of an oocyte microinseminated with a spermatid in an in vitro fertilization program. *Hum Reprod* 1995;10:502

34. Chen SU, Ho HN, Chen HF, *et al.* Fertilization and embryo cleavage after intracytoplasmic spermatid injection in an obstructive azoospermic patient with defective spermiogenesis. *Fertil Steril* 1996;66:157

35. Fishel S, Green S, Bishop M, *et al.* Pregnancy after intracytoplasmic injection of spermatid. *Lancet* 1995; 345:1641

36. Tesarik J, Mendoza C, Testart J. Viable embryos from injection of round spermatids into oocytes. *N Engl J Med* 1995;33:525

37. Antinori S, Versaci C, Dani G, *et al.* Fertilization with human testicular spermatids: Four successful pregnancies. *Hum Reprod* 1997;12:286

38. Antinori S, Versaci C, Dani G, *et al.* Successful fertilization and pregnancy after injection of frozen–thawed round spermatids into human oocytes. *Hum Reprod* 1997;12:554

39. Kimura Y, Yanagimachi R. Development of normal mice from oocytes injected with secondary spermatocyte nuclei. *Biol Reprod* 1995;53:855

40. Boue J, Boue A, Lazar P. Retrospective and prospective epidemiological studies of 1500 karyotyped human abortions. *Teratology* 1975;12:11

41. Plachot M. Cytogenetic analysis of oocytes and embryos. *Ann Acad Med Singapore* 1992;21:538

42. Plachot M. The human oocyte. Genetic aspects. *Ann Genet* 1997;40:115

43. Martin RH, Balkan W, Burns K, *et al.* The chromosome constitution of 1000 human spermatozoa. *Hum Genet* 1983;63:305

44. Schulman JD, Dorfmann A, Evans MI. Genetic aspects of in vitro fertilization. *Ann NY Acad Sci* 1985; 442:466

45. Palermo GD, Schlegel PN, Sills ES, *et al.* Birth after intracytoplasmic injection of sperm obtained by testicular extraction from men with nonmosaic Klinefelter's syndrome. *N Engl J Med* 1998;338:588

46. Staessen C, Coonen E, Van Assche E, *et al.* Preimplantation diagnosis for X and Y normality in embryos from three Klinefelter patients. *Hum Reprod* 1996;11:1650

5 The cleaving human preembryo

Two- to sixteen-cell stage

Cytokinesis

Cytoplasmic division following nuclear replication and segregation is a universal characteristic of all cells. Cleavage of the human preembryo involves a series of mitotic divisions of the cytoplasm every 12–18 h, with no discernible increase in overall size (Figure 5.1). Failing to progress to the first cleavage after forming two pronuclei is relatively uncommon, occurring in ≤5% of normally fertilized oocytes[1]. As with most mammals, except for some rodents, the centrosome of the human sperm controls the first mitotic divisions after fertilization has taken place[2].

As the first-cleavage mitosis reaches telophase, the cytoplasm of the zygote elongates and the surface contracts around the lesser circumference (Figures 5.2–5.4). This constriction continues until the zygote has divided into two blastomeres. The same process occurs throughout all subsequent mitotic cell divisions[3]. It has been estimated that mean blastomere volume is reduced by approximately 28.5% per division by the first three cleavages and that some diversity among the volumes of sister blastomeres is normal[4]. The two- to eight-cell conceptus depends largely on the translation of stored maternal RNA for cleavage.

Morphology

Many dividing preembryos have small anucleate cytoplasmic fragments within the perivitelline space or adhering to blastomeres. These arise because blastomeres constantly change shape, making and breaking cell contact during cleavage, thereby leaving cellular debris behind[5]. This constant, living motion is particularly apparent when specimens are viewed under time-lapse cinematography, which reveals the characteristic continuous pulsing formation of fragments and blebs, and cytoplasmic reorganization (personal observation). Human and primate preembryos may be more disposed to such activity as fragments are rarely seen in the conceptuses of other mammals. As preembryos flushed from the uterine cavity after fertilization *in vivo* also exhibit fragments, it may be deduced that *in vitro* culture methods are not solely responsible for this deviation.

Preembryos that exhibit large numbers of anucleate fragments tend to implant less frequently (see Chapter 6). This may be the result of a reduction in cytoplasm available for normal cell division which, in turn, leads to reduced cell numbers in the blastocyst. Alternatively, large numbers of fragments may interfere with the process of *compaction* by rendering intimate cell-to-cell contact difficult.

Cytoplasmic fragments often arise during the first cleavage. Studying the frequency of fragmentation 24 h after insemination reveals that, when excessive numbers of fragments are formed this early, the subsequent development of the preembryo is generally impaired. On the other hand, the development of small fragments after the first division usually has no detrimental effects on the cleaving conceptus.

Individual blastomeres remain distinct and totipotent (capable of developing independently to form a new organism) until approximately the eight-cell stage, when changes occur in both the structure and properties of their plasma membranes and cytoplasm. Cells at this point become less distinct as they adhere more tightly to one another during the process of compaction. After compaction, their development is committed towards becoming part of either the inner cell mass or the trophectoderm, with a resultant loss of totipotency.

Rate of cleavage

Two-cell conceptuses may be observed at any time from 20 h postinsemination onwards – usually after 24 h – and may persist until 42 h postinsemination. Viable four-cell preembryos are observed between 39–60 h postinsemination, and eight-cell stages are not generally seen until after 54 h, but usually before 72 h. In humans, three-, five-, and seven-cell preembryos are not an uncommon finding, particularly when the examination is carried out during mitotic cell division (Figures 5.5 and 5.6). This sometimes asynchronous division persists throughout cleavage of the early conceptus, and any number of blastomeres may be noted in a given observation (Figures 5.7–5.21). Interestingly, in some strains of mice and cows, male preembryos cleave faster than those which are female[6]. There have been reports suggesting that this may be true of human preembryos as well[7], although not all investigators have confirmed such a finding[8].

In normally fertilized specimens, retarded growth (no doubling within 24 h) often indicates reduced viability, but accelerated cleavage (doubling within 12 h) may not necessarily reflect a healthier conceptus[9]. Occasionally, a pregnancy may be established with a slow-growing preembryo, even one found to possess only six to eight blastomeres at 96 h. In the Cornell program, intrauterine transfer is postponed for one day whenever preembryos are observed to possess fewer than five blastomeres on day 3. If further cleavage occurs over the next 24 h, then the transfer is carried out but, if no further cleavage occurs, transfer is canceled. It has been surprising to note the number of pregnancies resulting from the transfer of six- or eight-celled preembryos on day 4.

A conceptus exhibiting three pronuclei may appear to cleave at an accelerated rate to the morula stage, when its development is usually arrested[1]. This is because many triploid zygotes split directly into three cells at the first cleavage as a result of possessing a tripolar spindle; subsequent divisions reflect the higher overall cell number in the conceptus, not more rapid growth. The cell doubling time in human preembryos at days 2–6 has been reported to be 31 h, with accelerated doubling noted after the first two divisions[10]. At first glance, these rates appear to be rather slow. During IVF treatment, doubling usually takes considerably less than 24 h (two cells by 24 h, four cells in less than 48 h, and eight or more cells within 72 h), probably averaging 18 h in healthy preembryos. However, it is not unreasonable to conclude that 31 h may represent the average doubling time if poor-quality and slow-growing (?arrested) preembryos are also calculated into the mean.

Compaction

Compaction is a process by which a cleaving preembryo changes from a collection of individual cells into a solid mass with indistinguishable cell membranes (Figure 5.22). Compaction is due to the formation of tight intercellular junctions causing blastomeres to become closely apposed. This positioning increases the extent of contact between blastomeres which is essential for subsequent development. In humans, this usually occurs at around the eight- or 16-cell stage[11]. Although compaction has been observed at earlier stages in human preembryos, it is not known whether this represents an abnormal occurrence. When compaction takes place, the cells lose their totipotency as a result of their interactions with one another. It is believed that the onset of compaction marks the beginning of embryonic DNA transcription. The formation of the morula and blastocyst quickly follows.

Morula and blastocyst

Morula

Morula literally means 'mulberry'. The preembryo is said to have become a morula when either the 16-cell stage is reached, because of its berry-like shape and appearance at that time, or compaction takes place. Normal compaction usually results in the formation of an outer layer of cells which evolve into the trophectoderm of the ensuant blastocyst; inner cells give rise to the inner cell mass (the inside / outside theory). Morulae have been seen to vacuolate *in vitro*, when they roughly approximate the appearance of a cavitating blastocyst. However, these soon become arrested in their development, fail to secrete hCG, and have fewer nuclei[12]. Human morulae may be seen as early as 72 h, but are more usually observed later than that, between days 3 and 4.

Blastocyst

Approximately 24 h after the morula has formed and compaction has taken place, the intercellular spaces begin to enlarge to create a central fluid-filled cavity called the blastocele (Figures 5.23 and 5.24). The cells of the developing human blastocyst form a spherical shell to enclose the blastocele, one pole of which is distinguished by a thicker accumulation of cells which becomes the inner cell mass. The outer ring of cells comprises the trophoblast. Whereas the inner cell mass gives rise to the embryo, the trophoblast gives rise to the placenta.

Early and late stages in blastocyst development may be identified by both the thickness of the zona pellucida and the overall size of the blastocyst. In early blastocyst formation, the zona is thick and the diameter of the conceptus is little changed; the blastocele begins to fill with fluid. At later stages, the blastocyst increases in overall size due to the accumulated fluid and a single ring of trophoblastic cells surrounds the cavity; the inner cell mass is clearly delineated and the zona stretches to become a mere thin outline (Figures 5.25 and 5.26). In culture, the blastocyst is seen to expand and contract during the later stages as it attempts to break free of the zona. It may remain in such an expanded state for 24 h or more before *hatching* from the zona pellucida[13] (Figures 5.27–5.30). As soon as it is free of its glycoprotein layer, the blastocyst is able to implant in the uterine wall.

The first report of an ongoing human pregnancy following the intrauterine transfer of day-6 zona-free blastocysts was presented in early 1997[14]. In this particular case, the patient had undergone eight previous transfers without success. The preembryos were cocultured on Vero cells until the blastocyst stage and their zonae removed using 0.5% pronase. It is hypothesized that the zona pellucida is required during early preembryonic development (two- to eight-cell stage), but may not be necessary after complete compaction.

Coculture techniques appear to be helpful in encouraging preembryos to reach blastocyst stages of development. Whether the coculture cells themselves impart factors favorable to support growth or whether they use unnecessary media components and / or absorb toxins is as yet not clearly ascertained. It may be that the cells are helpful for all of these reasons, especially under conditions where culture media or environmental factors are suboptimal. Despite the occasional study showing no differences in the results obtained after coculture *vs* conventional culture[15], there have been numerous published reports of enhanced rates of development after placing preembryos on various types of cell monolayers, in particular, Vero cells, autologous endometrial cells, autologous granulosa and cumulus cells, and bovine oviductal cells[16–23]. Similarly, there is increasingly more evidence to suggest high rates of blastocyst development after exposure of preembryos to culture medium components that are tailored to their precise stage of development[24].

Of interest is the fact that the blastocyst appears to have a built-in 'clock'. It has often been observed that a cavity will begin to coalesce in a day-4 or -5 preembryo regardless of the number of cells present or even after one-quarter of its cells have been removed at an earlier stage for biopsy. There is speculation that this internal clock may not necessarily be related to chronological age, but is instead associated with the number of nuclear divisions that have taken place. Cleaving preembryos have been treated experimentally with chemical agents to interrupt the cell cycle by disrupting microtubules and microfilaments. Although cell division is thus stopped, nuclear division continues. Once exposure to the drug is discontinued, compaction and blastocyst formation occur, although fewer cells than normal are present and many of these are multinucleated[25].

In related experiments by the same investigators, four-cell mouse preembryos were treated with cytochalasin-D to inhibit cytokinesis. On removal of the cytochalasin-D, although the preembryos were capable of forming 'blastocysts' at the same time as did the controls, they contained only four polyploid cells. They also possessed the ability to hatch and implant after intrauterine transfer, but none proved able to produce living young[26]. It is now generally accepted that the rate of cleavage is less important than the number of cells that eventually comprise the blastocyst.

In 1954, Hertig *et al.*[27] recorded counts of 158 and 107 cells in two blastocysts, respectively, collected at the time of hysterectomy. In 1972, Croxatto *et al.*[28] estimated 186 cells in a blastocyst obtained after uterine flushing. In retrospect, it becomes necessary to consider that either multinucleated cells accounted for the excessive distortion of cell number in these early reports or the current culturing systems *in vitro* are not producing the cell numbers that occur *in vivo*.

In 1989, nuclear fluorescent staining was used to obtain an average cell count in nine *in vitro*-derived blastocysts. In this study, only 58 ± 8.1 cells (?nuclei) were counted with a wide range of 24–90[29]. Similarly, in 1991, based on the examination results of 57 human specimens, Winston *et al.*[30] estimated that two-thirds of cavitated preembryos on day 5 comprise fewer than 32 cells and that a large proportion of these are often multinucleated. Furthermore, these last authors speculate that the majority of preembryos developing *in vitro* fail to complete sufficient cell cycles to produce a blastocyst with cell numbers adequate for normal differentiation of an inner cell mass. In the mouse, there is indeed evidence that more rapidly dividing blastomeres contribute to the inner cell mass of the blastocyst[31]. Clearly, there is a need to improve our culturing systems and to further define an accurate measurement for determining the viability of the conceptuses we so carefully nurture.

Blastocysts are generally observed *in vitro* after 110 h postinsemination. If left in culture for 5–6 days, 26–65% of preembryos will achieve this stage, depending on the method of culture and composition of the medium[12,32]. The results of exciting new research suggest that, in the near future, human blastocysts may be studied non-invasively using ultramicrofluorescence techniques to select those with the greatest potential for implantation[33]. In the mouse, an excellent correlation was found between blastocysts with a high glucose uptake / low lactate production (as an estimate of glycolytic activity) and fetal development. Such intriguing prospects have the potential to revolutionize laboratory techniques in the future.

References

1. Van Blerkom J, Motta P, eds. *Ultrastructure of Human Gametogenesis and Early Embryogenesis*. Boston: Kluwer Academic Publishers, 1989:125

2. Palermo G, Munne S, Cohen J. The human zygote inherits its mitotic potential from the male gamete. *Hum Reprod* 1994;9:1220

3. Austin CR. *The Mammalian Egg*. Oxford: Blackwell Scientific Publishers, 1961:78

4. Goyanes VJ, Ron-Corzo A, Costas E, Maneiro E. Morphometric categorization of the human oocyte and early conceptus. *Hum Reprod* 1990;5:613

5. Sathananthan AH, Trounson AO, Wood C. *Atlas of Fine Structure of Human Sperm Penetration, Eggs, and Embryos Cultured In Vitro*. New York: Praeger, 1986:158

6. Leese HJ, Edwards RG. The potential for preimplantation diagnosis by non-invasive methods. In: Edwards RG, ed. *Preconception and Preimplantation Diagnosis*. Cambridge, MA: Cambridge University Press, 1993:299

7. Ray PF, Conaghan J, Winston RM, Handyside AH. Increased number of cells and metabolic activity in male human preimplantation embryos following in vitro fertilization. *J Reprod Fertil (Engl)* 1995;104:165

8. Ng E, Claman P, Leveille MC, *et al.* Sex ratio of babies is unchanged after transfer of fast versus slow cleaving embryos. *J Assist Reprod Genet* 1995;12:566

9. Veeck LL. The morphological assessment of human oocytes and early concepti. In: Keel BA, Webster BW, eds. *Laboratory Diagnosis and Treatment of Infertility*. Boca Raton: CRC Press, 1990:353

10. Herbert M, Wolstenholme J, Merdoch AP, Butler TJ. Mitotic activity during preimplantation development of human embryos. *J Reprod Fertil* 1995;103:209

11. Hartshorne GM, Edwards RG. Early embryo development. In: Adashi EY, Rock JA, Rosenwaks Z, eds. *Reproductive Endocrinology, Surgery, and Technology*. New York: Lippincott–Raven, 1996:435

12. Dokras A, Sargent IL, Barlow DH. Human blastocyst grading: An indicator of developmental potential? *Hum Reprod* 1993;8:2119

13. Cohen J, Simons RF, Edwards RG, *et al.* Pregnancies following the frozen storage of expanding human blastocysts. *J In Vitro Fert Embryo Transf* 1985;2:59

14. Fong CY, Bongso A, Ng SC, *et al.* Ongoing normal pregnancy after transfer of zona-free blastocysts: Implications for embryo transfer in the human. *Hum Reprod* 1997;12:557

15. Van Blerkom J. Development of human embryos to the hatched blastocyst stage in the presence or absence of a monolayer of Vero cells. *Hum Reprod* 1993;8:1525

16. Barmat LI, Veeck LL, Liu HC, *et al.* Autologous endometrial coculture in patients with repeated failures of implantation after IVF (in preparation)

17. Desai NN, Kennard EA, Kniss DA, Friedman CI. Novel human endometrial cell line promotes blastocyst development. *Fertil Steril* 1994;61:760

18. Freeman MR, Whitworth CM, Hill GA. Granulosa cell coculture enhances human embryo development and pregnancy rate following in vitro fertilization. *Hum Reprod* 1995;10:408

19. Mansour RT, Aboulghar MA, Serour GI, Abbass AM. Coculture of human pronucleate oocytes with their cumulus cells. *Hum Reprod* 1994;9:1727

20. Menezo YJ, Sakkas D, Janny L. Coculture of the early human embryo: Factors affecting human blastocyst formation in vitro. *Microsc Res Tech (US)* 1995;32:50

21. Nieto FS, Watkins WB, Lopata A, *et al.* The effects of coculture with autologous cryopreserved endometrial cells on human in vitro fertilization and early embryo morphology: A randomized study. *J Assist Reprod Genet* 1996;13:386

22. Quinn P, Margalit R. Beneficial effects of coculture with cumulus cells on blastocyst formation in a prospective trial with supernumerary human embryos. *J Assist Reprod Genet* 1996;13:9

23. Wiemer KE, Hoffman DI, Maxson WS, *et al.* Embryonic morphology and rate of implantation of human embryos following coculture on bovine oviductal epithelial cells. *Hum Reprod* 1993;8:97

24. Gardner DK, Lane M, Calderon I, Leeton J. Environment of the preimplantation human embryo in vivo: Metabolite analysis of oviduct and uterine fluids and metabolism of cumulus cells. *Fertil Steril* 1996;65:349

25. Surani MAH, Barton SC, Burling A. Differentiation of 2-cell and 8-cell mouse embryos arrested by cytoskeletal inhibitors. *Exp Cell Res* 1980;125:275

26. Pratt H, Chakraborty J, Surani M. Molecular and morphological differentiation of the mouse blastocyst after manipulations of compaction with cytochalasin D. *Cell* 1981;26:279

27. Hertig AT, Rock J, Adams EC, Mulligan WJ. On the preimplantation stages of the human ovum: A description of four normal specimens ranging from the second to fifth day of development. *Contrib Embryol* 1954;35:199

28. Croxatto HB, Diaz S, Fuentealba G, *et al.* Studies on the duration of egg transport in the human oviduct. I. The time interval between ovulation and egg recovery from the uterus in normal women. *Fertil Steril* 1972;23:447

29. Hardy K, Handyside AH, Winston RML. The human blastocyst: Cell number and allocation during late preimplantation development in vitro. *Development* 1989;107:597

30. Winston NJ, Braude PR, Pickering SJ, *et al.* The incidence of abnormal morphology and nucleocytoplasmic ratios in 2-, 3-, and 5-day human preembryos. *Hum Reprod* 1991;6:17

31. Pedersen RA. Early mammalian embryogenesis. In: Knobil E, Neill J, eds. *The Physiology of Reproduction.* New York: Raven Press, 1988:187

32. Gardner DK, Lane M, Kouridakis K, Schoolcraft WB. Complex physiologically based serum-free culture media increase mammalian embryo development. In: Gomel V, Leung PCK, eds. *In Vitro Fertilization and Assisted Reproduction. Proceedings of the Tenth World Congress,* 1997:187

33. Gardner DK. Routine culture to blastocyst – The solution to high-order multiple pregnancy with IVF. *Syllabus. 10th Annual In Vitro Fertilization and Embryo Transfer.* Santa Barbara, CA, 1997:263

6 Preembryo grading and degree of cytoplasmic fragmentation

Preembryo morphology and correlation to pregnancy

The quality of preembryos produced after IVF is variable. Many contain multiple cellular fragments or blastomeres of unequal size, or exhibit slow cell-doubling times. The selection of viable preembryos for intrauterine transfer is considered an important factor in establishing pregnancy. It is assumed that the overall morphology and cleavage rate reflect, at least to some extent, the potential of the preembryo for continued growth and implantation.

Extensive cytoplasmic fragmentation has been associated with impending preembryo death. After studying fragmented preembryos and comparing them with non-fragmented controls, Jurisicova *et al.*[1] in 1996 concluded that the high incidence of condensed chromatin, degraded DNA, cell corpses, and apoptotic bodies commonly found in fragmented conceptuses almost certainly indicates a reduced potential for continued growth. This contention is supported by the experience of most embryologists and physicians working in assisted reproduction programs who have observed that somewhat lower implantation rates are associated with irregular blastomeres and excessive fragmentation, although some preembryos with these qualities retain the capacity for normal implantion[2].

Shulman *et al.*[3] in 1993 reported that the implantation potential of transferred preembryos may be directly correlated to morphological parameters and have suggested that the number of preembryos replaced be balanced against their grade to reduce multiple gestation.

Other reports have linked normal cell-doubling times to preembryo viability. Slow-growing conceptuses have demonstrated a markedly impaired capacity to implant after intrauterine transfer. In 1987, Claman *et al.*[4] reported that 21 of 23 ongoing IVF pregnancies arose from transfers in which at least one preembryo had reached the four-cell stage by 40 h postinsemination. Later reports similarly concluded that preembryos with slow cleavage rates (less than four blastomeres at 42–44 h postinsemination) were less likely to result in pregnancy[5,6].

Furthermore, it has been demonstrated in the hamster that faster-cleaving preembryos not only lead to more morulae and blastocysts in culture, but that subsequent *in vivo* development of faster-growing conceptuses is associated with a higher proportion of viable fetuses[7]. These last authors suggest that the timely completion of the third cell cycle (the eight-cell stage) is a critical and favorable factor for predicting successful embryogenesis in the hamster.

Regular cleavage to the eight-cell stage has also been noted as a favorable observation in humans, but has often proved to be an inexact means of predicting implantation success when used as an analytic parameter on its own. In spite of this, it has been proposed that the developmental rate may be more important than morphology when weighing individual factors for human intrauterine transfer[8].

Some investigators have reported that accelerated preembryonic growth combined with minimal fragmentation leads to increased pregnancy rates, and that these conditions are achieved more often through coculture systems[9]. Other studies have associated the occurrence of a timely first cleavage (within 25 h postinsemination) with an enhanced pregnancy outcome[10].

Factors other than fragmentation and growth rates have also been associated with the implantation potential of human preembryos. These include zona pellucida thickness and / or variation in its thickness, with thin and variable being more advantageous[11–13], as well as adequate blastomere expansion[12] and absence of multinucleation[14]. In addition, recent studies on follicular blood flow have demonstrated a high correlation between the dissolved oxygen content in the follicle (≥3%) and the subsequent normal development of the oocyte / preembryo[15–17].

Grading schemes

As a result of the reported correlations between morphology and pregnancy, embryologists generally use a grading scheme to document the presumptive quality of the transferred preembryos. Most of these schemes are related to the extent of observed cytoplasmic fragmentation and growth rate, but some include other factors, such as zona pellucida thickness or blastomere size and regularity. Usually, a grade is assigned to the transfer based on the morphology of the highest-grade preembryo in that group, with additional fractions added or subtracted for appropriate growth or for the concurrent transfer of other exceptional conceptuses.

Some groups will attempt to calculate an *average* score for the cohort of transferred preembryos based on the assigned grades of each individual preembryo, but these systems tend to be less informative when there is a wide disparity among the conceptuses, as this will distort the value of the final averaged figure.

In one early scoring system, a morphological grade of 1 through 4 was assigned to each preembryo and then combined with a grade developed from direct comparison to ideal growth rate. Using this two-stage system, the scores proved to be of value in predicting clinical success[18]. Similarly, in 1987, Puissant *et al.*[19] published the results of grading preembryos based on the number of anucleate fragments and rate of division. It was found that those preembryos with the higher grades contributed more often to pregnancy and multiple pregnancy. These authors suggested that, if grading scores are high in conjunction with optimal clinical parameters, then fewer preembryos should be transferred to offset high multiple-pregnancy rates.

A three-grade scoring system was evaluated by Erenus *et al.*[20] in 1991. Grade 1 preembryos represented those with equal-sized blastomeres and no fragmentation, grade 2 included preembryos with unequal-sized blastomeres, and grade 3 included preembryos associated with cytoplasmic fragmentation. In cycles where the best preembryo transferred was grade 1, 22% achieved clinical pregnancy compared with grades 2 and 3, which produced pregnancy rates of 13% and 0%, respectively. In addition, pregnancy rates increased with the transfer of multiple grade 1 preembryos (40% with three grade 1 preembryos).

In 1992, Steer *et al.*[21] developed a cumulative grading system in an attempt not only to predict pregnancy outcome, but also to reduce the potential for high-order multiple gestation in the Bourne Hall and Hallam programs. In this system, the morphological grade of each preembryo (1–4, with the higher number associated with better morphology) was multiplied by the number of blastomeres in the preembryo. The sum of the grades from all conceptuses transferred on day 2 after insemination represented the final score. Retrospective analysis showed that the pregnancy rates among women <36 years of age rose as the cumulative score increased to a maximum of 42. Continued increases beyond this number did not contribute further to establishing pregnancy, but did have an impact on the multiple-pregnancy rate. They estimated that, by using this system prospectively, 78% of triplet pregnancies and 100% of quadruplet pregnancies could have been predicted and avoided.

Using the same cumulative grading system, Visser and Fourie[22], in 1993, reported pregnancy rates of only 4% with scores of 1–10, but >35% with scores of 41–50. They also found more biochemical pregnancies, but not clinical pregnancy losses, with the lower scores. All triplet and quadruplet pregnancies were associated with scores >40.

Giorgetti *et al.*[23] devised a system whereby preembryos were assigned one point for each of the following parameters: cleavage; no fragmentation; no irregular cells; and four blastomeres on day 2. The idea for this system arose from a previous evaluation of 957 single preembryo transfers in which no ongoing pregnancies were established from the transfer of uncleaved preembryos or after delayed fertilization (99 transfers), and higher pregnancy rates were found with regular blastomeres and an absence of fragmentation (858 transfers). Applying this four-point scoring system retrospectively, they discovered that both clinical pregnancy and delivery rates correlated significantly to a higher score after single preembryo transfer, and each point corresponded to a 4% increase in pregnancy. Only maternal age (>38 years) had as great an impact as this simple morphological assessment.

In 1995, Tasdemir *et al.*[24] developed a system in which the degree of preembryo fragmentation and general morphology were assessed as either good (A) or poor (B). The outcomes of transfers with AA, BB, and AB double transfers, or AAA, BBB, AAB, and ABB triple transfers were then examined. When only good preembryos were transferred, the pregnancy rates in the double (AA) and triple (AAA) transfers were 41% and 43%, respectively. When only poor preembryos (BB and BBB) were transferred, the rates were 11% and 23%, respectively. AB transfers resulted in a 37% pregnancy rate and AAB / ABB transfers resulted in a 40% incidence. The authors concluded that, if at least one good preembryo is available for transfer, then double rather than triple transfer should be carried out; higher numbers should only be considered in cases of poor preembryo quality. After applying this policy for one year in patients <37 years of age, they compared their results to previous data generated from triple transfers. Although this prospective trial demonstrated a slightly lower pregnancy rate in the study group compared with the controls, the authors believe that the lower incidence of triplet gestations provides a practical compromise between high pregnancy rates and high-order gestations[25].

Figures 6.1–6.22 use a system wherein a grade is assigned to the morphology of the cleaving preembryos and the transfers are classified according to the highest score in each cohort of replaced conceptuses. With grade 1 representing perfect morphology, the grading system is:

Grade 1 Preembryo with blastomeres of equal size and no cytoplasmic fragmentation;

Grade 2 Preembryo with blastomeres of equal size and minor cytoplasmic fragmentation covering ≤10% of the preembryo surface;

Grade 3 Preembryo with blastomeres of distinctly unequal size and variable fragmentation;

Grade 4 Preembryo with blastomeres of equal or unequal size and moderate-to-significant cytoplasmic fragmentation covering >10% of the preembryo surface; and

Grade 5 Preembryo with few blastomeres of any size and severe fragmentation covering ≥50% of the preembryo surface.

At our institution, we have observed that transfers with at least one grade 1 or grade 2 preembryo have a greater potential for establishing pregnancy (Table 6.1). When the data are normalized for the number of preembryos transferred, this trend continues for all groups except single preembryo transfer, where the number of replacements is too

Table 6.1 Clinical pregnancy per transfer according to grade (April 1995–December 1997; $n = 2492$)

	Clinical pregnancy per transfer		*Multiple pregnancy per transfer*	
Grade	*All patients*	*Patients < 34 years old**	*All patients*	*Patients <34 years old**
1	63%	72%	31%	44%
2	54%	66%	22%	29%
3	39%	45%	11%	13%
4	36%	53%	9%	14%
5	29%	33%	8%	11%

*≤3 preembryos transferred

Table 6.2 Clinical pregnancy per transfer according to grade (April 1995–December 1997; $n = 2492$) normalized for the number of preembryos transferred

	Clinical pregnancy per transfer + (Multiple pregnancy per transfer)			
Grade	1 tr*	2 tr**	3 tr†	≥4 tr††
1	23% (0%)	45% (14%)	68% (39%)	62% (30%)
2	27% (0%)	40% (9%)	57% (27%)	57% (24%)
3	23% (0%)	27% (2%)	39% (12%)	47% (17%)
4	9% (0%)	23% (2%)	43% (7%)	43% (16%)
5	17% (0%)	11% (0%)	44% (11%)	36% (7%)

*Highly represented by women of all ages with poor ovarian response

**Highly represented by very young women or women of all ages with relatively poor ovarian response

†Highly represented by women with good ovarian response < 34 years old or older women having delivered previously

††Highly represented by women with good ovarian response 34–47 years old

tr, preembryos transferred

low for comparison and the group is highly represented by patients with poor ovarian response (Table 6.2). Clearly, transferring three or four preembryos of good quality produces the best clinical pregnancy rates, albeit with a concurrent increase in multiple implantations. Although a higher score (lower number) is favorable, pregnancy is still possible even in cycles with grade 4 or 5 morphology (unequal-sized blastomeres and moderate-to-severe cytoplasmic fragmentation). Of interest is the fact that the scores are remarkably repetitive for the same patient in successive cycles.

In the Cornell program, two or, most frequently, three preembryos are replaced in women < 34 years of age; four preembryos are recommended for women ages 34–39 years, and five preembryos are often replaced in women > 40 years of age, when and if the preembryos are available. More conceptuses may be considered in special circumstances in women > 43 years old. This strategy is based on the obstetrical outcomes of > 4000 IVF deliveries. Although the multiple-pregnancy rate is high when more than two preembryos are replaced, particularly in young women, the vast majority are twin gestations, acceptable to most infertile couples.

An attractive alternative currently under investigation at Cornell is to replace one less preembryo in cycles with grade 1 or 2 morphology. Such a procedure may result in continued acceptable pregnancy rates while reducing the occurrence of multiple births.

It has recently been reported that the idea of older women establishing fewer multiple pregnancies than younger women is a fallacy[26]. In a recent report, the authors suggest limiting the number of preembryos transferred to three, regardless of age. Our own data do not support a reduction of transfer numbers in this particular population. Examination of the replacement outcomes of 805 cycles during the last two-and-one-half years involving women >40 years of age has indicated a significantly higher clinical pregnancy rate per transfer when four or more preembryos are replaced compared with three (46% and 25%, respectively; $p<0.05$). Nonetheless, we have also found a slight difference in the incidence of multiple pregnancy per transfer of four or more *vs* three preembryos, although the numbers are relatively small (13% and 5%, respectively; $p<0.05$). However, on comparison of these results with those in younger women (<40 years), a much higher incidence of both clinical and multiple pregnancy was seen when three (mostly women <34 years old) or four (mostly women ages 34–39 years) preembryos were transferred (clinical pregnancy: 60% and 61%, respectively; multiple pregnancy: 30% and 29%, respectively). The difference between the incidence of multiple pregnancy in older compared with younger women is significant, despite the fact that none of the younger women had more than four preembryos replaced whereas many of the women >40 years of age did. In view of the current policy to replace more than three preembryos in older women whenever possible, those who received three represent women with poor ovarian response or limited oocyte reserve. This fact cannot be overlooked when weighing the comparisons. Nevertheless, transferring more than three preembryos to older patients did not appear to expose these women to either excessive or unacceptably high rates of multiple pregnancy.

In deciding how many preembryos to transfer in a given patient, it appears reasonable to weigh the risks of multiple pregnancy against age, previous history, preembryo morphology and development, the desires of the couple, and the delivery rates of the relevant clinic.

References

1. Jurisicova A, Varmuza S, Casper RF. Programmed cell death and human embryo fragmentation. *Mol Hum Reprod* 1996;2:93

2. Grillo JM, Gamerre M, Lacroix O, *et al.* Influence of the morphological aspect of embryos obtained by in vitro fertilization on their implantation rate. *J In Vitro Fert Embryo Transf* 1991;8:317

3. Shulman A, Ben-Nun I, Ghetler Y, *et al.* Relationship between embryo morphology and implantation rate after in vitro fertilization treatment in conception cycles. *Fertil Steril* 1993;60:123

4. Claman P, Armant DR, Seibel MM, *et al.* The impact of embryo quality and quantity on implantation and the establishment of viable pregnancies. *J In Vitro Fert Embryo Transf* 1987;4:218

5. Lewin A, Schenker JG, Safran A, *et al.* Embryo growth rate in vitro as an indicator of embryo quality in IVF cycles. *J Assist Reprod Genet* 1994;11:500

6. Zhu J, Meniru GI, Craft IL. Embryo developmental stage at transfer influences outcome of treatment with intracytoplasmic sperm injection. *J Assist Reprod Genet* 1997;14:245

7. McKiernan SH, Bavister BD. Timing of development is a critical parameter for predicting successful embryogenesis. *Hum Reprod* 1994;9:2123

8. Ziebe S, Petersen K, Lindenberg S, *et al.* Embryo morphology or cleavage stage: How to select the best embryos for transfer after in vitro fertilization. *Hum Reprod* 1997;12:1545

9. Wiemer KE, Dale B, Hu Y, *et al.* Blastocyst development in coculture: Development and morphological aspects. *Hum Reprod* 1995;10:3226

10. Shoukir Y, Campana A, Farley T, Sakkas D. Early cleavage of in vitro fertilized human embryos to the 2-cell stage: A novel indicator of embryo quality and viability. *Hum Reprod* 1997;12:1531

11. Cohen J, Inge KL, Suzman M, *et al.* Videocinematography of fresh and cryopreserved embryos: A retrospective analysis of embryonic morphology and implantation. *Fertil Steril* 1989;51:820

12. Morgan K, Wiemer K, Steuerwald N, *et al.* Use of videocinematography to assess morphological qualities of conventionally cultured and cocultured embryos. *Hum Reprod* 1995;10:2371

13. Garside WT, Loret de Mola JR, Bucci JA, *et al.* Sequential analysis of zona thickness during in vitro culture of human zygotes: Correlation with embryo quality, age, and implantation. *Mol Reprod Dev* 1997; 47:99

14. Kligman I, Benadiva C, Alikani M, Munne S. The presence of multinucleated blastomeres in human embryos is correlated with chromosomal abnormalities. *Hum Reprod* 1996;11:1492

15. Nargund G, Bourne T, Doyle P, *et al.* Associations between ultrasound indices of follicular blood flow, oocyte recovery, and preimplantation embryo quality. *Hum Reprod* 1996;11:109

16. Chui D, Pugh N, Walker S, Shaw R. Follicular vascularity – the predictive value of transvaginal Doppler ultrasonography in an in vitro fertilization programme: A preliminary study. *Hum Reprod* 1997;12: 191

17. Van Blerkom J. Can the developmental competence of early human embryos be predicted effectively in the clinical IVF laboratory? *Hum Reprod* 1997;12: 1610

18. Cummins JM, Breen TM, Harrison KL, *et al.* A formula for scoring human embryo growth rates in in vitro fertilization: Its value in predicting pregnancy and in comparison with visual estimates of embryo quality. *J In Vitro Fert Embryo Transf* 1986;3:284

19. Puissant F, Van Rysselberge M, Barlow P, *et al.* Embryo scoring as a prognostic tool in IVF treatment. *Hum Reprod* 1987;2:705

20. Erenus M, Zouves C, Rajamahendran P, *et al.* The effect of embryo quality on subsequent pregnancy rates after in vitro fertilization. *Fertil Steril* 1991; 56:707

21. Steer CV, Mills CL, Tan SL, *et al.* The cumulative embryo score: A predictive embryo scoring technique to select the optimal number of embryos to transfer in an in vitro fertilization and embryo transfer programme. *Hum Reprod* 1992;7:117

22. Visser DS, Fourie FR. The applicability of the cumulative embryo score system for embryo selection and quality control in an in vitro fertilization/ embryo transfer programme. *Hum Reprod* 1993;8: 1719

23. Giorgetti C, Terriou P, Auquier P, *et al.* Embryo score to predict implantation after in vitro fertilization: Based on 957 single embryo transfers. *Hum Reprod* 1995;10:2427

24. Tasdemir M, Tasdemir I, Kodama H, *et al.* Two instead of three embryo transfer in in vitro fertilization. *Hum Reprod* 1995;10:2155

25. Kodama H, Fukuda J, Karube H, *et al.* Prospective evaluation of simple morphological criteria for embryo selection in double embryo transfer cycles. *Hum Reprod* 1995;10:2999

26. Senoz S, Ben-Chetrit A, Casper RF. An IVF fallacy: Multiple pregnancy risk is lower for older women. *J Assist Reprod Genet* 1997;14:192

7 Preembryos with the ability to implant

Preembryos that develop into fetuses

Early demise of the human conceptus is a common event. Approximately 73% of natural single conceptions are lost before reaching week 6 of gestation and, of the remainder, approximately 90% survive to term[1]. IVF conceptions do nearly as well as natural pregnancies after clinical recognition, but compare poorly between the onset of fertilization and completion of implantation, presumably due to preclinical developmental arrest.

Which factors contribute to preembryo viability? Certainly, genetic health is a major prerequisite for the implantation and delivery of a healthy child. Unfortunately, little is known of the genetic constitutions of the preembryos within our incubators unless they are biopsied and examined. There is evidence to suggest that chromosomal abnormalities, both numerical and structural, are more often associated with fragmented and arrested preembryos, although many poor-quality preembryos retain the capacity to develop normally into healthy fetuses.

On the other hand, many preembryos from older women present with good morphology, yet possess lethal genetic aberrations[2]. This implies that, although grading systems may furnish clues which enhance our proficiency at choosing the best preembryos for transfer, these systems are severely limited in their ability to provide indisputable evidence for subsequent normal development. Thus, selection during very early preembryonic development remains, at least for the time being, a somewhat random exercise.

One comforting notion involves the fact that many genetically unhealthy preembryos may cease growth at the early cleavage stages. A progressive loss of chromosomally abnormal preembryos after pronuclear development through to at least the eight-cell stage has been suggested[3]. When preembryos of varying morphological grades were studied cytogenetically, investigators found a 65% incidence of abnormality at the pronuclear stage, a 55% incidence at the two- to four-cell stage, and a 27% incidence at the five- to eight-cell stage. Not surprisingly, cleaved preembryos with poor morphology (irregularly shaped blastomeres and severe extracellular fragmentation) demonstrated an almost three-fold increase in chromosomal anomalies compared with preembryos of good morphology.

From these data, it is logical to deduce that a form of natural selection continues to exert an influence beyond the eight-cell stage and perhaps into early fetal development. Thus, should we not expect such progressive natural selection to continue if culture times are extended beyond the standard two or three days? There is evidence to support this idea provided that culture systems capable of supporting prolonged *in vitro* growth are successfully developed[4]. Preliminary studies have already demonstrated significantly enhanced implantation rates when cavitating morulae are transferred on the fourth day[5], or when fully expanded blastocysts with clearly defined inner cell masses are replaced on the fifth day[6].

In addition to the need to improve culture medium components, some investigators have suggested that other laboratory factors, such as removing antibiotics from the media[7], reducing sperm exposure time to oocytes during insemination[8], and culturing preembryos in groups rather than singly[9,10], may contribute to normal *in vitro* growth of human conceptuses.

Figures 7.1–7.12 show preembryos that have implanted, produced a fetal heartbeat as determined by ultrasound, and most often resulted in a thriving healthy child. (Where this was not the case, the outcome has been indicated in the legend.)

Poor morphology and implantation

Figures 7.13–7.18, taken at the time of intrauterine transfer, represent cohorts of preembryos with poor morphology, one or more of which implanted and produced a fetal heartbeat as determined by ultrasound, and most often resulted in one or more healthy children. (Where this was not the case, the outcome has been indicated in the legend.) Although it is well established that poor preembryo morphology is often associated with chromosomal abnormality, this is clearly not an exact correlation[11]. Thus, young women <34 years of age never receive more than three preembryos at transfer, regardless of the morphology of their conceptuses.

Excellent morphology and failure to implant

Figures 7.19–7.26, taken at the time of intrauterine transfer, represent cohorts of preembryos with excellent morphology, none of which produced a viable pregnancy.

There is a clear correlation between advanced female age and a decline in fecundity. The excellent results following oocyte donation to older women have validated the hypothesis that this decline is related more to oocyte quality than to inadequate endometrial conditions. Extremely high pregnancy rates can be achieved in women >40 years of age upon receiving donated oocytes from a younger donor[12]. One recent report describes the delivery of a healthy female infant to a 63-year-old woman who falsely presented her age as 53 years when seeking treatment through oocyte donation[13].

Without oocyte donation, it has been observed that the potential for implantation decreases gradually past the age of 30 years and by more than two-thirds after 40 years of age[14]. It is possible that transferring blastocysts to older women may increase their opportunity for pregnancy (through the natural selection process already discussed), although many patients fail to produce adequate oocytes to offset the almost certain loss of developing preembryos during the preimplantation culture period[15].

As will be noted from the legends, some, but by no means all, of the preembryos shown in these figures (see pages 157–9) developed from the oocytes of women >40 years of age. In the cases of unsuccessful development, genetic competence, transfer technique, and uterine receptivity need to be considered as possible factors in the failure to give rise to pregnancy.

Application of coculture techniques to improve implantation

As already mentioned in Chapters 5 and 6, coculture techniques appear to be helpful in encouraging preembryos to develop into viable fetuses. Whether a monolayer of cells imparts factors favorable to support growth or whether the cells utilize unnecessary medium components and / or absorb toxins is not yet clearly ascertained. It is likely that the coculture cells are helpful for all of these reasons, especially under conditions in which culture media or environmental factors are less than optimal.

In the Cornell program, only homologous cell lines are used for coculture to ensure patient safety and protection. Although homologous granulosa and cumulus cells have been used, the currently favored protocol involves the use of an endometrial cell line (Figures 7.27–7.31). Briefly, endometrial cells are grown in culture after endometrial biopsy; a good mix of glands and stroma is preferred. The cells are frozen until the patient cycles for an IVF attempt; the cells are then thawed and plated. Three-quarters of a patient's fertilized conceptuses are placed on a monolayer of these cells on day 1 after harvest. Slightly enhanced growth and a slightly improved morphology have been noted in cocultured preembryos compared with controls. In addition, the rates of pregnancy thus far have been encouraging[16].

Outcomes of IVF pregnancies

Babies born through IVF procedures exhibit no greater incidence of congenital malformations nor developmental problems than do naturally conceived children in the general population when matched for plurality and gestation. Most adverse outcomes are related to the effects of multiple birth, and the most common difficulties are preterm labor and a low birth weight. Some reports suggest that even singleton IVF children exhibit slightly lower birth weights, but the literature is contradictory on this point. When twin gestations evolving from IVF are compared with twins conceived naturally or after intrauterine insemination (IUI), no significant differences are found except for one published report describing a greater likelihood of discordant birth weight.

The intelligence and behavior of IVF children fall within normal limits. As a group, social adaptation and language skills are satisfactory.

Higher-order multiple gestations are the largest single cause of poor obstetrical outcome and neonatal difficulties. Although multifetal pregnancy reduction to twins is an option in such cases, the procedure itself carries risk and the outcomes are not as favorable as those observed with spontaneously conceived twin pregnancies. Triplet and quadruplet pregnancies are associated with high incidences of preeclampsia, gestational diabetes, pregnancy-induced hypertension, preterm labor, low birth weight, and neonatal care. Despite these difficulties, however, many higher-order multiple pregnancies do well, probably because of early medical intervention and close monitoring. Congenital malformations are not increased in triplet and quadruplet pregnancies.

The follow-up of children conceived through intracytoplasmic sperm injection (ICSI) procedures similarly reveals no increase in the incidence of congenital malformations or chromosomal aberrations.

The cryopreservation process does not appear to adversely affect fetal development and no perinatal risk has been identified. Gestational age at delivery, Apgar scores, birth weights, incidence of malformations, and perinatal mortality have been found to be comparable to those of controls.

Children conceived through IVF procedures, even singleton births, tend to be delivered more often by Cesarean section. This was especially the case during the first decade of widespread use of the procedure and still occurs more often today than in naturally conceived pregnancies. The reason for this to be true in singleton deliveries is unclear; one possible speculation is that physicians are overly nervous about outcomes because of the dear price paid to achieve the pregnancies.

Despite the issues of low birth weight and the high incidence of multiple births (~25%), it may be concluded that neither IVF nor its closely related procedures are independent factors significantly affecting obstetrical or perinatal outcome.

(References 17–40 are the sources used in writing this section.)

References

1. Boklage CE. Survival probability of human conceptions from fertilization to term. *Int J Fertil* 1990;35:75

2. Munne S, Alikani M, Tomkin G, *et al.* Embryo morphology, developmental rates, and maternal age are correlated with chromosome abnormalities. *Fertil Steril* 1995;64:382

3. Almeida PA, Bolton VN. The relationship between chromosomal abnormality in the human preimplantation embryo and development in vitro. *Reprod Fertil Dev (Australia)* 1996;8:235

4. Gardner DK, Lane M, Spitzer A, Batt PA. Enhanced rates of cleavage and development for sheep zygotes cultured to the blastocyst stage in vitro in the absence of serum and somatic cells: Amino acids, vitamins, and culturing embryos in groups stimulate development. *Biol Reprod* 1994;50:390

5. Huisman GJ, Alberda AT, Leerentveld RA, *et al.* A comparison of in vitro fertilization results after embryo transfer after 2, 3, and 4 days of embryo culture. *Fertil Steril* 1994;61:970

6. Scholtes MC, Zeilmaker GH. A prospective, randomized study of embryo transfer results after 3 or 5 days of embryo culture in in vitro fertilization. *Fertil Steril* 1996;65:1245

7. Magli MC, Gianaroli L, Fiorentino A, *et al.* Improved cleavage rate of human embryos cultured in antibiotic-free medium. *Hum Reprod* 1996;11:1520

8. Gianaroli L, Magli MC, Ferraretti AP, *et al.* Reducing the time of sperm–oocyte interaction in human in vitro fertilization improves the implantation rate. *Hum Reprod* 1996;11:166

9. Moessner J, Dodson WC. The quality of human embryo growth is improved when embryos are cultured in groups rather than separately. *Fertil Steril* 1995;64:1034

10. Almagor M, Bejar C, Kafka I, Yaffe H. Pregnancy rates after communal growth of preimplantation human embryos in vitro. *Fertil Steril* 1996;66:394

11. Pellestor F, Dufour MC, Arnal F, Humeau C. Direct assessment of the rate of chromosomal abnormalities in grade IV human embryos produced by in-vitro fertilization procedure. *Hum Reprod* 1994;9:293

12. Navot D, Bergh PA, Williams MA, *et al.* Poor oocyte quality rather than implantation failure as a cause of age-related decline in female fertility. *Lancet* 1991; 337:1375

13. Paulson RJ, Thornton MH, Francis MM, Salvador HS. Successful pregnancy in a 63-year-old woman. *Fertil Steril* 1997;67:949

14. Hull MG, Fleming CF, Hughes AO, McDermott A. The age-related decline in female fecundity: A quantitative controlled study of implanting capacity and survival of individual embryos after in vitro fertilization. *Fertil Steril* 1996;65:783

15. Janny L, Menezo YJ. Maternal age effect on early human embryonic development and blastocyst formation. *Mol Reprod Dev* 1996;45:31

16. Barmat LI, Veeck LL, Liu HC, *et al.* Autologous endometrial coculture in patients with repeated failures of implantation after IVF. (in preparation)

17. Alsalili M, Yuzpe A, Tummon I, *et al.* Cumulative pregnancy rates and pregnancy outcome after in vitro fertilization: > 5000 cycles at one center. *Hum Reprod* 1995;10:470

18. Bernasko J, Lynch L, Lapinski R, Berkowitz RL. Twin pregnancies conceived by assisted reproductive techniques: Maternal and neonatal outcomes. *Obstet Gynecol* 1997;89:368

19. Bonduelle M, Legein J, Derde MP, *et al.* Comparative follow-up study of 130 children born after intracytoplasmic sperm injection and 130 children born after in vitro fertilization. *Hum Reprod* 1995;10:3327

20. Brandes JM, Scher A, Itzkovits J, *et al.* Growth and development of children conceived by in vitro fertilization. *Pediatrics* 1992;90:424

21. Cederblad M, Friberg B, Ploman F, *et al.* Intelligence and behavior in children born after in vitro fertilization treatment. *Hum Reprod* 1996;11:2052

22. Ezra Y, Schenker JG. Appraisal of in vitro fertilization. *Eur J Obstet Gynecol Reprod Biol* 1993;48:127

23. Gonzalez P, Hanna L, Thomas N, *et al.* Triplet and quadruplet pregnancy: Management and perinatal outcome. *Rev Chil Obstet Ginecol* 1994; 59:361

24. Groutz A, Yovel I, Amit A, *et al.* Pregnancy outcome after multifetal pregnancy reduction to twins compared with spontaneously conceived twins. *Hum Reprod* 1996;11:1334

25. Harrison RF, Hennelly B, Woods T, *et al.* Course and outcome of IVF pregnancies and spontaneous conceptions within an IVF setting. *Eur J Obstet Gynecol Reprod Biol* 1995;59:175

26. Howe RS, Sayegh RA, Durinzi KL, Tureck RW. Perinatal outcome of singleton pregnancies conceived by in vitro fertilization: A controlled study. *J Perinatol* 1990;10:261

27. Melgar CA, Rosenfeld DL, Rawlinson K, Greenberg M. Perinatal outcome after multifetal reduction to twins compared with nonreduced multiple gestations. *Obstet Gynecol* 1991;78:763

28. Morin NC, Wirth FH, Johnson DH, *et al.* Congenital malformations and psychosocial development in children conceived by in vitro fertilization. *J Pediatr* 1989;115:222

29. Olivennes F, Kadhel P, Rufat P, *et al.* Perinatal outcome of twin pregnancies obtained after in vitro fertilization: Comparison with twin pregnancies obtained spontaneously or after ovarian stimulation. *Fertil Steril* 1996;66:105

30. Olivennes F, Kerbrat V, Rufat P, *et al.* Follow-up of a cohort of 422 children aged 6 to 13 years conceived by in vitro fertilization. *Fertil Steril* 1997;67:284

31. Petersen K, Hornnes PJ, Ellingsen S, *et al.* Perinatal outcome after in vitro fertilization. *Acta Obstet Gynecol Scand* 1995;74:129

32. Pons JC, Nekhlyudov L, Dephot N, *et al.* Management and outcomes of 65 quadruplet pregnancies: Sixteen years' experience in France. *Acta Genet Med Gemellol (Rome)* 1996;45:367

33. Reubinoff BE, Samueloff A, Ben-Haim M, *et al.* Is the obstetric outcome of in vitro fertilized singleton gestations different from natural ones? A controlled study. *Fertil Steril* 1997;67:1077

34. Saunders K, Spensley J, Munro J, Halasz G. Growth and physical outcome of children conceived by in vitro fertilization. *Pediatrics* 1996;97:688

35. Seoud MA, Toner JP, Kruithoff C, Muasher SJ. Outcome of twin, triplet, and quadruplet in vitro fertilization pregnancies: The Norfolk experience. *Fertil Steril* 1992;57:825

36. Skupski DW, Nelson S, Kowalik A, *et al.* Multiple gestations from in vitro fertilization: Successful implantation alone is not associated with subsequent preeclampsia. *Am J Obstet Gynecol* 1996;175:1029

37. Tanbo T, Dale PO, Lunde O, *et al.* Obstetric outcome in singleton pregnancies after assisted reproduction. *Obstet Gynecol* 1995;86:188

38. Tarlatzis BC. Report on the activities of the ESHRE Task Force on intracytoplasmic sperm injection. European Society of Human Reproduction and Embryology. *Hum Reprod* 1996;11(Suppl 4):160

39. Wada I, Macnamee MC, Wick K, *et al.* Birth characteristics and perinatal outcome of babies conceived from cryopreserved embryos. *Hum Reprod* 1994;9: 543

40. Wennerholm UB, Hamberger L, Nilsson L, *et al.* Obstetrical and perinatal outcome of children conceived from cryopreserved embryos. *Hum Reprod* 1997;12:1819

8 Abnormal morphology of the human oocyte and conceptus

Abnormal fertilization

It is not uncommon to observe oocytes with three or more pronuclei after IVF; the reported incidence of *polyploidy* ranges from 1–30% in the literature, with most programs reporting around 5%[1–8]. After the first cleavage, triploid or tetraploid conceptuses often demonstrate cleavage patterns indistinguishable from those of two-pronuclear origin. For this reason, it is extremely important to assess correctly the number of pronuclei before the prezygote enters syngamy.

Evaluation of the prezygote should be carried out with care. The number and size of pronuclei must be recorded, and the nucleoli in each one identified. Vacuolar structures which have the ability to move within the cytoplasm and become juxtaposed with true pronuclei have been erroneously reported as pronuclei in some instances[9]. Use of a high-resolution inverted microscope and careful examination for the presence of nucleoli should eliminate the potential of inaccurate identification due to such *pseudopronuclei*.

Haploidy (one pronucleus)

Oocytes can be artificially activated under experimental protocols to produce haploid prezygotes capable of undergoing rudimentary cleavage[10–16]. Similarly, haploid conceptuses can be produced by the removal or inactivation of one pronucleus in a diploid prezygote[17,18]. Accidental activation of an oocyte by heat, cold, biochemical, osmotic or mechanical means often leads to extrusion of the first polar body and the development of a single haploid gynogenic pronucleus. Purposeful oocyte activation is remarkably easy in some species, but tends to be more difficult in humans[19].

It has been suggested that all inseminated oocytes displaying a single pronucleus should be rechecked within 2–6 h to confirm pronuclear status. A report in which investigators did this revealed that 25% of second repeat observations led to the visualization of two pronuclei rather than one[20]. Such a finding suggests that developmental asynchrony between male and female pronuclei may not be a rare event.

A single pronucleus can form and persist after *in vitro* insemination or sperm injection, resulting in a gynogenic or, rarely, androgenic haploid prezygote (Figures 8.1–8.5). Human oocytes displaying a single pronucleus have been observed to continue growth to blastocyst stages, some of which have been shown to be diploid. One such study describes removing pronuclei from single-pronucleate oocytes after conventional insemination. Of 16 pronuclei examined, six were diploid, four of which contained XY chromosomes[21]. This suggests that sperm and oocyte nuclei can associate to form a single diploid pronucleus rather than being simply asynchronous in development. It has further been shown that preembryos developing from single-pronucleate oocytes after IVF insemination are usually diploid and most often fertilized whereas those from activated intracytoplasmic sperm injection (ICSI) oocytes are almost always haploid parthenotes[20–23]. For this reason, preembryos which develop from inseminated oocytes displaying one pronucleus may be replaced; those developing after ICSI should not be transferred. As diploid pronuclei are often described as being larger than usual due to their doubled amount of DNA[24], this characteristic may be favorable in single-pronucleate oocytes after *in vitro* insemination.

An interesting observation is that a nuclear envelope may form around the M II chromosome group in an *unpenetrated* oocyte, resulting in a digynic prezygote with two pronuclei. This is commonly seen in some lower lifeforms where parthenogenesis occurs naturally, and has been noted in humans after oocyte cryopreservation and thawing with 1,2-propanediol. However, whether this occurs naturally in humans, or has the potential for subsequent development, is unknown.

Triploidy (three pronuclei)

Triploidy (Figures 8.6 and 8.7) may arise through several different mechanisms, some of which are well documented in humans. Although advanced maternal age is not implicated, the production of meiotically incompetent or unhealthy oocytes can lead to triploid conditions. Oocytes that lack an effective block to polyspermy or fail to segregate chromosomes properly during meiosis are often associated with this abnormality.

Four circumstances frequently account for triploid fertilization (the first two listed here are the most often observed):

(1) **Penetration of an oocyte by two spermatozoa.** This may lead to the formation of one maternal and two paternal pronuclei. The usual chromosome complements of the resulting diandric preembryos are 69,XXX or 69,XXY. For reasons that remain obscure, 69,XYY is rarely observed;

(2) **Retention of the first or second polar body chromosomes.** Retention of either the first (rarely) or second polar body during oocyte meiotic maturation may lead to the formation of two maternal pronuclei and one paternal pronucleus. The resulting digynic preembryos – 69,XXX or 69,XXY – are responsible for most late term triploid fetuses and live triploid births[25–27];

(3) **Penetration of an oocyte by a binucleate spermatozoon.** This may lead to the development of one maternal and two paternal pronuclei. Only 0.5% of human spermatozoa have been reported to be diploid;

(4) **Penetration of a binucleate oocyte by a single spermatozoon.** Penetration of a binucleate oocyte may lead to the formation of two maternal pronuclei and one paternal pronucleus.

Giant and binucleate oocytes

An occasional observation is oocytes that are much larger than those routinely seen (Figures 8.8–8.10). They may exhibit up to twice the volume of normal oocytes and are presumed to have arisen through failure of cytoplasmic division of oogonia. Consistent with this assumption is the fact that most are binucleate, possessing diploid amounts of DNA. Some have been observed to extrude two polar bodies at the end of meiosis I. On exposure to spermatozoa, large oocytes may be expected to develop into triploid preembryos. Through the use of fluorescence in-situ hybridization (FISH) techniques on four giant oocytes, triploidy and triploid mosaicism has been confirmed[28].

A binucleate oocyte of normal size may be the result of suppression of the first polar body. Suppression of the second polar body results in a binucleate prezygote (sperm-penetrated oocyte) destined for triploidy. Normal-sized, binucleate, germinal vesicle-bearing oocytes arise through abnormal division of oogonia (Figure 8.11).

Pronuclear size in triploid specimens

Triploid conditions may be present in prezygotes displaying two pronuclei if one overly large pronucleus contains a diploid number of chromosomes.

Fertilization involving mononucleate, but diploid, oocytes or spermatozoa may be the cause of this occurrence. Such gametes arise through failure of both cytoplasmic and nuclear divisions of oogonia or spermatogonia.

Pronuclear size is generally altered in the triploid specimen (Figure 8.12). It has been reported that the formation of multiple pronuclei results in an overall reduction in size for each[24].

Triploid development

Preembryos developing from triploid prezygotes often appear to undergo more rapid cleavage than diploid preembryos, perhaps because many cleave directly into three blastomeres at the first division due to a tripolar spindle (Figures 8.13 and 8.14). Three patterns of cleavage have been documented in triploid prezygotes:

(1) Direct cleavage into three blastomeres, resulting in variable and abnormal karyotypes which display near-diploid complements (62%);

(2) Cleavage into two blastomeres, resulting in uniform triploid karyotypes (24%); and

(3) Cleavage into two blastomeres plus a small extrusion mass, resulting in diploid karyotypes in each blastomere and a probable haploid complement in the extrusion mass (14%; Figure 8.15)[29].

Given this information, an interesting correlation emerges between the pattern of cleavage and subsequent chromosomal complement of the preembryo. Furthermore, it suggests that some triploid preembryos, albeit a low percentage, are capable of self-regulation and potentially normal development (Figures 8.16–8.18).

Triploidy is implicated in approximately 20% of spontaneous abortions in humans. Although fetuses affected by this disorder rarely survive to term, when they do, they exhibit severe physical abnormalities and mental retardation.

The centrosome in triploid conditions

Associated with the organization of spindle fibers, which function during mitosis and meiosis, the centrosome replicates before cell division. There is convincing evidence that the human sperm centrosome controls the first mitotic divisions after fertilization and that the maternal centrosome is probably inactive[30,31].

Studies with human conceptuses have demonstrated that dispermic prezygotes often form abnormal tripolar spindles because they possess two functional centrosomes, both contributed by the sperm. These prezygotes divide directly into three cells at the first cleavage, and exhibit abnormal karyotypes and mosaicism. On the other hand, digynic prezygotes form bipolar spindles because of the one functional centrosome contributed by a single sperm, and the resultant preembryos are uniformly triploid. In one fascinating study, it was found that removing one pronucleus in a dispermic prezygote before syngamy did not prevent the formation of a tripolar spindle, indicating that an extranuclear factor, the second active paternal centrosome, was responsible[32]. When one pronucleus from a digynic prezygote was removed, however, the expected bipolar spindle formed and the resultant preembryo was diploid rather than triploid. These data confirm the importance of the sperm centrosome and suggest a mechanism to explain why parthenogenesis is not compatible with embryonic development in humans.

Correction of triploidy

In 1996, Feng and Gordon[33] demonstrated that, in the mouse, the supernumerary male pronucleus of a mammalian dispermic triploid prezygote was removable, thereby allowing normal development which could result in live birth. In effect, an abnormal conceptus was rescued and restored to a diploid state. In light of the finding in humans that abnormal karyotypes and mosaicism follow the removal of one male pronucleus (see above), initially there appears to be a contradiction. The different results probably stem from the fact that, unlike humans and most other mammals, the mouse zygote does not rely on paternal centrosomes for early cleavage. There have been reports that the centrosome is maternally inherited from cytoplasmic sites in the mouse oocyte[34–36].

As with the mouse, attempts have been made to alter the ploidy of triploid human prezygotes[37–39]. Although it has been shown that a third pronucleus can be removed successfully without apparent damage to the oocyte, children have yet to be born as a result of this procedure. Based on the current evidence regarding the role of the sperm centrosome, the technique should prove most successful in digynic triploid prezygotes produced after ICSI.

One potential problem involves the current inability to choose easily the most appropriate pronucleus for removal. It is uncertain what the fate of a 46,XX preembryo would be if all the genetic material were maternally derived. Thus far, such preembryos have never implanted successfully. On the other hand, the incorrect removal of the maternal pronucleus of a dispermic prezygote may potentially place a woman at risk for the development of a hydatidiform mole (all genetic material paternally derived) after intrauterine transfer. Approximately 95% of complete hydatidiforn moles have a 46,XX paternal chromosome constitution[40].

Indeed, if proficiency at removing the supernumerary pronucleus in triploid prezygotes were to be achieved (Figure 8.19), the procedure would have a positive impact on the number of preembryos available for transfer or freezing. In the Cornell program alone, >700 triploid oocytes are seen each year, some from women with a total of only one or two oocytes collected at harvest. It is estimated that, in the USA and Canada, as many as 14 000 triploid conceptuses are seen in IVF programs each year[33]. Making these conceptuses available for clinical use would be of great benefit in certain cases.

Tetra- (four pronuclei) or higher ploidy

Tetraploid conceptuses are known to arise through suppression of the first cleavage or after penetration of an oocyte by three sperm. When four pronuclei are seen in the prezygote (Figure 8.20), each pronucleus is generally smaller than average (as with triploidy). Thus, there is an inverse correlation between pronuclear number and size. As the number increases, the size decreases. The combined pronuclear volume, however, remains relatively constant.

As also with triploidy, maternal age is not associated with an increased incidence of tetraploidy. Conceptuses developing from these prezygotes are not commonly encountered and rarely proceed beyond two or three weeks *in utero*[41]. As most aborted tetraploid fetuses exhibit an XXXX or XXYY karyotype, their likely origin is failed cytokinesis at the first cleavage. Tetraploidy is seen relatively frequently in some somatic cell cultures, but this is thought to be mostly artifactual, due to a culture system that is unable to support the molecular requirements for cytokinesis in a large number of growing cells.

Five, six, seven or more pronuclei (Figures 8.21 and 8.22) have been observed in human oocytes after IVF.

Monosomy and trisomy

Monosomic and *trisomic* conditions cannot be recognized by any morphologic criteria used in the IVF laboratory, but are easily identified with the use of FISH techniques (see Chapter 12). Autosomal trisomies represent the largest single class of chromosomal complements found in cytogenetically abnormal spontaneous abortions[41].

Nondisjunction, leading to monosomy and trisomy, results when two members of a chromosome pair fail to segregate properly during the anaphase of cell division. Studies of liveborn trisomic offspring have shown that the vast majority of trisomies arise during maternal meiosis I[42]. Advanced maternal age is associated with most, but not all, trisomic abortuses. In particular, trisomy 16 does not appear to be related to *in vivo* aging of oocytes[43]. Many trisomies, and most monosomies other than those involving sex chromosomes, are incompatible with life, and death occurs during early preembryonic or embryonic development. Some of these deaths are associated with placental fragmentation, cord stumps, blighted ova, or empty gestational sacs.

If nondisjunction occurs during the first mitotic cleavage, then two separate abnormal cell lines are established with different chromosome numbers, resulting in affliction of all subsequent cells. The resulting preembryo is termed a *mosaic*. Nondisjunction at the time of second cleavage results in three cell lines with 50% of the subsequent cells being abnormal and, at the third cleavage, 25% of the resultant cells are abnormal. These ratios extend through each succeeding division. Usually, monosomic cell lines are underrepresented in karyotypic analysis of mosaic subjects, presumably due to the monosomic cell tendency for an early demise.

Children born with mosaic Down syndrome exhibit trisomy 21 in some, but not all, of their cells and, thus, usually present with a milder form of the disorder. Monosomy involving the X chromosome results in Turner's syndrome; 70% of the fetuses thus afflicted die *in utero*. Some, but not all, of the survivors are mosaics with some normal cells. Another notable feature of Turner's syndrome is that, in 75% of cases, the nondisjunction event is of paternal origin.

In all, approximately 50% of human conceptions are chromosomally abnormal. Most of these will have been lost by term, although around 0.5% survive to birth.

Multinucleated blastomeres

Multinucleated blastomeres are not an uncommon observation in cleaving preembryos and blastocysts[44] (Figures 8.23–8.26). The high incidence of multinucleation both *in vivo* and *in vitro* has led investigators to question its role in early embryogenesis; it may perhaps serve as a mechanism for ridding the preembryo of defective blastomeres. Indeed, most events in nature occur for a reason (?a means to an end). This idea notwithstanding, the general consensus is that these cells most likely represent random failures of cytokinesis and that their presence is detrimental rather than purposeful. Up to 70% of preimplantation preembryos exhibit multinucleated blastomeres[45,46]. Not surprisingly in view of such a high incidence, multinucleated blastomeres have been observed in preembryos associated with ongoing pregnancy[47,48]. Based on chromosome analyses, however, there is sufficient evidence to dissuade embryologists from preferentially replacing these preembryos even when cell number and preembryo morphology is good[49].

Nuclear / pronuclear fragmentation

Nuclei and pronuclei are capable of breaking up into multiple smaller structures called *subnuclei* which contain scattered membrane-bound chromatin. Similarly, unfertilized oocytes may develop subnuclei with chromatin that has become disconnected from spindle microtubules during meiosis[24,50]. It is to be expected that the chromosomes within these fragments are unable to participate in meiotic or mitotic events. Aged oocytes *in vitro* appear to be more prone to developing subnuclei.

Irregularities of polar bodies

Variation in the size of the first polar body (overly large or small) may represent an abnormal condition. The factor determining the size of the polar body is probably the position of the meiotic spindle in relation to the surface of the oocyte. In this case, inward displacement of the spindle results in a polar body of atypically large size. Through this mechanism, aged oocytes are reported to extrude larger polar bodies in some circumstances[24]. Descriptions of *immediate cleavage* and *parthenogenic division* may be related to this type of unequal distribution of ooplasm at the end of meiosis I. Truly enormous polar bodies are not commonly seen in human oocytes and many of those described as such are, in fact, large cytoplasmic fragments (Figure 8.27).

Oocytes with very small first polar bodies are associated with reduced fertilization and increased triploidy[51]. It is postulated that chromosomes destined for the first polar body may remain entirely in the oocyte or be incompletely expelled, thereby giving rise to a small empty first polar body and subsequent triploidy in the oocyte after sperm penetration.

Oocytes with fragmented and / or flattened first polar bodies (Figures 8.28–8.32) may demonstrate a reduced potential for development. Oocyte post-maturity and *in vitro* aging are often associated with these oocytes, and the incidence of triploid fertilization is somewhat higher than normal[52]. A recently published report has correlated the morphology of the first polar body to the fertilization rate after ICSI. It was also determined that the presence of a fragmented polar body, particularly in conjunction with a large perivitelline space and the presence of cytoplasmic inclusions, was associated with reduced fertilization and subsequent poor preembryo quality[53]. Furthermore, oocytes with flattened, fully attached, first polar bodies ('immature' polar bodies) demonstrated little potential for either fertilization or cleavage beyond the two-cell stage (Figure 8.33).

Cytoplasmic fragmentation

Preembryos are frequently capable of undergoing a series of spontaneous cytoplasmic divisions, often in a manner that superficially resembles cleavage. Such divisions are caused by disorganized fragmentation of the cytoplasm (Figures 8.34 and 8.35). Fragments may contain DNA, but are more likely to contain no nuclear material whatsoever. In the Cornell program, approximately 80% of all replacements involve preembryos exhibiting some degree of cytoplasmic fragmentation (from mild to severe) and 16% involve significant fragmentation. Preembryos developed from aging oocytes – those with too long an interval between maturation and fertilization – exhibit high rates of fragmentation[54–56].

Fragments often develop before or during the first cleavage and persist throughout the culture period. When they arise before pronuclei have disappeared, this is termed early fragmentation (Figures 8.36–8.38). Furthermore, they appear in different forms. Fragments may be localized or scattered, free or bound to blastomeres and / or small or large in size (for more details on fragmentation, see Chapter 11).

Irregularities of the zona pellucida

The zona pellucida is the prime controller of interspecific fertilization. This structure prevents non-species sperm from passing through and contacting the oolemma. In humans, the zona pellucida is a relatively thick (approximately 17–18 μm), transparent, acellular vestment that surrounds the oocyte and perivitelline space[44]. During follicular growth, the mucopolysaccharide-rich zona layer is deposited in patches between the surfaces of the oocyte and its surrounding cells. As the follicle grows, these patches enlarge and coalesce to form a continuous layer that separates most of the follicular cells from the oocyte surface. The cumulus cell processes remaining in contact with the oocyte surface become attenuated. Whether the material that makes up the zona is a product of the cumulus cells, the oocyte, or both, is as yet undetermined[57].

Ultrastructural studies of the zona have demonstrated two types of surface: smooth and compact; and mesh-like and porous[58]. The smooth type is commonly associated with immature and atretic oocytes; the mesh-like one is typical of mature, fertilizable oocytes. Spermatozoa are better able to bind to a porous zona, suggesting enhanced exposure or heightened development of binding sites. It may be that, in some unsuccessful IVF trials, the outer zona lacked this porosity.

The inner zona is an effective barrier to polyspermy. After penetration by one sperm, others are generally blocked from further entry.

On LM, the healthy zona of an unfertilized oocyte appears to be clear and continuous, with little variation in thickness, and usually displays a slightly speckled aspect. Excessive break-up of the zona within a dispersed matrix of granular material is associated with aging and deterioration. After fertilization, the zona often exhibits variation in thickness.

The zona pellucida is thought to protect the preembryo during its journey to the uterus. At approximately 6 days after sperm penetration, the preembryo undergoes a hatching process, during which it expands and enlarges until it breaks free of the zona and becomes capable of implantation[59].

Atypical color, thickness or composition

Some zonae present a yellowish-brown or dark brown color. Preembryos with dark zonae are candidates for assisted-hatching (AHA) procedures (Figures 8.39 and 8.40; see Chapter 11).

A zona diameter that is $>25\,\mu m$ or $<10\,\mu m$ is rarely observed (Figure 8.41). It has been recommended that ICSI be carried out on oocytes with zonae $>21\,\mu m$ in diameter[60] (for more details, see Chapter 11).

An oocyte possessing a detritus-laden perivitelline space may be associated with inner zona pellucida deterioration and shedding (Figure 8.42). Such a finding has been termed *perivitelline debris*. When the debris is excessive, the potential for normal fertilization after insemination may be impaired, although ICSI appears to be helpful in overcoming this problem. Cumulus cells are sometimes seen trapped under zona investments. These may be removed by microsurgery (Figures 8.43–8.45).

Bilayering / distortion

The term *bilayered* is perhaps inappropriate as it has already been determined that the healthy zona pellucida normally possesses both a compact and a porous layer. However, when used to describe an aberrant finding, the term denotes either irregular separation or visible thickening in one or both of the zona layers (Figures 8.46–8.50). A significant number of oocytes collected for IVF possess zonae with a bilayer defect. In some instances, an ICSI procedure may be rendered more difficult because of abnormal zona thickening. Whenever thickening is observed in a preembryo destined for intrauterine transfer, AHA is carried out to enhance subsequent blastocyst escape within the uterus.

Shape distortion

Because of irregularities in the shape and composition of the zona pellucida, oocytes, prezygotes, and preembryos occasionally exhibit extraordinary cytoplasmic contours. Two oocytes may share a common zona (Figure 8.51) and yet be disparate in maturation. Oval, comma-like, teardrop, and hourglass configurations have been observed in oocytes at harvest and in developing preembryos (Figures 8.52–8.55). Amazingly, many of the oddest forms retain the ability to undergo monospermic fertilization and subsequent cleavage. Some of these unique shapes arise through bilayer defects whereas others appear to be the longlasting effect of simple compression and distortion of the zona by tightly packed surrounding cells.

Minor breaches

Occasionally, oocytes are observed to have minute breaks in continuity of the zona which allow herniation of part of the ooplasm. The oocyte remains viable if surrounded by an intact oolemma[61]. The breaches are usually the result of excessive negative pressure during handling procedures. Depending on the location of the meiotic spindle, either the intra- or extrazonal segment of cytoplasm may exhibit pronuclei during fertilization. Because the effective zona block to polyspermy is altered, abnormal fertilization often occurs.

If the breach occurs after fertilization, one or all blastomeres may escape the zona pellucida, leading to a theoretical reduction of implantation potential. It is thought that early-cleavage-stage preembryos, before compaction, are unable to develop properly in culture without the protection and molding assistance of the zona. However, this assumption may not be true, as human oocytes have been observed to undergo compaction and blastocyst formation in the absence of a zona (Figures 8.56 and 8.57).

Complete absence

Under normal conditions, synthesis of zona glycoproteins is initiated shortly after the primary oocyte has begun to grow and is completed by the time the oocyte reaches full size. It is extremely rarely that a fully grown oocyte is found to be capable of being fertilized normally without the presence of a zona. In one such case, a patient was initially diagnosed with idiopathic infertility and sought treatment at our clinic in New York. She was found to produce oocytes lacking a zona in both natural and stimulated IVF cycles. In her first stimulated cycle, all of the *zonaless* oocytes were damaged by the negative pressure used during oocyte collection. A subsequent attempt with the negative pressure greatly reduced resulted in the harvest of 11 zonaless oocytes, five of which appeared to be intact after removal of the surrounding cumulus cells using a weak hyaluronidase solution.

ICSI was performed with particular care on these oocytes to avoid damage to the ooplasmic membrane. Four of the oocytes later demonstrated normal fertilization (Figures 8.58–8.60). After cleavage to the two- to four- cell stages, these were transferred to empty donor zonae. All four preembryos were allowed to grow one more day than usual before intrauterine transfer was carried out. Despite the large gaps in the donor zonae, the preembryos remained intact, developed well, and showed good blastomere adherence. Disappointingly, however, an early pregnancy was established and lost.

The patient returned for a third attempt and, this time, received no medication in a natural cycle. A single zonaless oocyte was injected. Normal fertilization ensued and led to a preembryo which exhibited poor blastomere adherence. At the time of intrauterine transfer, one blastomere was seen to be partially extruded through the gap in the donated zona. No pregnancy was established.

A fourth attempt yielded 13 zonaless oocytes and one immature oocyte that appeared unhealthy, but possessed a thin rudimentary zona pellucida. Nine intact oocytes were injected (Figure 8.61). Six of these were normally fertilized and placed within donor zonae on day 2. These preembryos developed well over the next 24 h; four were then replaced and two were frozen. No pregnancy resulted from either fresh or thawed transfer.

The patient returned for yet another attempt and became pregnant on her first transfer with donor oocytes. She is now the happy mother of twins.

In research applications, experimental protocols have been designed to remove the zona pellucida enzymatically or mechanically to provide free blastomeres. These can then be used to study preimplantation growth, evaluate blastomere totipotency at early stages, and produce chimeric fusion in animal models. Although zona-free aggregated blastomeres have the potential to continue development through to the morula or blastocyst stage, as a general rule, they usually do not respond well to *in vitro* culture conditions[62].

Excessive granularity / mottled cytoplasm

Moderate to excessive cytoplasmic granularity (Figure 8.62) does not appear to be associated with a reduced developmental potential. Fertilization rates are similar for granular and non-granular oocytes, although triploid fertilization is marginally higher in the granular group[51,52]. Similarly, pregnancy potential is not reduced because of granular cytoplasm in oocytes or blastomeres of preembryos (Figures 8.63–8.66). Some commercially available culture media appear to intensify granulation of cultured oocytes and preembryos, sometimes to the point of producing a mottled appearance. Although this was initially assumed to be a negative finding and an indication of reduced viability, the clinical pregnancy rate after transfer is completely unaffected.

Unlike simple granularity, an oocyte or blastomere exhibiting an excessively darkened and granular center together with a wide acytoplasmic peripheral ring is usually destined for degeneration or a reduced developmental potential. In such cases, it is assumed that the intense granularity represents fundamental necrotic changes (Figure 8.67).

Vacuoles and inclusions

Cytoplasmic vacuolization generally indicates a poor prognosis for optimal development. Vacuoles form by dilatation and coalescence of vesicular elements of smooth endoplasmic reticulum, by aggregation and fusion of preexisting smaller vacuoles, or as the result of aberrant endocytosis due to oolemma instability[47]. On LM, vacuoles are noticeably membrane-bound and apparently vacant or empty. Although very small vacuolar structures (<5 µm) are relatively common and may not affect overall developmental potential, large vacuoles (>25 µm) are likely to interfere significantly with subsequent growth (Figures 8.68–8.74).

The term *inclusion* describes several different morphological features. Technically, a vacuole is an inclusion. Other common inclusions include refractile bodies (small light-refractive structures composed of lipid material and dense granules associated with poor fertilization after conventional insemination), minute areas of cytoplasmic necrosis, and clustered organelles (Figures 8.75 and 8.76).

Cytoskeletal abnormalities

With monoclonal antibodies, it is possible to obtain a submicroscopic view of the human prezygote and zygote. Cytoskeletal assessment using fluorescent antibodies against antitubulin antibodies reveals the tubulin architecture of the fertilized oocyte, often exposing the sperm aster or meiotic spindle. Simultaneous counterstaining of chromatin with propidium iodide provides insight into the phases of pronuclear formation and eventual syngamy (Figures 8.77 and 8.78). Nuclear and cytoskeletal staining of unfertilized or abnormally fertilized oocytes may provide information which may either complement or contradict the assessment using LM. Oocytes presumed to be unfertilized may reveal sperm; single-pronucleate prezygotes may exhibit two dyssynchronous pronuclei. As more relevant monoclonal antibodies become available, it may eventually be possible to completely ascertain the dynamics involved in the processes of fertilization, syngamy, and the first mitotic division.

References

1. Dandekar PV, Martin MC, Glass RH. Polypronuclear embryos after in vitro fertilization. *Fertil Steril* 1990; 53:510
2. Englert Y, Puissant F, Camus M, *et al.* Factors leading to tripronucleate eggs during human *in vitro* fertilization. *Hum Reprod* 1986;1:117
3. Michelmann HW, Bonhoff A, Mettler L. Chromosome analysis of polyploid human embryos. *Hum Reprod* 1986;1:243
4. Motta PM, Nottola SA, Micara G, Familiari G. Ultrastructure of human unfertilized oocytes and polyspermic embryos in an IVF-ET program. *Ann NY Acad Sci* 1988;541:367
5. Plachot M, Mandelbaum J, Junca AM, *et al.* Impairment of human development after abnormal in vitro fertilization. *Ann NY Acad Sci* 1985;442:336
6. Rudak E, Dor J, Mashiach S, *et al.* Chromosome analysis of multipronuclear human oocytes fertilized in vitro. *Fertil Steril* 1984;41:538
7. Van der Ven HH, Al-Hasani S, Diedrich K, *et al.* Polyspermy in in vitro fertilization of human oocytes: Frequency and possible causes. *Ann NY Acad Sci* 1985;442:88
8. Wramsby H, Fredga K, Liedholm P. Ploidy in human cleavage stage embryos after in vitro fertilization. *Hum Reprod* 1987;2:223
9. Van Blerkom J, Bell H, Henry G. The occurrence, recognition and developmental fate of pseudo-pronuclear eggs after in vitro fertilization of human oocytes. *Hum Reprod* 1987;2:217
10. Chang MC. Development of parthenogenetic rabbit blastocysts induced by low temperature storage of unfertilized ova. *J Exp Zool* 1954;125:127
11. Fulton BP, Whittingham DG. Activation of mammalian oocytes by intracellular injection of calcium. *Nature* 1978;273:149
12. Kaufman MH, Surani MAH. The effect of osmolarity on mouse parthenogenesis. *J Embryol Exp Morph* 1974;31:513

13. Komar A. Parthenogenetic development of mouse eggs activated by heat-shock. *J Reprod Fert* 1973; 35:433

14. Muechler EK, Graham MC, Huang KE, *et al.* Parthenogenesis of human oocytes as a function of vacuum pressure. *J In Vitro Fert Embryo Transf* 1989; 6:335

15. Pincus G, Shapiro H. Further studies on the parthenogenetic activation of rabbit eggs. *Proc Nat Acad Sci* 1940;26:163

16. Uehara T, Yanagimachi R. Activation of hamster oocytes by pricking. *J Exp Zool* 1977;199:269

17. Edwards RG. The experimental induction of gynogenesis in the mouse. I. Irradiation of the sperm by X-rays. *Proc R Soc Lond, Series B* 1957;146:469

18. Surani MAH, Barton SC. Development of gynogenetic eggs in the mouse: Implications for parthenogenetic embryos. *Science* 1983:222:1034

19. Abramczuk JK, Lopata A. Resistance of human follicular oocytes to parthenogenetic activation: DNA distribution and content in oocytes maintained in vitro. *Hum Reprod* 1990;5:578

20. Staessen C, Janssenswillen C, Devroey P, Van Steirteghem AC. Cytogenetic and morphological observations of single-pronucleated human oocytes after in vitro fertilization. *Hum Reprod* 1993;8:221

21. Levron J, Munne S, Willadsen S, *et al.* Male and female genomes associated in a single pronucleus in human zygotes. *Biol Reprod (US)* 1995;52:653

22. Sultan KM, Munne S, Palermo GD, *et al.* Chromosomal status of unipronuclear human zygotes following in vitro fertilization and intracytoplasmic sperm injection. *Hum Reprod* 1995;10:132

23. Palermo GD, Munne S, Colombero LT, *et al.* Genetics of abnormal human fertilization. *Hum Reprod* 1995;10(Suppl):120

24. Austin CR. *The Mammalian Egg.* Oxford: Blackwell Scientific Publications, 1961:34(subnuclei);38(single pronucleus);46(pronuclear size);73(polar body size)

25. Dietzsch E, Ramsay M, Christianson AL, *et al.* Maternal origin of external haploid set of chromosomes in third trimester triploid fetuses. *Am J Med Genet* 1995;58:360

26. McFadden DE, Pantzar JT. Placental pathology of triploidy. *Hum Pathol* 1996;27:1018

27. Miny P, Koppers B, Dworniczak B, *et al.* Parental origin of the extra haploid chromosome set in triploidies diagnosed prenatally. *Am J Med Genet* 1995;57:102

28. Munne S, Alikani M, Cohen J. Monospermic polyploidy and atypical embryo morphology. *Hum Reprod* 1994;9:506

29. Kola I, Trounson A, Dawson G, Rogers P. Tripronuclear human oocytes: Altered cleavage patterns and subsequent karyotypic analysis of embryos. *Biol Reprod* 1987;37:395

30. Sathananthan AH, Kola I, Osborne J, *et al.* Centrioles in the beginning of human development. *Proc Natl Acad Sci USA* 1991;88:4806

31. Sathananthan AH. Mitosis in the human embryo: The vital role of the sperm centrosome (centriole). *Histol Histopathol* 1997;12:827

32. Palermo G, Munne S, Cohen J. The human zygote inherits its mitotic potential from the male gamete. *Hum Reprod* 1994;9:1220

33. Feng YL, Gordon JW. Birth of normal mice after removal of the supernumerary male pronucleus from polyspermic zygotes. *Hum Reprod* 1996;11:341

34. Sathananthan AH, Tatham B, Dharmawardena V, *et al.* Inheritance of sperm centrioles and centrosomes in bovine embryos. *Arch Androl* 1997;38:37

35. Schatten G, Simerly C, Schatten H. Maternal inheritance of centrosomes in mammals? Studies on parthenogenesis and polyspermy in mice. *Proc Natl Acad Sci USA* 1991;88:6785

36. Sutovsky P, Hewitson L, Simerly C, Schatten G. Molecular medical approaches for alleviating infertility and understanding assisted reproductive technologies. *Proc Assoc Am Physicians* 1996;108:432

37. Rawlins RG, Binor Z, Radwanska E, Dmowski WP. Microsurgical enucleation of tripronuclear human zygotes. *Fertil Steril* 1988;50:266

38. Gordon JW, Grunfeld L, Garrisi GJ, *et al.* Successful microsurgical removal of a pronucleus from tripronuclear human zygotes. *Fertil Steril* 1989;52:367

39. Malter H, Cohen J. Embryonic development after microsurgical repair of polyspermic human oocytes. *Fertil Steril* 1989;52:373

40. Szulman AE, Surti U. The syndromes of hydatidiform mole. II. Cytogenetic and morphologic correlations. *Am J Obstet Gynecol* 1978;131:665

41. Simpson JL. The genetic factor. In: Adashi EY, Rock JA, Rosenwaks Z, eds. *Reproductive Endocrinology, Surgery, and Technology.* New York: Lippincott–Raven, 1996:2245

42. Antonarakis SE. Parental origin of the extra chromosome in trisomy 21 as indicated by analysis of DNA polymorphisms. Down's Syndrome Collaborative Group. *N Engl J Med* 1991;324:872

43. Ginsberg N, Strom DC, Applebaum M, *et al.* Ultrasound correlation and karyotype analysis of 94 missed abortions in the first trimester. *Am J Hum Genet* 1992;51:A409

44. Sathananthan AH, Trounson AO, Wood C. *Atlas of Fine Structure of Human Sperm Penetration, Eggs, and Embryos Cultured In Vitro.* New York: Praeger, 1986:44,46,82(vacuoles);70(zona pellucida);16(multinucleated blastomeres)

45. Tesarik J, Kopecny V, Plachot M, Mandelbaum J. Ultrastructural and autoradiographic observations on multinucleated blastomeres of human cleaving embryos obtained by in vitro fertilization. *Hum Reprod* 1987;2:127

46. Winston NJ, Braude PR, Pickering SJ, *et al.* The incidence of abnormal morphology and nucleocytoplasmic ratios in 2-, 3-, and 5-day human preembryos. *Hum Reprod* 1991;6:17

47. Van Blerkom J. Developmental failure in human reproduction associated with preovulatory oogenesis and preimplantation embryogenesis. In: Van Blerkom J, Motta PM, eds. *Ultrastructure of Human Gametogenesis and Early Embryogenesis.* Boston: Kluwer Academic Publishers, 1989: 169(vacuoles, pseudopronuclei);171(multinucleated blastomeres)

48. Balakier H, Cadesky K. The frequency and developmental capability of human embryos containing multinucleated blastomeres. *Hum Reprod* 1997;12:800

49. Kligman I, Benavida C, Alikani M, Munne S. The presence of multinucleated blastomeres in human embryos is correlated with chromosomal abnormalities. *Hum Reprod* 1996;11:1492

50. Sathananthan AH, Trounson AO. The human pronuclear ovum: Fine structure of monospermic and polyspermic fertilization in vitro. *Gamete Res* 1985; 12:385

51. Veeck LL. Pregnancy rate and pregnancy outcome associated with laboratory evaluation of spermatozoa, oocytes, and preembryos. In: Mashiach S, Ben-Rafael Z, Laufer N, Schenker JG, eds. Advances in Assisted Reproductive Technologies. *Proceedings of the Sixth World Congress on In Vitro Fertilization and Embryo Transfer.* Jerusalem, 1990:745

52. Veeck LL. The morphological assessment of human oocytes and early concepti. In: Keel BA, Webster BW, eds. *Laboratory Diagnosis and Treatment of Infertility.* Boca Raton: CRC Press, 1990:353

53. Xia P. Intracytoplasmic sperm injection: Correlation of oocyte grade based on polar body, perivitelline space, and cytoplasmic inclusions with fertilization rate and embryo quality. *Hum Reprod* 1997;12:1750

54. Bomsel-Helmreich O. The aging of gametes, heteroploidy, and embryonic death. *Int J Gynaecol Obstet* 1976;14:98

55. Ortiz ME, Salvatierra AM, López J, Fernandéz-Croxatto HB. Postovulatory aging of human ova: I. Light microscopic observations. *Gamete Res* 1982; 6:11

56. Peluso JJ, England-Charlesworth C, Hutz R. Effect of age and of follicular aging on the preovulatory oocyte. *Biol Reprod* 1980;22:999

57. Familiari G, Sayoko M, Motta PM. The ovary and ovulation: A three-dimensional ultrastructural study. In: Van Blerkom J, Motta PM, eds. *Ultrastructure of Human Gametogenesis and Early Embryogenesis*. Boston: Kluwer Academic Publishers, 1989:87

58. Familiari G, Nottola SA, Petrillo S, *et al.* The application of electron microscopy in the evaluation of in vitro unfertilized human oocytes. In: Spera G, de Kretser DM, eds. *Morphological Basis of Human Reproductive Function.* New York, London: Plenum Press (Rome: Acta Medica), 1987:99

59. O'Rahilly R, Müller F. *Developmental Stages in Human Embryos, Publication 637*. Washington, DC: Carnegie Institution of Washington, 1987:17

60. Bertrand E, Van den Bergh M, Englert Y. Does zona pellucida thickness influence the fertilization rate? *Hum Reprod* 1995;10:1189

61. Veeck LL. *Atlas of the Human Oocyte and Early Conceptus, Vol I*. Baltimore: Williams & Wilkins, 1986: 322

62. Edwards RG. *Conception in the Human Female.* New York: Academic Press, 1980:677

9 Cryopreservation

It has been only 15 years since the world's first pregnancy from a frozen and thawed conceptus was reported[1]. Since then, most IVF programs have embraced cryobiology as a means to augment the opportunity for pregnancy from a single ovarian-stimulation cycle. As ovulation-induction protocols have improved to allow the recruitment of multiple healthy oocytes, so has the need grown for responsible management of their numbers. It is not unusual today to collect >10 mature oocytes from one woman, and often substantially more. Before freezing techniques were routinely used in the laboratory, a woman producing so many gametes had either to limit the number inseminated or risk having to discard healthy preembryos, as only three or four preembryos could be transferred safely to the uterus after fertilization. Neither was an attractive option.

Today, it has been demonstrated that the pregnancy potential after thawing is nearly equal to that with fresh preembryos, at least in some programs. When the cumulative effect of adding thawed pregnancies (only from cycles failing to generate pregnancy after fresh transfer) to fresh pregnancies is examined, delivery outcomes are significantly enhanced[2]. In addition, patients at risk of ovarian hyperstimulation syndrome (OHSS) may be managed more effectively by freezing all conceptuses at the outset, thereby reducing, although not eliminating, the likelihood of adverse clinical symptoms following pregnancy[3]. Furthermore, the clinical pregnancy rate after thawing for patients having all conceptuses frozen is relatively high, exceeding 60%.

Nevertheless, national and worldwide statistics have not reflected comparable results for thawed and fresh cycles. The 1995 Centers for Disease Control Assisted Reproductive Technology Fertility Clinic Report (United States)[4] indicated that, of 7465 cycles with thawed conceptuses (excluding donor oocyte cycles), only 15% delivered a child. This discouraging rate is almost identical to the 1994 data published by the Society for Assisted Reproductive Technology in 1996[5], and is lower than the 25% delivery per transfer and the 21% delivery per cycle reported after fresh transfer from these same data sources. Moreover, it appears that the French programs are not faring any better with regard to freezing. A recent report detailing the status of preembryo cryopreservation in France over a 9-year period states that only 3.5% of transferred thawed conceptuses led to a live birth[6]. World data indicate a clear need to improve current cryotechnology.

Techniques

Freezing

The primary goal of a freezing program is to do as little damage as possible while exposing gametes and preembryos to non-physiologic ultralow temperatures. The protocols in use today are essentially *freeze-dry* techniques that involve dehydration of the cell to prevent the formation of intracellular ice.

The formation of intracellular ice crystals may cause mechanical damage to oocytes and conceptuses by disrupting and displacing organelles, or by slicing through membranes. This is why freezing techniques are based on the need for cryoprotective agents and controlled ice formation at critical temperatures. It has been shown that, when human cells are placed in a medium containing an intracellular cryoprotective agent, intracellular water readily leaves the cell as a result of the higher extracellular concentration of cryoprotectant. This causes the cell to shrink until osmotic equilibrium is reached by the slower diffusion of the cryoprotectant into the cell[7]. Once equilibrium is reached, the cell resumes its normal appearance. The rate of permeation of cryoprotectant and water is dependent on temperature; equilibrium is achieved faster at higher temperatures. For this reason, oocytes and preembryos are usually added to cryoprotective media at room temperature. However, as some cryoprotectants, such as dimethylsulfoxide (DMSO), are toxic at elevated concentrations, these are often used at lower temperatures to reduce adverse effects.

Cryoprotectants are also beneficial because of their ability to lower the freezing point of a solution. Solutions may remain unfrozen at −5° to −15° C because of *supercooling* (cooling to well below the freezing point without extracellular ice formation). When solutions are supercooled, cells do not dehydrate appropriately as there is no increase in osmotic pressure with the formation of extracellular ice crystals. To prevent supercooling, an ice crystal is introduced in a controlled process called *seeding*. This contributes to intracellular dehydration as water leaves the cell to achieve equilibrium with the extracellular environment[7,8]. If the rate of cooling is too rapid, water cannot pass quickly enough from the cell and, as the temperature continues to drop, a point is reached where the intracellular solute concentration is not high enough to prevent the formation of ice crystals. Mammalian oocytes and preembryos, which possess relatively low ratios of surface area to unit volume and contain substantial amounts of intracellular water, are usually cooled at slow rates (0.1°–1° C / min) to permit adequate dehydration.

Membrane permeability by cryoprotectants differs between the oocyte, preembryo, and blastocyst. It has thus been found that different cryoprotective agents are more suitable for certain stages of gamete and preembryo development. DMSO and 1,2-propanediol (PROH) are frequently used for freezing early-cleavage-stage preembryos, and propylene glycol (glycerol) is commonly used for blastocysts. All three intracellular agents have fairly small molecules that are able to permeate cell membranes easily. In addition to these agents, there are several extracellular substances that help dehydrate and protect cells. The most frequently used is sucrose, which possesses large non-permeating molecules and exerts an osmotic effect to aid in accelerated cell dehydration. Sucrose cannot be used alone and is often used in conjunction with standard permeating intracellular cryoprotectants.

Thawing

If cooling is terminated at relatively high temperatures (≥ −30° C), the cell then carries more intracellular ice than if cooled for a longer period of time to lower temperatures (≤ −80° C). To protect the cell in the former situation, thawing must be carried out rapidly to induce rapid ice dispersal. Conversely, samples cooled to ≤ −80° C should be thawed more slowly to allow for gradual rehydration[9]. If water reenters the cell too rapidly, the cell may swell or burst. Thus, thawed specimens are usually exposed to progressively lower dilutions of cryoprotectant to gently and slowly remove it from the cell.

Vitrification

The purpose of vitrification is to protect the cell by completely avoiding all ice crystal formation. To accomplish this, cryoprotective solutes must be increased to 40% (wt / vol) or higher. DMSO is frequently used, although PROH, glycerol, and other agents have been tested. Because high concentrations of cryoprotectant are toxic at room temperature, preembryos are exposed to such agents at 0° C. Samples may be plunged directly into liquid nitrogen (LN_2) without first introducing a 'seed'; the viscosity is so great that solutions solidify into a glasslike state. Vitrified specimens must be thawed in iced water, which may be inconvenient[10–12]. Thus far, most trials using this technique have been carried out in animal models.

Ultrarapid freezing

Vitrification and ultrarapid freezing are, in fact, similar techniques. If no ice crystals form during the latter process, the result is vitrification[13]. However, one difference is that specimens are handled at room temperature rather than in ice baths.

With ultrarapid freezing, specimens are exposed for short periods (2–3 min) to relatively high concentrations of DMSO (3.5 M) and sucrose (0.25 M), followed by direct plunging into LN_2. Specimens are then thawed rapidly in a 37°C waterbath with removal of cryoprotectant in a single step[14]. Using these simple and rapid techniques, a number of children have been born. Gordts *et al.*[15], as early as 1990, reported four pregnancies after ultrarapid freezing of pronuclear stage oocytes. In that study, an improved survival was noted for pronuclear oocytes compared with cleaved preembryos, a finding that has also been reported by other investigators[16]. In contrast, Lai *et al.*[17] in 1996 reported an 83% survival rate (at least one blastomere intact) and a 16% birthrate for ultrarapid-frozen cleaved preembryos. Mitochondrial distribution and overall subcellular structure are described as normal after this method of freezing[18].

Oocytes

Oocytes are easily frozen if they contain a nucleus (Figure 9.1). Studies using human germinal vesicle-bearing oocytes collected from both stimulated and unstimulated cycles have demonstrated that this stage yields acceptable survival and maturation rates after thawing[19,20]. Furthermore, it has been shown that the percentage of frozen / thawed germinal vesicle-bearing oocytes with normal meiotic spindles is similar to that with non-frozen controls. This finding is not supported by the significantly lower percentage of normal spindles observed in frozen / thawed M II oocytes[21] (Figure 9.2). Other abnormalities described in thawed mature oocytes include: disruption of the plasma membrane; extensive disorganization of the ooplasm; subnuclei; and frequent triploidy[22,23]. Nevertheless, concern over potential aneuploidy has been the primary factor in discouraging most clinical programs from actively pursuing techniques using mature oocytes.

These concerns notwithstanding, a handful of pregnancies have been reported after the freezing and thawing of mature oocytes[24–29], although few pregnancies have been described in the last 10 years. It is hoped that the development of ultrarapid freezing will improve future results.

The ability to freeze unfertilized human oocytes would be invaluable in some cases. A young woman about to undergo radiation treatment or facing the loss of her ovaries could benefit greatly. Similarly, an older woman wishing to store multiple oocytes before losing ovarian function could be aided by this technology. Donor oocyte banks could be created in much the same way as sperm banks have been to assist the evergrowing population of women requesting donor eggs. It is a pity that, despite the considerable interest in the development of reliable oocyte freezing methods, only a limited success has thus far been achieved.

Prezygotes

Sperm-penetrated oocytes represent a completely different treatment option. Freezing success with this cell stage has spanned more than a decade and culminated in thousands of births (Figures 9.3–9.10). It is thought that the prezygote's lack of a spindle is largely responsible for its excellent survival and potential for implantation. Being single-celled, it is easy to determine whether or not a prezygote has survived thawing. When the membrane is not intact, the cell appears to be flattened and is usually dark in color. Left in culture for 15–24 h, the healthy pronucleate oocyte enters syngamy, completes the fertilization process, and proceeds to the first cleavage. Cell division is the true indicator of survival after thawing; $<5\%$ of prezygotes which appear to be healthy after thawing fail to follow this pattern.

Despite the good results achieved after freezing at this stage, there are certain disadvantages. Because prezygotes are frozen before cleavage occurs, there are no standard morphological parameters to aid in selection. Consequently, prezygotes with poor developmental potential are sometimes frozen. It is disappointing to freeze a large number of prezygotes only to find that those not frozen arrest in culture or exhibit abnormal morphological characteristics after two or three days. In such cases, the patient might have been better served if freezing had been delayed for one or two days. However, it is important to freeze the prezygote before the breakdown of pronuclei, as waiting too long has negative effects on the results. The urgency to begin freezing may be inconvenient for some programs which lack adequate scientific staff.

The morphology of thawed prezygotes is generally similar to their prefrozen appearance but, occasionally, the cytoplasm is clearer and organelle accumulation around pronuclear structures is reduced. After thawing, nucleoli are often seen scattered within pronuclei despite their previous alignment at pronuclear junctions before freezing. An interesting observation (made several times by the author) is where two pronuclei have coalesced into one large pronucleus during these procedures.

Preembryos

The first reported birth following cryopreservation and thawing developed from a frozen preembryo[1] (Figures 9.11–9.24). As with pronuclear oocytes, cleaving preembryos do well after thawing and contribute to pregnancy at acceptable rates. Almost any cleavage stage can be successfully frozen, from two-cell to blastocyst. Freezing the preembryo is convenient because, unlike the prezygote, there are no time constraints. In addition, both the morphology and growth rate are known, allowing selection of potentially viable conceptuses. It is becoming more common to choose the best preembryos for fresh transfer and to freeze all others with good morphology only after fresh selection has been made.

Survival is sometimes difficult to evaluate because not all blastomeres survive the rigors of freezing and thawing. Dying blastomeres may be scattered among those which are alive, but are easily removed during AHA procedures. In general, a preembryo possessing >50% viable blastomeres upon thawing is considered a survivor. There is no convincing evidence that the loss of one or two blastomeres is overtly detrimental to preembryos very early in their development[30–33]. Despite this, it has been reported that fully intact human preembryos demonstrate a higher implantation rate than do those which are partially intact[34].

Blastocysts

Blastocysts have generated a great deal of interest in recent years. There may well be a growing tendency towards routine culture to this stage and, as a consequence, to routine freezing of expanded blastocysts (Figure 9.25). Several groups have reported successful freezing with subsequent live births, and many of these used coculture systems to support preembryo growth[35–38]. Surprisingly, most reports of ongoing pregnancy in the range of 10–20% per transfer do not demonstrate significantly higher rates compared with USA statistics on freezing at earlier stages, but this may perhaps be related to the lower number of blastocysts being transferred or an indication of asynchrony between the blastocyst and uterus. One study has described an admirable 100% survival rate with frozen blastocysts, but the pregnancy rate was only 16% per transfer. Although the pregnancy rate for blastocysts was higher than that with thawed preembryos at earlier stages (6%), it is difficult to determine the reasons for the low incidence of pregnancy in the latter group[39].

Cryopreservation strategy

The Cornell program has developed the following strategy for determining when and how many conceptuses to freeze:

(1) Never freeze only one conceptus unless the patient has others in cryostorage or will not be receiving a fresh transfer. Twelve years of experience indicate that single preembryo transfer results

after freezing and thawing are too poor to justify the cost to the patient and workload on laboratory staff (clinical pregnancy rate of 14% / transfer). Attempt to freeze at least three conceptuses whenever possible. After thawing, the best outcomes occur when a patient has more than two preembryos replaced (clinical pregnancy rate of 50% per transfer).

(2) Where applicable, continue to culture all preembryos deemed unsuitable for transfer and freezing (>20% fragmentation, <6 cells on day 3) for 3 days. Document daily observations of cell number and morphology. Freeze any developing blastocysts on day 5 or 6 if two or more appear to be healthy (infrequent).

Patients <40 years of age

(1) If the patient's previous history includes preembryos with good morphology, then hold five to seven of these in culture (depending on exact age) and freeze the remainder at the pronuclear stage. Plan to freeze the remainder on day 3 provided that the morphology is good.

(2) If the patient's previous history demonstrates that the preembryos are likely to possess moderate-to-poor morphology or if the patient has no history to evaluate, then hold seven to ten of these in culture and freeze the remainder at the pronuclear stage. Plan to freeze additional preembryos on day 2 or 3 if two or more exhibit <20% fragmentation and normal cleavage.

(3) If the patient's previous history indicates poor morphology or developmental arrest, then wait until day 3 before considering freezing.

Patients ≥40 years of age

(1) Do not freeze at the pronuclear stage unless >10 prezygotes are available and previous history includes preembryos with good morphology.

(2) Freeze after cleavage only if two or more preembryos possessing excellent morphology and regular cleavage are available over the number required for transfer.

(3) Consider transferring five fresh preembryos in patients 41–43 years of age and six in patients >43 years (with the agreement of both the patient and physician).

References

1. Trounson AO, Mohr L. Human pregnancy following cryopreservation, thawing and transfer of an eight-cell embryo. *Nature* 1983;305:707

2. Veeck LL, Amundson CH, Brothman LJ, *et al.* Significantly enhanced pregnancy rates through cryopreservation and thaw of pronuclear stage oocytes. *Fertil Steril* 1993;59:1202

3. Queenan JT Jr, Veeck LL, Toner JP, *et al.* Cryopreservation of all prezygotes in patients at risk of severe hyperstimulation does not eliminate the syndrome, but the chances of pregnancy are excellent with subsequent frozen-thaw transfers. *Hum Reprod* 1997;12:1573

4. Centers for Disease Control and Prevention. *1995 Assisted Reproductive Technology Success Rates: National Summary and Fertility Clinic Reports.* Atlanta, GA: US Department of Health and Human Services, 1998

5. Society for Assisted Reproductive Technology. Assisted reproductive technology in the United States and Canada: 1994 results generated from the American Society for Reproductive Medicine / Society for Assisted Reproductive Technology Registry. *Fertil Steril* 1996;66:697

6. Federation of BLEFCO. Embryo freezing: Status survey in France (1985–1993). *Contracept Fertil Sex* 1996; 24:674

7. Mazur P. Freezing of living cells: Mechanisms and implications. *Am J Physiol* 1984;247(*Cell Physiol* 16):C125

8. Whittingham DG. Some factors affecting embryo storage in laboratory animals. *Ciba Found Symp* 1977; 52:97

9. Schneider U. Cryobiological principles of embryo freezing. *J In Vitro Fert Embryo Transf* 1986;3:3

10. Friedler S, Shen E, Lamb EJ. Cryopreservation of mouse 2-cell embryos and ova by vitrification: Methodologic studies. *Fertil Steril* 1987;48:306

11. Friedler S, Giudice LC, Lamb EJ. Cryopreservation of embryos and ova. *Fertil Steril* 1988;49:743

12. Quinn P, Kerin JFP. Experience with the cryopreservation of human embryos using the mouse as a model to establish successful techniques. *J In Vitro Fert Embryo Transf* 1986;3:40

13. Quinn P. Cryopreservation of embryos and oocytes. In: Keye WR Jr, Chang RJ, Rebar RW, Soules MR, eds. *Infertility: Evaluation and Treatment.* Philadelphia: WB Saunders Co., 1995:821

14. Trounson A, Sjoblom P. Cleavage and development of human embryos in vitro after ultrarapid freezing and thawing. *Fertil Steril* 1988;50:373

15. Gordts S, Roziers P, Campo R, Noto V. Survival and pregnancy outcome after ultrarapid freezing of human embryos. *Fertil Steril* 1990;53:469

16. Ciriminna R, Schillaci R, Cefalu E, Agrifoglio V. What is the most idoneous developmental stage for embryo-freezing? *Acta Eur Fertil* 1994;25:173

17. Lai AC, Lin BP, Chang CC, *et al.* Pregnancies after transfer of ultrarapidly frozen human embryos. *J Assist Reprod Genet* 1996;13:625

18. Noto V, Campo R, Roziers P, *et al.* Mitochondrial distribution after fast embryo freezing. *Hum Reprod* 1993;8:2115

19. Toth TL, Baka SG, Veeck LL, *et al.* Fertilization and in vitro development of cryopreserved human prophase I oocytes. *Fertil Steril* 1994;61:891

20. Toth TL, Lanzendorf SE, Sandow BA, *et al.* Cryopreservation of human prophase I oocytes collected from unstimulated follicles. *Fertil Steril* 1994;61:1077

21. Baka SG, Toth TL, Veeck LL, *et al.* Evaluation of the spindle apparatus of in vitro matured human oocytes following cryopreservation. *Hum Reprod* 1995;10: 1816

22. Sathananthan AH, Trounson A, Freeman L. Morphology and fertilizability of frozen human oocytes. *Gamete Res* 1987;16:343

23. Trounson A. Preservation of human eggs and embryos. *Fertil Steril* 1986;46:1

24. Al-Hasani S, Diedrich K, van der Ven H, *et al.* Cryopreservation of human oocytes. *Hum Reprod* 1987;2:695

25. Chen C. Pregnancy after human oocyte cryopreservation. *Lancet* 1986;i:884

26. Chen C. Pregnancies after human oocyte cryopreservation. *Ann NY Acad Sci* 1988;541:541

27. Van Uem JFHM, Siebzehrübl ER, Schuh B, *et al.* Birth after cryopreservation of unfertilized oocytes. *Lancet* 1987;i:752

28. Porcu E, Fabbri R, Seracchioli R, *et al.* Birth of a healthy female after intracytoplasmic sperm injection of cryopreserved human oocytes. *Fertil Steril* 1997;68:724

29. Tucker M, Wright G, Morton P, *et al.* Preliminary experience with human oocyte cryopreservation using 1,2-propanediol and sucrose. *Hum Reprod* 1996;11:1513

30. Hartshorne GM, Wick K, Elder K, Dyson H. Effect of cell number at freezing upon survival and viability of cleaving embryos generated from stimulated IVF cycles. *Hum Reprod* 1990;5:857

31. Rulicke T, Autenried P. Potential of two-cell mouse embryos to develop to term despite partial damage after cryopreservation. *Lab Anim* 1995;29:320

32. Veiga A, Calderon G, Barri PN, Coroleu B. Pregnancy after the replacement of a frozen-thawed embryo with less than 50% intact blastomeres. *Hum Reprod* 1987;2:321

33. Willadsen SM. The viability of early cleavage stages containing half the normal number of blastomeres in the sheep. *J Reprod Fertil* 1980;59:357

34. Van den Abbeel E, Camus M, Van Waesberghe L, *et al.* Viability of partially damaged human embryos after cryopreservation. *Hum Reprod* 1997;12:2006

35. Cohen J, Simons RF, Edwards RG, *et al.* Pregnancies following the frozen storage of expanding human blastocysts. *J In Vitro Fert Embryo Transf* 1985;2:59

36. Hartshorne GM, Elder K, Crow J, *et al.* The influence of in vitro development upon post-thaw survival and implantation of cryopreserved human blastocysts. *Hum Reprod* 1991;6:136

37. Kaufman RA, Menezo Y, Hazout A, *et al.* Cocultured blastocyst cryopreservation: Experience of more than 500 transfer cycles. *Fertil Steril* 1995;64:1125

38. Menezo YJ, Ben Khalifa M. Cytogenetic and cryobiology of human cocultured embryos: A 3-year experience. *J Assist Reprod Genet* 1995;12:35

39. Freitas S, Le Gal F, Dzik A, *et al.* Value of cryopreservation of human embryos during the blastocyst stage. *Contracept Fertil Sex* 1994;22:396

10 Assisted fertilization by intracytoplasmic sperm injection (ICSI)

Gianpiero Palermo, MD

Background

Since the time of the first human birth as a result of IVF in 1978, the procedure has been used extensively in the alleviation of infertility. However, because the spermatozoa in many cases of male-factor infertility are unable to fertilize, a number of supplementary techniques have been developed to overcome this inability; these are generally referred to as *assisted fertilization*, *microsurgical fertilization* or, simply, *micromanipulation*. The application of micromanipulation to human gametes has not only allowed fertilization in cases of severe oligozoospermia and even by defective spermatozoa, it has provided a powerful tool for a better understanding of the basic elements of oocyte maturation, fertilization, and early development. Micromanipulation techniques also now permit the diagnosis, and sometimes even the correction, of genetic anomalies as well as optimization of implantation rates in certain cases.

When sperm density, motility or morphology are inadequate, various techniques have been used to bypass the zona pellucida. The practical use of micromanipulation for these purposes burst onto the scene in the mid-1980s with *zona drilling (ZD)* and *partial zona dissection (PZD)*. Since then, this field has undergone such a rapid evolution that these early approaches have largely been abandoned in favor of intracytoplasmic sperm injection (ICSI), with the use of ZD confined to the four- to sixteen-cell preembryo stage (AHA) in an effort to promote implantation. Nevertheless, as several of the techniques used initially are of interest from the standpoint of recent history, these are first briefly discussed to maintain some perspective in that regard.

ZD was first reported by Gordon and Talansky[1], and involves the creation of a circumscribed opening in the zona pellucida by the application of AT (acid Tyrode's) solution (pH 2.35) through a fine glass micropipette. After insemination, more than one spermatozoon frequently enters these drilled zonae. Moreover, AT solution has a deleterious effect on the single-celled oocyte – an effect not seen to the same extent in four- to sixteen-cell preembryos using an AHA procedure (see Chapter 11). At the same time as ZD was being tested, mechanical *cutting* of a hole in the zona pellucida was introduced as another technique, but for nuclear manipulation of fertilized eggs[2]. Alternative, but similar, procedures were similarly investigated, including *zona cracking* in which the zona is breached mechanically with the use of two fine glass hooks controlled by a micromanipulator[3], and *zona softening* wherein oocytes are briefly exposed to trypsin[4] or pronase. PZD, used extensively for a while in cases of fertilization failure, involved cutting the zona with glass pipettes just before incubation of the treated oocytes with spermatozoa[5].

With each of these techniques, spermatozoa had to be progressively motile and had to have undergone, or at least possess the potential for, an acrosome reaction. These procedures also carried a distinct risk of injury to the oocytes related to the need to produce an opening of optimal size in the zona. Localized laser photoablation of the zona has also been used to produce a gap of precise dimensions, and this has resulted in healthy offspring[6,7]. However, not only did all of these early procedures generate only a moderate rate of fertilization, with PZD being the most successful in that regard, but all were associated with a significant incidence of polyspermy.

Mechanical insertion of spermatozoa directly into the perivitelline space – termed *subzonal sperm injection (SUZI)*[8] – was soon introduced as another means to overcome inadequacies of sperm concentration and motility, and proved to be more effective than either ZD or PZD, particularly following previous induction of the acrosome reaction[9,10]. However, SUZI required that spermatozoa be normal, capacitated, and even hyperactivated or acrosome-reacted. Thus, this technique remained limited by an inability to overcome acrosomal abnormalities or disjunction of the sperm–oolemma fusion process and, ultimately, by unacceptably low fertilization rates.

Intracytoplasmic sperm injection (ICSI)

As ICSI involves the insertion of a single selected spermatozoon directly into the oocyte, this method bypasses all of the preliminary steps of fertilization. The technique was pioneered in animals, initially by Hiramoto[11] in the sea urchin, then by Lin[12] in mammalian (mouse) oocytes. Later, Uehara and Yanagimachi[13] observed relatively high rates of sperm nuclear decondensation after microinjection of human or golden hamster spermatozoa into hamster eggs. Subsequently, ICSI was used to study the determinants of male pronucleus formation[14,15]. However, even this technique may cause oocyte injury and lysis[16] and, in early studies, only around 30% of injected mouse eggs survived the procedure, even when fine micropipettes (4–6 μm in diameter) were used under ideal conditions[17].

Because the fusion step of fertilization is bypassed in ICSI, pronucleus development generally requires oocyte activation in most species tested. This may be provoked by energetic suction of cytoplasm immediately before or during sperm nucleus insertion[18]. In the hamster[19] and bovine[20] oocyte, exposure to a calcium ionophore (for example, A23187) appeared to further increase the likelihood of oocyte activation.

The first live offspring using ICSI were obtained in the rabbit, following the transfer of sperm-injected eggs into the oviduct of a pseudopregnant female[21]. Soon after, the first ICSI live birth was reported in the cow[22]. Although applied to human gametes a few years earlier[23], the first human pregnancies with ICSI were seen only as recently as in 1992[24]; since then, thousands of babies have been born as a result of this procedure (Figures 10.1–10.6)[25].

Methodology

The pipettes are made from borosilicate glass capillary tubes (Drummond Scientific, Broomall, PA, USA) that are 0.97 mm in external diameter, 0.69 mm in internal diameter, and 78 mm in length. Cleaning the capillary tubes involves:

(1) Soaking overnight in MilliQ water (Millipore Corp., Bedford, MA, USA);

(2) Sonication;

(3) Rinsing at least 30 times in MilliQ water before drying in a hot-air oven; and

(4) Heat sterilization.

Pipettes are formed by drawing the thin-walled glass capillary tubes using a horizontal microelectrode puller (Model 753, Campden Instruments Ltd., Loughborough, UK). The holding pipette is cut and fire-polished on a microforge (Narishige Co. Ltd, Tokyo, Japan) to a final outer diameter of 60 μm and an inner diameter of 20 μm. To prepare the injection pipette, a pulled capillary tube is opened and sharpened on a grinder (Narishige Co. Ltd), with a bevel angle of 30°, an outer diameter of approximately 7 μm, and an inner diameter of approximately 5 µm. A spike is made on the injection pipette using a microforge, and both pipettes are bent to an angle of approximately 35 °at a point positioned horizontally 1 mm from the edge, allowing injection in a plastic Petri dish (Model 1006, Falcon).

Immediately before injection, 1 µl of sperm suspension is diluted with 4 µl of a 10% polyvinylpyrrolidone solution (PVP-K 90; MW 360 000; ICN Biochemicals, Cleveland, OH, USA) in HTF-Hepes medium placed in the middle of the Petri dish. The viscosity of PVP, which is used as it comes from the manufacturer, decelerates the aspiration and prevents sperm cells from sticking to the injection pipette. If <500 000 spermatozoa are available in an ejaculate, then these are usually concentrated in approximately 5 µl of ejaculate and transferred directly into the injection dish. A spermatozoon is then aspirated from the concentrated 5-µl sperm suspension and transferred into the central drop containing PVP solution to remove debris and facilitate aspiration control.

After the spermatozoa are washed and prepared, oocytes are placed in protein-supplemented 5-µl droplets of HTF-Hepes medium surrounding the central drop containing the sperm suspension / PVP. They are then covered with lightweight paraffin oil (BDH Limited, Poole, UK). The droplets in each dish are used only once to avoid dilution of the buffered medium during transport of the oocyte.

The injection is performed at ×400 magnification using Hoffman Modulation Contrast optics on the heated stage (Eastreach Laboratory, Centereach, NY, USA) of a Nikon Diaphot inverted microscope equipped with two motor-driven coarse control manipulators and two hydraulic micromanipulators (MM-188 and MO-109, Narishige Co. Ltd). The micropipettes are fitted to a tool holder controlled by two IM-6 microinjectors (Narishige Co. Ltd).

When the 1-µl sperm suspension is added to the drop containing PVP, the motile spermatozoa are able to swim into the viscous medium whereas the debris (other cells, bacteria, and immotile spermatozoa) floats in the PVP at its interface with the paraffin oil. It is important to emphasize that the presence of too many spermatozoa in the PVP drop may favor adherence of debris to the injection pipette and thereby contaminate the injection medium. In addition to deceleration of the spermatozoon, the high viscosity of the PVP highlights its movement patterns in three dimensions. This not only facilitates sperm aspiration into the pipette – difficult with even slowly moving cells at ×400 – but, to some extent, also aids in the selection of normal-shaped spermatozoa, as determined by their form, light refraction, and motility patterns highlighted by such a medium.

The spermatozoa chosen for injection are those that tend to stick to the bottom of the Petri dish by their heads, usually becoming immotile after displaying short periods of simple vibration patterns. In general, these are located along the edges of the droplet. Paradoxically, the ICSI technique is more successful with spermatozoa that are immotile rather than motile in the final stage. Thus, active spermatozoa must first be immobilized. This is accomplished by gently compressing the midregion of the sperm flagellum against the bottom of the dish with the tip of the injection pipette[26] (Figure 10.7).

Once spermatozoa are immobilized, it is essential to lift them from the bottom of the dish by gentle suction with the injection pipette. Once free, the sperm cell should finally be drawn, tail first, into the injection pipette. Following this, the injection needle is lifted slightly by turning the knob of the joystick clockwise to avoid damaging the needle spike by inadvertently scratching it against the surface of the dish. It is important to note that, as the needle is then redirected by moving the microscope stage to the droplet containing the oocyte, the differences in medium consistency (PVP *vs* culture medium) may promote loss of the spermatozoon from the pipette.

As the holding pipette is lowered into the droplet, the oocyte is slowly rotated to locate and identify both the polar body and its associated area of cortical rarefaction (polar granularity), at one time presumed to be the site from which the first polar body is extruded. Although the polar body is not a wholly reliable reference point for chromosome location, as it may move within the perivitelline space, the area nearest to it as well as any clearly granular area should be avoided during injection.

The depth of the holding pipette is adjusted so that its internal opening and the equator of the oocyte are both in focus. This allows greater support of the holding pipette in a position opposite the injection point. The inferior pole of the oocyte should touch the bottom of the dish as this stabilizes it during the procedure. The injection pipette is lowered and focused together with the outer right border of the oolemma on the equatorial plane at the three-o'clock position.

The spermatozoon within the injection pipette is then slowly advanced to lie close to the beveled opening, which is pushed against and through the zona, then further against the oolemma (Figures 10.8 and 10.9). A break in this membrane is indicated by a sudden quivering of its surface (at the site of invagination) above and below the needle. Penetration of the oolemma also brings an important flow of ooplasm up into the pipette, causing the spermatozoon to back up with it; this retrograde movement is encouraged to a point approximately 60 μm from the tip by active aspiration. To counteract the flow of ooplasm involved, which is important for oocyte activation, the spermatozoon is then ejected back with the ooplasm (Figure 10.10), thereby avoiding a tendency to inject any significant volume of medium into the oocyte.

The physical characteristics of the oolemma may vary from particularly soft to elastic, according to the maturity of the oocyte or the time spent *in vitro*[27]. In instances where the oolemma is very elastic, it may be necessary to withdraw the pipette slightly and slowly repeat the procedure, hooking the upper or lower border of the invagination with the spike to allow penetration of the oocyte in a line parallel to its equatorial plane. Once entry is confirmed, the spermatozoon should be ejected into the ooplasm well beyond the tip of the pipette as it is withdrawn. Any surplus medium is also removed at this time to promote association of the injected sperm with oocyte cytoplasmic organelles and final closure of the funnel-shaped opening at the three-o'clock position (Figure 10.11). If the surface of the oolemma becomes everted, cytoplasmic organelles may leak out and the oocyte may lyse. Thus, the penetration point is checked to ensure that the border of the opening maintains a funnel-like shape with the vertex pointing into the oocyte (see Figure 10.11). The average time required to inject a spermatozoon into an oocyte is ≤ 1 min.

Indications for ICSI

Despite agreement on some aspects of the ICSI procedure, there are as yet no universal standards for patient selection; this lack of standardized criteria has complicted attempts to quantify the therapeutic value of ICSI. There is a general consensus, however, that ICSI should certainly be performed following fertilization failure during standard IVF using oocytes with properly established nuclear maturity and using an appropriate sperm concentration, even when microdroplets are used. Also, in many instances, the performance of immotile spermatozoa may be improved by the addition of kinetic stimulators such as pentoxifylline.

Although oocytes which have failed to fertilize with standard IVF techniques may be reinseminated, this introduces the risk of fertilizing aged eggs[28]. In our own limited experience, six out of eight pregnancies established by micromanipulation of such oocytes miscarried, and cytogenetic studies performed on the aborted fetuses provided evidence of chromosomal abnormalities. Thus, in spite of a recent report of normal pregnancy[29], the reinsemination of unfertilized oocytes is currently performed at the Cornell clinic primarily for research purposes, and only when oocyte maturity is questionable.

With regard to sperm numbers, when the original count is $<5\times10^6$ / ml, the likelihood of fertilization with routine IVF procedures is significantly reduced, regardless of etiology[30]. A couple is considered unsuitable for standard IVF if the sperm concentration of progressively motile spermatozoa in the initial ejaculate is $<500\,000$ / ml, with

<4% being normal forms (strict criteria). Moreover, fertilization between apparently mature oocytes and motile spermatozoa may occasionally fail to occur[31]. One potential cause may be spontaneous hardening of the zona pellucida after *in vitro* culture[32], or an inherently impenetrable zona around oocytes that often reveal ooplasmic inclusions[33,34]. The rare sperm abnormality that prevents sperm fusion with the oolemma[35] also justifies sperm injection. In many instances, however, failure of fertilization is due to multiple sperm abnormalities in severe oligo-, astheno-, or teratozoospermia, as defined by the WHO[36]. There is now a clear consensus as to the value of micromanipulation in those cases where IVF pregnancy rates drop to <10%[37], with ICSI then being the only treatment option[25].

ICSI with mature spermatozoa

How effective is ICSI using ejaculated spermatozoa in cases judged *a priori* as unsuitable for standard IVF? The ICSI procedure performed at Cornell since early 1995 has involved 1718 such cases, with 76% of oocytes becoming normally fertilized, 96% of patients receiving good-quality preembryos, and a 49% clinical pregnancy rate (44% with unambiguous fetal heart), including 4 ectopic pregnancies and 135 miscarriages. The ongoing >20 weeks / delivery rate was 39% per oocyte retrieval and 41% per replacement (all data, including women >40 years old who represent more than one-fourth of the population). These results with ICSI were not related to the source of the spermatozoon (fresh or cryopreserved, or obtained by masturbation or electroejaculation) and, although an increased concentration of motile spermatozoa in the ejaculate positively influenced the fertilization rate ($p<0.001$), the pregnancy rate was unaffected compared with controls. Thus, the clinical outcome with ICSI is comparable to the outcome with IVF in couples who have no sperm abnormalities.

ICSI with immature or abnormal germ cells

Early experience showed that isolated nuclei of testicular, caput, and cauda epididymal hamster spermatozoa decondensed soon after injection into mature hamster oocytes, and were transformed into pronuclei in activated eggs[13]. Although conventional and standard IVF of human oocytes has often been accomplished in humans using functional epididymal spermatozoa[38,39], only with the advent of ICSI has it been possible to obtain normal preembryos with surgically retrieved immature epididymal spermatozoa[40–42]. Using ICSI, a clinical pregnancy rate of 71% was achieved with fresh spermatozoa collected microsurgically from the epididymis, and 56% of 111 couples became pregnant after ICSI using frozen epididymal sperm.

However, the therapeutic possibilities of ICSI go even further, as testicular spermatozoa and even spermatids have been successfully used (Figures 10.12–10.16). Testicular biopsies have been employed as a source of sperm cells from men who have a scarred epididymis and no possibility of sperm retrieval[43–45]. In 75 cycles where such testicular germ cells were used, the fertilization rate was 62%, and 39 (56%) clinical pregnancies / transfer were obtained with spermatozoa that were either totally immotile or only twitching slightly.

A few men form only round-headed (acrosomeless) spermatozoa which can neither bind to nor penetrate zona-free hamster oocytes[23]. After ICSI using such acrosomeless spermatozoa, 15 / 45 oocytes were fertilized, 10 preembryos were replaced in four cycles, and three pregnancies were established[46].

Future perspectives

It is now clear in principle that round spermatids can be used to create normal mammalian preembryos[47]. It is of further theoretical interest that even secondary spermatocytes are able to 'haploidize', at least within the mouse oocyte, and create normal offspring[48]. Nevertheless, only two term pregnancies have thus far been reported with round spermatids recovered from ejaculates produced by azoospermic men[49], and only one baby has been born after using round spermatids retrieved from testicular tissue[50].

An additional and perhaps final step could be the cryopreservation of spermatogonia for their future transfer and maturation in a recipient testis. This type of transfer has been performed successfully in the rat[51] and may have clinical applications to humans in the future. Men who are likely to lose their germ cells (for example, by undergoing chemotherapy) may have their spermatogonia cryopreserved for later recolonization in the irradiated testis. Although the hoped-for result is normal spermatogenesis, if this is not the case, it may prove possible to at least harvest haploid products for use in the ICSI procedure. On the other hand, it still remains difficult to select the appropriate round spermatids in humans with much certainty and, as already noted, their use so far has brought no more than modest results in the clinical setting.

Nuclear transplantation

Although the preembryo may carry chromosomal defects which may interfere with its development, several such abnormalities related to gamete defects have been corrected for or overcome with the use of micromanipulation techniques.

The oocyte may display a variety of defects, ranging from single chromosomal aneuploidy to complete diploidy. Diploid oocytes, in addition to being larger, often extrude two first polar bodies on activation. However, the most common abnormality of the oocyte is either retention or loss of both representatives of a particular chromosome during meiosis, an abnormality that appears increasingly with age. One solution to this problem involves transplantation of a germinal vesicle (GV) from an egg of the older patient to an enucleated immature young oocyte[52]. In this way, the genome of the older oocyte is able to use the cytoplasmic infrastructure to haploidize normally. A type of manipulation that also involves this principle is the transfer of 'young' ooplasm to putatively defective eggs[53].

Nuclear transfer in human oocytes has a number of potential benefits, ranging from avoidance of aneuploidy by correcting spindle behavior and nuclear division in oogonia or GV-stage oocytes to mitochondrial transfer for promotion of preembryo growth. This may be performed by either fusion, injection of selected organelles or transfer of anucleated cytoplasm (cytoplasmic transfer or donation). Such experimental reconstitution of oocytes and zygotes not only provides new therapeutic procedures, but also may prove useful in the study of fundamental processes.

Control of nucleus behavior by the cytoplasm has been demonstrated by nuclear transplantation and cytoplasmic transfer in several animal species[54,55] (Figures 10.17–10.20). Specific cell cycle-related events associated with cytoplasmic regulatory factors include GV breakdown[56,57], chromosomal decondensation[17], and metaphase arrest[58,59]. The capability of ooplasm to cause sperm nucleus decondensation depends upon the stage of oocyte maturation[60,61]. Several other studies addressing the importance of cytoplasmic factors and organelles during meiosis and cleavage have shown that mitochondria are closely associated with the mitotic spindle in normally dividing blastomeres, but are absent in those which are arrested. In such cases, the resumption of normal mitosis and mitochondrial distribution occurred after the transfer of G2 cytoplasm from normal blastomeres[62]. That the cytoplasmic factor(s) essential for developmental competence is(are) absent in primate GV oocytes is suggested by their normal fertilization and development only after becoming recipients of mature oocyte cytoplasm[63].

In three couples with previous implantation failure, nuclear transfer in donor cytoplasm was performed by electrofusion prior to ICSI, followed by 4 days of coculture of the preembryos with epithelial cells[64]. When 21 / 22 recipient oocytes were fused successfully with donor cytoblasts and then subjected to ICSI, 14 showed evidence of fertilization. At least three such preembryos were transferred to each patient, but none implanted. Two patients who returned for frozen donor preembryos became pregnant, but one miscarried. The authors concluded that electrofusion of human oocytes with M II cytoplasm may favor normal fertilization, cleavage and development. Among the many issues that still need to be resolved in this area is the possibility that preembryos may be affected by the gaps in their zonae or by other unknown side-effects of these treatments. Moreover, optimal timing of the procedure, and the ideal amount and precise handling of the material transferred, have yet to be determined.

Procedure

A GV is removed from the oocyte of an older woman using a glass tool similar to that used for the collection of cytoplasts after exposure to cytochalasin-B. After mechanical breach of the zona pellucida, the oocyte nucleus, which is surrounded by a small amount of cytoplasm (karyoplast), is gently sucked out with an aspiration pipette (30 μm in inner diameter). At the same time, the genomic material from a young oocyte is removed using the same technique.

The GV karyoplast (from the aged oocyte) is introduced into the perivitelline space of the enucleated young oocyte. Subsequently, the assembled oocyte, in a medium containing sucrose, is aligned and subjected to electrical (AC) pulses of 100 V / cm for 10 s, followed by a single DC pulse of 1.3 KV / cm for 70 μs, delivered by a BTX ECM 200 generator (Genetronics Inc., San Diego, CA). The treated oocyte is then rinsed in fresh medium and cultured for approximately 15–30 min to allow fusion. The success of the procedure is confirmed by examination of the extruded first polar body, which demonstrates the haploidization of the reconstituted oocyte.

Conclusions

Among the different techniques designed to overcome the inability of spermatozoa to fertilize *in vitro*, ICSI is, by far, the most effective as it leads to high rates of fertilization and pregnancy despite very low sperm number or extreme defects in sperm motility and morphology. The only requirement is sperm viability, usually reflected by some form of sperm motion (although the sperm should be immobilized at the time of injection). Because of the nature of the technique, ICSI initially raised some justifiable concerns. However, several studies have demonstrated that babies born as a consequence of ICSI have a neonatal malformation rate within the range observed with newborns from standard IVF[65,66]. As it permits high rates of fertilization and pregnancy, and has clearly proved safe, ICSI is now being used increasingly for non-male-factor situations where any aspect of gamete function is in doubt.

The correction of meiotic abnormalities by transplantation of oocyte nuclei and / or cytoplasm is an attempt to overcome age-related aneuploidy. These and other related procedures which, until recently, were considered science fiction now present a credible foundation for successful cloning from an adult mammal[67].

References

1. Gordon JW, Talansky BE. Assisted fertilization by zona drilling: A mouse model for correction of oligospermia. *J Exp Zool* 1986;239:347

2. Tsunoda Y, Yasui T, Nakamura K. Effect of cutting the zona pellucida on the pronuclear transplantation in the mouse. *J Exp Zool* 1986;240:119

3. Odawara Y, Lopata A. Zona cracking: A new technique for assisted fertilization. *Proceedings of the Australian Fertility Society Meeting.* Sydney, 1987:73

4. Gordon JW, Grunfeld J, Garrisi GJ, *et al.* Fertilization of human oocytes by sperm from infertile males after zona pellucida drilling. *Fertil Steril* 1988;50:68

5. Cohen J, Malter H, Wright G, *et al.* Partial zona dissection of human oocytes when failure of zona pellucida penetration is anticipated. *Hum Reprod* 1989;4:435

6. Feichtinger W, Strohmer H, Fuhrberg P, *et al.* Photoablation of oocyte zona pellucida by erbium-YAG laser for in-vitro fertilisation in severe male infertility. *Lancet* 1992;i:811

7. Antinori S, Versaci C, Fuhrberg P, *et al.* Seventeen live births after the use of an erbium-yttrium-aluminum-garnet laser in the treatment of male factor infertility. *Hum Reprod* 1994;9:1891

8. Laws-King A, Trounson A, Sathananthan H, Kola I. Fertilization of human oocytes by microinjection of a single spermatozoon under the zona pellucida. *Fertil Steril* 1987;48:637

9. Palermo G, Van Steirteghem AC. Enhancement of acrosome reaction and subzonal insemination of a single spermatozoon in mouse eggs. *Mol Reprod Dev* 1991;30:339

10. Palermo G, Joris H, Devroey P, Van Steirteghem AC. Induction of acrosome reaction in human spermatozoa used for subzonal insemination. *Hum Reprod* 1992;7:248

11. Hiramoto Y. Microinjection of live spermatozoa into sea urchin eggs. *Exp Cell Res* 1962;27:416

12. Lin TP. Microinjection of mouse eggs. *Science* 1966; 151:333

13. Uehara T, Yanagimachi R. Microsurgical injection of spermatozoa into hamster eggs with subsequent transformation of sperm nuclei into male pronuclei. *Biol Reprod* 1976;15:467

14. Perreault SD, Wolf RA, Zirkin B. The role of disulfide bond reduction during mammalian sperm nuclear decondensation in vivo. *Dev Biol* 1984;101:160

15. Naish SJ, Perreault SD, Zirkin BJ. DNA synthesis following microinjection of heterologous sperm and somatic cell nuclei into hamster oocytes. *Gamete Res* 1987;18:109

16. Markert C. Fertilization of mammalian eggs by sperm injection. *J Exp Zool* 1983;228:195

17. Thadani VM. *A study of oocyte interactions using in vitro fertilization and sperm microinjection*. New Haven, CN: Yale University, 1981 (PhD thesis)

18. Perreault SD, Zirkin BR. Sperm nuclear decondensation in mammals: Role of sperm-associated proteinase in vivo. *J Exp Zool* 1982;224:252

19. Hoshi K, Yanagida K, Sato A. Pretreatment of hamster oocytes with Ca^{2+} ionophore to facilitate fertilization by ooplasmic microinjection. *Hum Reprod* 1992;7:871

20. Younis AI, Keefer CL, Brackett BG. Fertilization of bovine oocytes by sperm injection. *Theriogenology* 1989;31:276

21. Iritani A. Current status of biotechnological studies in mammalian reproduction. *Fertil Steril* 1988;50:543

22. Goto K, Kinoshita A, Takuma Y, Ogawa K. Fertilization by sperm injection in cattle. *Theriogenology* 1990;33:238

23. Lanzendorf S, Maloney M, Ackerman S, *et al.* Fertilizing potential of acrosome-defective sperm following microsurgical injection into eggs. *Gamete Res* 1988; 19:329

24. Palermo G, Joris H, Devroey P, Van Steirteghem AC. Pregnancies after intracytoplasmic injection of single spermatozoon into an oocyte. *Lancet* 1992;340:17

25. Palermo GD, Cohen J, Rosenwaks Z. Intracytoplasmic sperm injection: A powerful tool to overcome fertilization failure. *Fertil Steril* 1996;65:899

26. Palermo GD, Schlegel PN, Colombero LT, *et al.* Aggressive sperm immobilization prior to ICSI with immature spermatozoa improves fertilization and pregnancy rates. *Hum Reprod* 1996;11:1023

27. Palermo GD, Alikani M, Bertoli M, *et al.* Oolemma characteristics in relation to survival and fertilization patterns of oocytes treated by intracytoplasmic sperm injection. *Hum Reprod* 1996;11:172

28. Nagy ZY, Staessen C, Liu J, *et al.* Prospective, auto-controlled study on reinsemination of failed-fertilized oocytes by intracytoplasmic sperm injection. *Fertil Steril* 1995;64:1130

29. Morton PC, Yoder CS, Tucker MJ, *et al.* Reinsemination by intracytoplasmic sperm injection of 1 day old oocytes after complete conventional fertilization failure. *Fertil Steril* 1997;68:488

30. Yovich JL, Stanger JD. The limitations of in-vitro fertilization from male with severe oligospermia and abnormal sperm morphology. *J In Vitro Fert Embryo Transf* 1984;1:172

31. Chia CM, Sathananthan H, Ng SC, *et al.* Ultrastructural investigation of failed in-vitro fertilisation in idiopathic subfertility. *Proceedings of the 18th Singapore–Malaysia Congress of Medicine*. Singapore: Academy of Medicine, 1984:52

32. De Felici M, Siracusa G. "Spontaneous" hardening of the zona pellucida of mouse oocytes during in-vitro culture. *Gamete Res* 1982;6:107

33. Bedford JM, Kim HH. Sperm / egg binding patterns and oocyte cytology in retrospective analysis of fertilization failure in vitro. *Hum Reprod* 1993;8:453

34. Van Blerkom J, Henry G. Oocyte dysmorphism and aneuploidy in meiotically mature human oocytes after ovarian stimulation. *Hum Reprod* 1992;3:379

35. Lalonde L, Langalis H, Antaki P, *et al.* Male infertility associated with round-headed acrosomeless spermatozoa. *Fertil Steril* 1988;49:316

36. World Health Organization. Task Force on the Diagnosis and Treatment of Infertility: Towards more objectivity in diagnosis and management of male infertility. (Prepared by Comhaire FH, de Kretser D, Farley TMM, Rowe PJ.) *Int J Androl* 1987;7(Suppl):1

37. De Kretser DM, Yates CA, McDonald J, *et al.* The use of in-vitro fertilization in the management of male infertility. In: Rolland R, Heineman MJ, Hillier SG, Vener M, eds. *Gamete Quality and Fertility Regulation.* Amsterdam: Elsevier Science Publishers BV, 1985:213

38. Temple-Smith PD, Southwick GJ, Yates CA, *et al.* Human pregnancy by in-vitro fertilization (IVF) using sperm aspirated from the epididymis. *J In Vitro Fert Embryo Transf* 1985;2:119

39. Silber SJ, Ord T, Borrero C, *et al.* New treatment for infertility due to congenital absence of the vas deferens. *Lancet* 1987;ii:850

40. Silber SJ, Devroey P, Nagy Z, *et al.* ICSI with testicular and epididymal sperm. *Proceedings of the ESHRE Workshop.* Brussels, 1994:36

41. Tournaye H, Devroey P, Liu J, *et al.* Microsurgical epididymal sperm aspiration and intracytoplasmic sperm injection: A new effective approach to infertility as a result of congenital bilateral absence of vas deferens. *Fertil Steril* 1994;61:1045

42. Palermo GD, Cohen J, Alikani M, *et al.* Intracytoplasmic sperm injection: A novel treatment for all forms of male factor infertility. *Fertil Steril* 1995;63:1231

43. Craft I, Bennett V, Nicholson N. Fertilising ability of testicular spermatozoa. *Lancet* 1993;342:864

44. Schoysman R, Vanderzwalmen P, Nijs M, *et al.* Pregnancy after fertilization with human testicular spermatozoa. *Lancet* 1993;342:1237

45. Fishel S, Green S, Bishop M, *et al.* Pregnancy after intracytoplasmic injection of spermatid. *Lancet* 1995; 345:1641

46. Liu J, Nagy Z, Joris H, *et al.* Successful fertilization and establishment of pregnancies after intracytoplasmic sperm injection in patients with globozoospermia. *Hum Reprod* 1995;10:626

47. Ogura A, Matsuda J, Yanagimachi R. Birth of normal young after electrofusion of mouse oocytes with round spermatids. *Proc Natl Acad Sci USA* 1994;91: 7460

48. Kimura Y, Yanagimachi R. Development of normal mice from oocytes injected with secondary spermatocyte nuclei. *Biol Reprod* 1995;53:855

49. Tesarik J, Mendoza C, Testart J. Viable embryos from injection of round spermatids into oocytes. *N Engl J Med* 1995;333:525

50. Schoysman R, Vanderzwalmen P, Zech H, *et al.* Results of spermatid injection in human oocytes in relation to previous testis biopsy and oocyte treatment. *Fertil Steril* 1996;(Suppl):S529

51. Avarbock MR, Brinster CJ, Brinster RL. Reconstitution of spermatogenesis from frozen spermatogonial stem cells. *Nat Med* 1996;2:693

52. Zhang J, Grifo J, Blaszczyk A, *et al.* In vitro maturation (IVM) of human preovulatory oocytes reconstructed by germinal vesicle (GV) transfer. *Fertil Steril* 1997;(Suppl):S1

53. Cohen J, Scott R, Schimmel T, *et al.* Birth of an infant after transfer of anucleate donor oocyte cytoplasm into recipient eggs. *Lancet* 1997;350:186

54. Willadsen SM. Nuclear transplantation in sheep embryos. *Nature* 1986;320:63

55. Willadsen SM. Cloning of sheep and cow embryos. *Genome* 1989;31:956

56. Masui Y, Markert CL. Cytoplasmic control of behavior during meiotic maturation of frog oocytes. *J Exp Zool* 1971;177:129

57. Kishimoto T. Microinjection and cytoplasmic transfer in starfish oocytes. In: Prescott DM, ed. *Methods in Cell Biology*. London: Academic Press, 1986:1379

58. Meyerhof PG, Masui Y. Properties of a cytostatic factor from *Xenopus laevis* eggs. *Dev Biol* 1979;72:182

59. Muggleton-Harris A, Whittingham DG, Wilson L. Cytoplasmic control of preimplantation development in-vitro in the mouse. *Nature* 1982;299:460

60. Thibault C, Gerard M. Cytoplasmic factor necessary for formation of male pronucleus in rabbit oocytes. *CR Acad Sci Hebd Seances Acad Sci D* 1970;270:2025

61. Usui N, Yanagimachi R. Behavior of hamster sperm incorporated into eggs at various stages of maturation, fertilization, and early development. The appearance and disappearance factors involved in sperm chromatin decondensation in egg cytoplasm. *J Ultrastruct Res* 1976;57:276

62. Muggleton-Harris AL, Brown JG. Cytoplasmic factors influence mitochondrial reorganization and resumption of cleavage during culture of early mouse embryos. *Hum Reprod* 1988;3:1020

63. Flood JT, Chillik CF, Van Uem JF, *et al.* Ooplasmic transfusion: Prophase germinal vesicle oocytes made developmentally competent by microinjection in metaphase II egg cytoplasm. *Fertil Steril* 1990;53:1049

64. Cohen J, Levron J, Schimmel T, Willadsen S. Cytoplasmic transfer. *Proceedings of the 9th Annual In Vitro Fertilization and Embryo Transfer Congress.* Santa Barbara, CA, July 21–24, 1996

65. Bonduelle M, Hamberger L, Joris H, *et al.* Assisted reproduction of intracytoplasmic sperm injection: An ESHRE survey of clinical experiences until December 1993. *Hum Reprod Update* 1995;1:3 (CD-ROM)

66. Palermo GD, Colombero LT, Schattman G, *et al.* Evolution of pregnancies and initial follow-up of newborns delivered after intracytoplasmic sperm injection. *J Am Med Assoc* 1996;276:1893

67. Wilmut I, Schieke AE, McWhir J, *et al.* Viable offspring derived from fetal and adult mammalian cells. *Nature* 1997;385:810

11 Assisted hatching and fragment removal

Nikica Zaninovic, MS

Background

Development of assisted-hatching techniques

The assisted-hatching (AHA) procedure was first introduced in the late 1980s. The observation that preembryos which developed after PZD (partial zona dissection) possessed a somewhat higher rate of implantation compared with conventionally inseminated preembryos led to the idea of artificially creating a gap in the zona pellucida before intrauterine transfer[1].

In 1989, the first clinical trial of AHA was performed by Reproductive Biology Associates of Atlanta, GA. Using a PZD-type technique, the zonae of test preembryos were pierced and torn to create a small slit. Although initial results were promising, with a moderate increase in the implantation rate of mechanically hatched preembryos, subsequent trials failed to demonstrate a statistically significant difference between test and control groups. Later analysis of this means of creating small gaps in the mouse zona revealed that abnormal hatching was often the result. The hole caused the mouse zona to fail to become thinned in the usual way as the blastocysts expanded; thus, the blastocysts were often observed to be partially trapped within the zona midway through the hatching process[1]. It was then postulated that larger, more open, gaps might better facilitate *in vivo* hatching and, as a consequence, promote implantation.

To create a larger hole in the zona, AT (acidic Tyrode's) medium was tested. This medium had previously been used for a technique called *zona drilling* wherein holes were dissolved in the zonae of oocytes before insemination in an attempt to assist the fertilization process[2]. Although AT medium was shown to exert a mild toxic effect when used on the zonae of unfertilized human oocytes, its effects were observed to be less detrimental to cleaving preembryos. For some time, the use of AT was considered dangerous before fertilization, and it was rarely used in association with oocytes. Recently, however, AT has regained a certain popularity for use with oocytes specifically as a result of its successful application in procedures for first-polar-body removal[3].

In addition to these PZD and AT techniques, other methods for facilitating the hatching process have been investigated. These include invasive (creating a gap in the zona) as well as non-invasive (thinning and softening of the zona) techniques[4]. Invasive techniques include mechanical tearing with PZD, chemical digestion with AT, burning a hole using a laser and, recently, piezomanipulation. As already mentioned, PZD techniques have been virtually abandoned for this application because of its association with preembryo trapping. Acidic digestion is probably the most well established and commonly used procedure[5,6]. With the introduction of laser techniques, it is clearly possible to create an opening in the zona of a uniform size; however, clinical efficacy, safety concerns, and cost issues have yet to be addressed[7–9]. Finally, recent procedures using a piezomanipulator have been encouraging. The device appears to be very effective in zona pellucida manipulation (Thomas Huang, personal communication).

Non-invasive techniques involve thinning and / or softening of the zona by culturing the preembryo for a short time in the presence of a weak acidic solution or protease[10,11]. However, these techniques have yet to be proven effective in human preembryos.

AHA may be performed on preembryos of any cleavage stage, from two-cell to blastocyst[12]. The optimal stage of development has not yet been determined. Most groups perform the procedure on the day of intrauterine transfer at 65–72 h post-insemination.

AT medium was successfully applied with AHA in human preembryos in 1991 at Cornell University Medical Center, NY[13]. Rates of implantation in the AHA group were slightly higher than in the zona-intact group, but these differences were not statistically significant. Retrospective analysis revealed that some patients benefited greatly by having their preembryos manipulated whereas others did not. It was eventually determined that preembryos with thick zonae (> 15 µm), preembryos from women with elevated serum follicle-stimulating hormone (FSH) levels, and preembryos from women > 38 years of age were best served by AHA. Preembryos from younger women with or without an appreciable zona thickness, were better left alone. This led to the application of selective AHA on a patient-by-patient basis after measuring zona thickness and considering the clinical characteristics of the woman[14].

When non-selective AHA is performed, all preembryos designated for transfer are manipulated[15]. Selective hatching protocols require that certain criteria be evaluated before determining whether or not a preembryo is a candidate for the procedure. These include: female age; female basal FSH; number of previous attempts without implantation; degree of preembryo fragmentation; preembryo growth rate; zona pellucida thickness; zona uniformity; and zona color. Inclusion criteria may vary from one IVF center to another.

Zona pellucida structure and function

The zona pellucida is the glycoprotein coat that surrounds the oocyte. This non-cellular structure is believed to be produced by both the oocyte and its surrounding cells during early follicular development. The human zona pellucida appears to consist of two layers: a thick outer layer that is easily dissolved during AHA; and a thin inner layer that is more difficult to penetrate[16]. During *in vitro* culture, the zona becomes brittle and loses its elasticity by a process called *zona hardening*[17]. This process may play a role in the block to polyspermic fertilization by providing a mechanism for protecting the preembryo. On the other hand, hardening may impair the hatching process and thereby decrease the chances for implantation.

The zona pellucida fulfils a number of important functions during oogenesis and early preembryo development (known so far):

♦ The zona is a physical barrier that serves to protect oocytes and preembryos from antigens during the preimplantation period;

♦ The zona is important during sperm / oocyte interaction because of sperm receptors on its surface; zonae with non-functional sperm receptors may inhibit sperm binding, thus resulting in fertilization failure (an indication for ICSI);

♦ The zona of a healthy oocyte prevents penetration by additional spermatozoa once one has fused with the oolemma (block to polyspermy); thus, oocytes fertilized in the absence of a zona demonstrate polyspermia; and

♦ The zona preserves the three-dimensional structure and integrity of the preembryo.

After fulfilling its role during oocyte maturation, fertilization, and early preembryo development, the zona pellucida is shed; *in vivo* hatching of the blastocyst (thinning and rupturing of the zona, followed by escape of the blastocyst) is essential for successful preembryo implantation. Abnormalities in the structure and function of this complex glycoprotein structure may result in impaired fertilization and decreased preembryo viability, and a poor prognosis for implantation. Creating an artificial hole in its surface before implantation (AHA) appears to facilitate natural hatching and may be effective in rescuing preembryos with poor implantation potential.

Indications for assisted hatching

Overtly thick zonae pellucidae

Zona pellucida thickness and rigidity is influenced by the preovulatory hormonal environment; variations may be associated with basal FSH and rising estradiol levels[18]. The thickness of the zona varies during oocyte and preembryo development. Thinning begins during the first and second cleavages, and progressively continues during blastocyst formation. At the expanded-blastocyst stage, the zona is so thin as to break under pressure, thereby allowing the blastocyst to hatch. Zona thinning is regulated by trypsin-like proteases produced by cleaving preembryos and blastocysts[19,20].

In the absence of thinning, possibly as a result of insufficient production of proteases, the preembryo may become trapped within the zona shell, effectively abolishing any potential for implantation. The fact that the zonae of some preembryos, particularly those with poor morphology, do not thin properly has been postulated as one reason for pregnancy failure after IVF. As already described, creating an artificial hole in thick zonae (>15 μm) may promote natural hatching and implantation of the preembryo. On the other hand, preembryos with thin zonae (<13 μm) may receive no benefit or even be adversely affected after AHA using AT medium[14].

Abnormal zona pellucida / preembryo shape

Oval-shaped oocytes and preembryos are not unusual. However, the ability of oddly shaped morulae to undergo compaction, further development, and *in vitro* hatching has been observed to be somewhat lower than that with normal, rounded, conceptuses. Oddly shaped preembryos are usually associated with an abnormal zona pellucida that may be completely or partially bilayered. Such bilayering usually occurs early in oocyte development within the follicle. AHA may help to promote appropriate cell-to-cell contact, compaction, and hatching in these abnormal preembryos (see Chapter 8).

Abnormal zona pellucida color

Dark (brownish / yellowish) zonae are sometimes observed *in vitro*. It has been noted that the zonae of some oocytes, particularly those determined to be postmature at harvest, progressively darken and deteriorate with prolonged culture (personal observation). When such a morphological characteristic is noted, the preembryo is considered to be a candidate for AHA (see Chapter 8).

Cytoplasmic fragmentation

Formation of anuclear cytoplasmic blebs or fragments during early preembryo development *in vitro* is frequently observed and appears to be limited primarily to human conceptuses. Except for monkeys, other species do not produce cytoplasmic fragments under normal conditions (Benjamin Bracket, personal communication).

Cytoplasmic fragments are membrane-bound components of cytoplasm which are expelled from the surface of fertilized oocytes or blastomeres of the preembryo. Fragments show different surface-membrane characteristics compared with blastomeres, and do not contain DNA[21]. Preembryos with excessive fragmentation (>20%) have lower implantation rates than those without fragments. The decreased implantation potential of these preembryos may be the result of a reduction in available cytoplasm for normal cell division which eventually leads to an overall lower blastomere number[22]. In addition, numerous fragments may affect compaction and subsequent blastocyst development.

Analysis of preembryos during a 72-h period (from insemination to transfer) indicates that the majority of cytoplasmic fragments develop between the pronuclear stage, and the first and second cleavage divisions. When fragmentation occurs very early (by 24 h after insemination), subsequent development is greatly impaired. In the present author's experience, >70% of preembryos with early minor fragmentation demonstrate excessive fragmentation (>20% of the preembryo surface) by day 3 in culture. This early cytoplasmic fragmentation may indicate *in vitro* injury to, or intrinsic abnormality of, preembryonic DNA.

Fragment formation occurring after the first cleavage tends to be less excessive and may not impair subsequent preembryo development. These fragments develop just before blastomere division as multiple small blebs on the cell membrane. As cleavage proceeds, some blebs are reincorporated into daughter blastomeres whereas others become true membrane-bound fragments. Occasionally, individual blastomeres may break up entirely into multiple fragments, an indication of cell death.

Why does fragmentation occur? Hypothetically, various intrinsic and extrinsic factors may be responsible. Culture conditions, cytoplasmic competence, genetic integrity, chromosomal imbalance, disorders of karyokinesis and cytokinesis, and other factors may contribute to cytoplasmic fragmentation. Programmed cell death and resultant apoptosis are observed in fragmented and arrested preembryos, although the conditions and factors causing these changes are not known.

Chromosome analysis of fragmented preembryos by FISH (fluorescence in-situ hybridization) indicates that >50% of these preembryos are abnormal, which may well account for their lower implantation rate[23]. It is interesting to note, however, that there is no relationship between cytoplasmic fragmentation and female age despite the increased incidence of chromosomal abnormalities in preembryos from women >40 years of age.

On days 2 and 3 of *in vitro* culture (48–72 h after insemination), totally different fragment patterns may be observed in different preembryos. Fragments may vary in size, position, composition, and number, with some preembryos showing no fragmentation in contrast to others which are so fragmented that counting individual blastomeres is impossible. Different patterns are often seen in the cohort of preembryos produced from one woman, suggesting that some preembryos are preprogrammed in their developmental potential. As fragmentation occurs at different stages of early development (pronuclear, zygotic, and cleavage), and demonstrates diverse patterns and localization, it is likely that various underlying mechanisms may lead to fragment formation.

Mild fragmentation (≤10% of the preembryo surface) is usually characterized by small fragments, may include polar body components, and is generally localized to one area. Preembryos with mild fragmentation have high rates of implantation. AHA is not indicated in these cases unless other clinical factors, such as female age or history, suggest that it may be useful.

Moderate fragmentation (10–20% of the preembryo surface) is usually associated with the presence of blastomeres of irregular size and shape. If the fragments are localized to one area, they may be due to the death of a single blastomere. Preembryos with moderate fragmentation may become excessively fragmented during prolonged culture. AHA and fragment removal are indicated as these preembryos possess a lower implantation potential.

Excessive fragmentation (≥20% of the preembryo surface) correlates to a very low incidence of implantation. Some women express this degree of fragmentation in all of their preembryos. Depending on the localization and type of fragments, there is growing evidence that some of these conceptuses may be salvaged by AHA and fragment removal. In addition to the general extent of fragmentation, there are other, more precise, variables which contribute to a given pattern of fragment development: Fragments may be localized or scattered, free or bound to blastomeres, and / or small or large in size.

Fragments localized to one area indicate origin due

to polar body disintegration or single blastomere death; unless excessive, pregnancy potential is not reduced. Such fragments may be easily and satisfactorily removed during AHA.

Scattered fragments may either lie free in the perivitelline space or be bound to blastomeres. If excessive in number and bound, they may impair cell-to-cell apposition, blastomere compaction, and implantation; if few and free, they may be completely removed during AHA. Scattered fragments originate during mitotic divisions (cleavage) and may increase in number with each subsequent division. The position of the blastomere cleavage plane may determine the locations of scattered fragments.

Preembryos possessing multiple fragments that are large and irregular have a relatively low implantation rate. Large fragments are often difficult to distinguish from cleaving blastomeres unless nuclei can be seen, as true blastomeres become smaller with each successive mitotic division. Preembryos with these abnormal characteristics have a poor prognosis for implantation due to their impaired cytokinesis and reduced viability in culture. Aggressive fragment removal may be attempted in these conceptuses, but results are generally poor.

Poor preembryo growth rate / morphology

Slow-growing preembryos, defined as <6 cells on day 3 (68–72 h after insemination) implant in the uterus at higher rates after AHA treatment compared with similarly slow-growing non-AHA-treated preembryos[13]. It is speculated that the hole in the zona pellucida may promote easier transport of nutrients as well as facilitate *in vivo* hatching. Other characteristics of the preembryo that may be indications for AHA are an irregular blastomere size and shape (implicated in abnormal cytokinesis), mottled and unhealthy-looking cytoplasm, cytoplasmic inclusions and vacuoles, and other abnormalities visible by light microscopy.

Previous reproductive history

Careful study of previous medical histories and analysis of earlier results helps to determine the best treatment options for couples undergoing IVF. The majority of women produce preembryos of remarkably similar quality throughout multiple treatment cycles. This allows a prospective, albeit not infallible, prediction of preembryo quality in subsequent cycles. If preembryo quality has been poor in the past, then ovarian-stimulation protocols may be altered accordingly, protein sources for culture media may be changed, coculture techniques may be attempted, or AHA may be considered, even in younger women. More than two attempts and failures to become pregnant, regardless of female age, is a clear indication for AHA.

Female age

Female age is clearly associated with implantation success and pregnancy outcome. With the application of IVF, it is now evident that implantation rates diminish drastically in infertile women >40 years of age. For this reason, AHA is indicated on the basis of age alone (irrespective of preembryo morphology) for women approaching or past their fourth decade of life.

In addition to the well-understood decrease in the number of genetically healthy oocytes from older women, it is possible that preembryos developed from aging oocytes lose their ability to implant because of an altered zona pellucida-thinning capacity and / or in response to altered endocrine system factors. Thus, all preembryos from older women need to undergo AHA regardless of morphology. Conversely, as preembryos from younger patients (<30 years) frequently implant, AHA is not deemed necessary unless there is a history of multiple implantation failure or very poor conceptus quality. There is a tendency to apply AHA more liberally as female age increases. In the Cornell program, in which one-quarter to one-third of the patient population is ≥40 years of age and virtually all consenting patients >40 years have all or most of their preembryos manipulated before intrauterine transfer, the clinical pregnancy rate for these women (pregnancy confirmed by ultrasound) per transfer exceeds 35%. Although this proportion is much lower than that for younger patients, it is high compared with worldwide IVF statistics involving pregnancy rates from women of such more advanced ages.

Other indications

Elevated FSH (>15 mIU / ml) on day 3 of the menstrual cycle indicates poor ovarian reserve and altered ovarian physiology. These changes may affect the oocyte and zona pellucida environment within the follicle[18]. It has been shown that patients with elevated basal FSH levels benefit from AHA, with doubling of implantation rates compared with non-hatched controls[14].

In specific cases, patients with no clear medical indications may request AHA to enhance their chances of becoming pregnant. Results from our program during the last 3 years suggest that AHA exerts no adverse effects on subsequent preembryo development (as far as is now known), even in younger patients with conceptuses that exhibit good morphology.

Methodology

Techniques involving the use of AT medium (pH 2.35) are most frequently used for AHA. In this procedure, a minute quantity of the acidic solution is used to dissolve a very small portion of the zona pellucida. If exposure to the solution is brief, no negative effects ensue.

Equipment and supplies

In the Cornell program, the procedure is performed on the warming stage of a Nikon Diaphot inverted microscope equipped with two motor-driven coarse-control manipulators and two hydraulic micromanipulators (MM-188 and MO-109, Narishige Co. Ltd, Tokyo, Japan). Micropipettes are fitted to a tool-holder controlled by two IM-6 microinjectors (Narishige Co. Ltd). AHA is performed at ×400 magnification using Hoffman Modulation Contrast optics.

Culture medium

HTF-Hepes medium supplemented with 6% human plasma protein fraction (Plasmanate™) is used to make working droplets in a shallow Petri dish (Falcon 1006). A single drop of AT medium is added to the dish and circled in red to distinguish it from the droplets that will contain preembryos. All droplets (10 µl) are covered with equilibrated light mineral oil (BDH Ltd, Poole, UK). Before starting the procedure, the Petri dish is tightly capped because of the Hepes in the medium and placed in an incubator until needed. Up to four preembryos may be manipulated at a time with one preembryo per working droplet (Figure 11.1).

Microtools

Micropipettes for holding and hatching are made from sterilized borosilicate glass capillary tubes (Drummond Scientific, Broomall, PA, USA) with a 0.97 mm external diameter, a 0.69 mm internal diameter, and 78 mm length. Pipettes are made by drawing the thin-walled glass capillary tubes with a horizontal microelectrode puller (Model 753, Campden Instruments Ltd, Loughborough, UK). The holding micropipette is cut and fire-polished on a microforge (Narishige Co. Ltd) to a final outer diameter of 60–80 µm and an inner diameter of 20 µm. The hatching micropipette is prepared in a similar way, but with an outside diameter of approximately 10 µm. Both micropipettes are bent to an angle of 30°. The micropipettes are then positioned closely to one other (Figure 11.2) and focused before use.

Procedure

Using ×200 magnification, the AHA micropipette is front-loaded with AT solution before each hatching procedure by inserting only the tip of the micropipette into the AT medium. Once it is filled, the micropipette is moved away from the dish. A working droplet containing the preembryo is then moved to the center of the dish, and the preembryo visualized. The preembryo is then positioned on the holding micropipette so that the AHA micropipette is aligned with either empty perivitelline space between blastomeres or an area containing cytoplasmic fragments (three-o'clock position).

Using a ×400 magnification, the AHA micropipette is lowered into the working droplet to a point where the zona pellucida and micropipette tip are both in focus. With the AHA micropipette gently touching the zona, the AT solution is carefully expelled over a small (20–30 μm) area. Small circular and / or up-and-down movements assist the rapid dissolution of the proteinaceous shell whereas the inner layer may prove more difficult to dissolve. However, as soon as the zona is penetrated, AT expulsion should be stopped immediately and followed by gentle suction to remove any acidic solution from the area. Excess AT solution is also removed from the perivitelline space and zona surface using small circular motions. Finally, the preembryo is moved to the far (opposite) edge of the droplet before returning to the site of the hole to further clear the area of AT medium by aspiration. Rapid and thorough removal of AT solution is essential to protect the preembryo from pH changes which are, in fact, difficult to observe. When in doubt, non-toxic dyes may be added to the AT solution to enhance its visibility.

The zonae of different preembryos may respond differently to the acidic solution. In general, however, an opening is usually easily made within a few seconds although, occasionally, some difficulty may be encountered. In some cases, the zona is extremely elastic or appears to be connected to the blastomeres.

The size of the hole in the zona should not be too small (<20 μm); apertures which are inadequate in size have been implicated in cases of impaired hatching, trapped blastocysts, and monozygotic twinning. Conversely, too large a hole may result in blastomere loss if intrauterine transfer is difficult.

If no fragments need to be removed, the preembryo is released from the holding micropipette and AT medium is reloaded to repeat the procedure on the next preembryo (Figures 11.3–11.5). It is not necessary to change micropipettes between preembryos from a single patient. On completion of AHA, all preembryos are washed with at least four droplets of fresh medium before being returned to their culture dishes.

Fragment removal

Cytoplasmic fragments can be removed by gentle suction after a hole has been made in the zona pellucida (Figures 11.6 and 11.7). When carried out properly, there is no evidence that removing fragments interferes with subsequent preembryo development; indeed, doing so may be beneficial[24,25]. Certain types of fragments are easily removed, particularly those lying free in the perivitelline space. On the other hand, fragments that are bound to blastomeres or incompletely expelled from the blastomere surface should be left alone.

Constant refocusing on the fragment membrane and tip of the micropipette are required for successful and safe fragment removal. Carefully controlled suction is also important during manipulation, especially when the micropipette is inside the zona and suction is being applied to draw out the fragments. The safest method is to remove one fragment at a time, aspirating them into the micropipette once outside the zona. Fragment removal may be time-consuming and requires great patience, but every fragment need not be removed; an end-result of 5–10% of the fragments remaining should be sufficient.

To facilitate fragment visualization and removal, preembryos may be rotated on the holding micropipette (Figure 11.8). This allows complete fragment removal in one area. If fragments are scattered, then constant rotation and repositioning of the preembryo is necessary.

Our program paperwork describes fragments that are free in the perivitelline space and easily removable as *free* or *extra* whereas those appearing as masses in one location and / or firmly attached to blastomeres or to one another are termed *clumped*. Individual fragments dispersed throughout are called *scattered*, and hard fragments, which are difficult to aspirate and remove (? hardening polar bodies), are termed *rigid*.

On rare occasions (<1% of manipulated preembryos), blastomeres are damaged during fragment removal. When this occurs, the damaged blastomere should be removed. Good pregnancy rates after blastomere biopsy suggest that subsequent development is not impaired by the loss of a single blastomere.

During AHA, bound corona cells, granulosa cells, and sperm may be removed from the outermost surface of the zona pellucida. This is desirable as such cells undergo apoptotic changes after prolonged *in vitro* culture. The cleaned preembryo has a markedly improved morphological appearance after fragment removal (Figures 11.9 and 11.10).

Assisted hatching on day 2

In special cases where excessive fragments (>20%) are present in all preembryos on day 2 (42–46 h after insemination), AHA may be performed early to optimize preembryo developmental potential. Removal of degenerating and space-consuming fragments may allow more room for growth and encourage better cell-to-cell contact. However, fragment removal on day 2 is more difficult because of the greater amount of clumped fragments and degree of fragment–blastomere binding (Figures 11.11–11.14). In addition, damage to even one blastomere when so few are available may impair subsequent preembryo development. Nevertheless, in spite of the difficulty and stress of the procedure, it has proved to be of benefit to subsequent preembryo development compared with control sibling preembryos without day 2 AHA (manuscript in preparation).

Assisted hatching on cryopreserved / thawed preembryos

During preembryo freezing and thawing, one or more blastomeres may lyse and die (Figure 11.15). The resultant degenerative material may be removed following AHA. This will ensure that only preembryos cleared of material that may impair development are transferred. Dead or dying blastomeres and fragments are removed immediately after thawing.

The zona pellucida changes in consistency after exposure to ultralow temperatures; it is thought that the ensuing increased rigidity may impair the hatching process. Thus, AHA is indicated in this particular circumstance. Special care is required when removing degenerative blastomeres due to the reduced elasticity of the zona (Figures 11.16 and 11.17) and its tendency to collapse, and the fragility of the blastomere membrane. If cracks are noted in the zona after thawing, an effort should be made to use the existing hole for removal of the degenerative material as multiple holes may impair the natural hatching process[26]. Studies of AHA procedures show increased implantation rates in thawed preembryos with, compared with those without, AHA[27,28].

Assisted hatching on blastocysts

AHA may be performed at the blastocyst stage[29,30]. Some expanded blastocysts are unable to hatch naturally, as observed during *in vitro* culture. AHA is able to rescue such blastocysts and prevent their collapse. However, the use of AT solution is not recommended due to the thinness of the zona and lack of perivitelline space. Use of a PZD type of technique or other mechanical treatment is preferable at this stage of development.

Discussion and future perspectives

The major advantages of AHA include a potentially higher implantation rate in some patients, and the salvage of preembryos with abnormalities of the zona pellucida and excessive cytoplasmic fragmentation. Furthermore, it has been demonstrated that hatched preembryos implant earlier than zona-intact preembryos, which may account for the closer conceptus / uterus synchronization during the implantation period[31].

Immunosuppression of the patient before intrauterine transfer of hatched preembryos is a preventative measure designed to reduce the possible contact of immune cells in the uterus to exposed preembryos[32].

Preembryo fragmentation represents one of the main factors for IVF failure. Fragmentation reduces the amount of cytoplasm available for blastomere division[22] and anuclear fragments may undergo an apoptotic process that is potentially detrimental to viable blastomeres. For these reasons, it is thought that early fragment removal helps some preembryos to continue to develop beyond their given capacity. Fragment removal may mimic the natural elimination of apoptotic cells by the immune system (assisted apoptotic cell removal) as preembryos and fragments express early apoptotic membrane markers which physiologically signal their impending removal. The role of the apoptotic process during human preembryo development requires further investigation.

The introduction of novel techniques, such as laser ablation and piezomanipulation, has provided new and exciting directions for AHA. Piezomanipulation is especially promising as it is a mechanical technique involving no chemical exposure. Technical advances will eventually allow improvements in control of gap size and blastomere protection.

AHA has proved successful when applied to preembryos with a poor prognosis for implantation[33], and may be combined with coculture[34]. However, too small a gap created in the zona leads to impairment of the natural hatching process and promotion of monozygotic twinning[29,35,36]. Conversely, too large a gap may lead to blastomere loss during preembryo transfer. AT solution, with its low pH, may have adverse effects on blastomere viability[37], but only if handled improperly. Finally, as human preembryos do not express polarization during compaction, the site along the zona where natural hatching is likely to take place cannot be identified. Consequently, the optimal site of the artificial hole or, indeed, whether the location is of any importance, has yet to be ascertained.

Identifying the preembryos that are most likely to implant (using a preembryo 'fingerprint') will enable selection of the best preembryos for AHA and transfer. Determination of the causes of preembryo death *in vitro*, and the application of non-invasive techniques to detect apoptotic blastomeres will allow their selective removal (Figure 11.18). Determination of preembryo viability using vital non-toxic dyes and genetic markers will permit the transfer of only healthy conceptuses, thereby improving the rate of implantation.

In conclusion, AHA is not a miracle technique, although there is growing evidence that its application is of particular benefit to specific patients. It is absolutely safe when performed by an experienced embryologist. Whereas the technique itself is still controversial and its results vary from one center to another[38], these differences are probably due to the use of different culture systems, different AHA procedures, and different levels of experience.

References

1. Cohen J, Elsner C, Kort H, *et al.* Impairment of the hatching process following IVF in the human and improvement of implantation by assisting hatching using micromanipulation. *Hum Reprod* 1990;5:7

2. Gordon JW, Talansky BE. Assisted fertilization by zona drilling: A mouse model for correction of oligospermia. *J Exp Zool* 1986;239:347

3. Smith SE, Morton PC, Tucker MJ, *et al.* Birth after polar body biopsy using acidified Tyrode's medium followed by ICSI. *Proceedings of the ASRM Meeting.* Cincinnati, OH, 1997

4. Katayama KP. Assisted hatching: The current status and future projections. *Assist Reprod Rev* 1994;4:33

5. Chao KH, Chen SU, Chen HF, *et al.* Assisted hatching increases the implantation and pregnancy rate of in vitro fertilization (IVF)-embryo transfer (ET), but not that of IVF-tubal ET in patients with repeated IVF failures. *Fertil Steril* 1997;67:904

6. Castellotti DS, Da Motta ELA, Alegretti AR, *et al.* Successful birth after intrafallopian transfer of micro-hatched embryos. *Fertil Steril* 1997;68:367

7. Strohmer H, Feichtinger W. Successful clinical application of laser for micromanipulation in an in vitro fertilization program. *Fertil Steril* 1992;58:212

8. Tadir Y, Neev J, Berns MW. Lasers in micromanipulation of preimplantation embryos and gametes. *Semin Reprod Endocrinol* 1994;12:169

9. Antinori S, Selman HA, Caffa B, *et al.* Zona opening of human embryos using a non-contact UV laser for assisted hatching in patients with poor prognosis of pregnancy. *Hum Reprod* 1996;11:2488

10. Gordon JW, Dapunt U. Restoration of normal implantation rates in mouse embryos with a hatching impairment by the use of a new method of assisted hatching. *Fertil Steril* 1993;59:1302

11. Lee JE, Lee DR, Paik HR, *et al.* Application of biochemical assisted hatching (BAH) by proteases in a human assisted reproductive technology program. *Proceedings of the ASRM Meeting.* Cincinnati, OH, 1997

12. Barnes FL, Crombie A, Gardner DK, *et al.* Blastocyst development and birth after in vitro maturation of human primary oocytes, intracytoplasmic sperm injection and assisted hatching. *Hum Reprod* 1995; 10:3243

13. Cohen J. Assisted hatching of human embryos. *J In Vitro Fert Embryo Transf* 1991;8:179

14. Cohen J, Alikani M, Trowbridge J, Rosenwaks Z. Implantation enhancement by selective assisted hatching using zona drilling of human embryos with poor prognosis. *Hum Reprod* 1992;7:685

15. Hu Y, Hoffman DI, Maxson WS, Ory SJ. Clinical application of nonselective assisted hatching of human embryos. *Fertil Steril* 1996;66:991

16. Dunbar BS, Maresh GA, Washenick K. Ovarian development and the formation of the mammalian zona pellucida. In: Dietl J, ed. *The Mammalian Egg Coat – Structure and Function.* Berlin: Springer-Verlag, 1989:38

17. Schiewe MC, Araujo Jr E, Asch RH, Balmaceda JP. Enzymatic characterization of zona pellucida hardening in human eggs and embryos. *J Assist Reprod Genet* 1995;12:2

18. Loret de Mola JR, Garside WT, Bucci J, *et al.* Analysis of the human zona pellucida during culture: Correlation with diagnosis and the preovulatory hormonal environment. *J Assist Reprod Genet* 1997; 14:332

19. Perona RM, Wassarman PM. Mouse blastocysts hatch in vitro by using a trypsin-like proteinase associated with cells of the mural trophectoderm. *Dev Biol* 1986;114:42

20. Swada H, Yamazaki K, Hoshi M. Trypsin-like hatching protease from mouse embryos: Evidence for the presence in culture medium and its enzymatic properties. *J Exp Zool* 1990;254:83

21. Dale B, Tosti E, Iaccarino M. Is the plasma membrane of the human oocyte reorganized following fertilization and early cleavage? *Zygote* 1995;3:31

22. Xu K, Rosenwaks Z. The importance of cytoplasm in early embryonic development. *J Assist Reprod Genet* 1996;13:1

23. Munne S, Alikani M, Tomkin G, *et al.* Embryo morphology, developmental rates, and maternal age are correlated with chromosome abnormalities. *Fertil Steril* 1995;64:382

24. Cohen J, Alikani M, Reing AM, *et al.* Selective assisted hatching of human embryos. *Ann Acad Med* 1992;21: 565

25. Cohen J, Alikani M, Liu HC, Rosenwaks Z. Rescue of human embryos by micromanipulation. *Baillière's Clin Obstet Gynaecol* 1994;8:95

26. Cohen J, Feldberg D. Effects of the size and the number of zona pellucida openings on hatching and trophoblast outgrowth in the mouse embryo. *Mol Reprod Dev* 1991;30:70

27. Check JH, Hoover L, Nazari A, *et al.* The effect of assisted hatching on pregnancy rates after frozen embryo transfer. *Fertil Steril* 1996;65:254

28. Tao J, Tamis R. Application of assisted hatching for 2-day-old, frozen-thawed embryo transfers in a poor-prognosis population. *J Assist Reprod Genet* 1997;14:128

29. Nijs M, Vanderzwalmen P, Segal-Bartin G, *et al.* A monozygotic twin pregnancy after application of zona rubbing on a frozen-thawed blastocyst. *Hum Reprod* 1993;8:127

30. Dokras A, Ross C, Gosden B, *et al.* Micromanipulation of human embryos to assist hatching. *Fertil Steril* 1994;61:514

31. Liu HC, Cohen J, Alikani M, *et al.* Assisted hatching facilitates earlier implantation. *Fertil Steril* 1993; 60:871

32. Cohen J, Malter H, Elsner C, *et al.* Immunosuppression supports implantation of zona pellucida dissected human embryos. *Fertil Steril* 1990;53:662

33. Schoolcraft WB, Schlenker T, Gee M, *et al.* Assisted hatching in the treatment of poor prognosis in vitro fertilization candidates. *Fertil Steril* 1994;62:551

34. Wiemer KE, Garrisi J, Steuerwald N, *et al.* Beneficial aspects of coculture with assisted hatching when applied to multiple-failure in vitro fertilization patients. *Hum Reprod* 1996;11:2429

35. Alikani M, Noyes N, Cohen J, Rosenwaks Z. Monozygotic twinning in the human is associated with the zona pellucida architecture. *Hum Reprod* 1994;9:1318

36. Slotnick RN, Ortega JE. Monoamniotic twinning and zona manipulation: A survey of U.S. IVF centers correlating zona manipulation procedures and high-risk twinning frequency. *J Assist Reprod Genet* 1996; 13:381

37. Van Golde R, Grossmann M, Egozcue J, *et al.* *Abstract book: Annual Meeting of ESHRE.* Maastricht, 1996 (Abstr 147)

38. Hellebaut S, De Sutter P, Dozortsev D, *et al.* Does assisted hatching improve implantation rates after in vitro fertilization or intracytoplasmic sperm injection in all patients? A prospective randomized study. *J Assist Reprod Genet* 1996;13:19

12 Preimplantation genetic diagnosis (PGD)

Kangpu Xu, PhD

Background

From an historical point of view, preimplantation genetic diagnosis (PGD) may be regarded as an extension of prenatal genetic diagnosis. The genetic diagnosis of gametes and conceptuses before implantation in the human uterus is possible only because of recent developments in the field of IVF. In much the same way as when IVF was first introduced to the world, the application of PGD has generated considerable controversy. Nonetheless, subsequent to reports of the first pregnancies with the use of PGD[1], the number of cases has steadily increased. As of 1997, there have been more than one hundred healthy babies brought into this world because of this new technology.

PGD is a technically challenging procedure which requires a good understanding of embryology and molecular biology. During IVF, oocytes and early cleavage-stage preembryos are readily accessible, thereby allowing one or a series of biopsies to be taken from oocytes, prezygotes, or preembryos. However, the amount of genetic material that may be safely obtained for testing is still restricted, thus limiting confirmational analysis. When further confounded by the fact that current protocols require transfer to a synchronized uterus, the permitted 'window of opportunity' in which to complete this relatively costly genetic analysis is very small indeed. Yet, in spite these drawbacks, PGD is rapidly becoming an integral part of many IVF programs (Figure 12.1). At present, there are more than 30 centers around the world which offer PGD to selected patients.

Thus far, three major aspects of PGD have been successfully applied:

(1) The sex of a preembryo can now be reliably determined by FISH (fluorescent in-situ hybridization) using specific probes for the X and Y chromosomes, or by specific sex chromosome sequence analysis using the polymerase chain reaction (PCR) technique. Thus, severe sex-linked disorders can be identified and avoided;

(2) Enumeration of chromosome composition can be achieved by FISH, thus allowing the exact ploidy of the preembryo to be determined concurrent with the diagnosis of certain common aneuploidies. In women of advanced maternal age, this reduces or even eliminates the risk of delivering a child with a chromosomal trisomy such as Down syndrome (trisomy 21). FISH may also be used to detect structural chromosomal abnormalities in cases of balanced translocations; and

(3) Single-gene defects (such as cystic fibrosis, sickle cell anemia, Tay–Sachs disease) and other commonly occurring genetic disorders may be detected by PCR.

Figures 12.2 and 12.3 (see pages 194–5) illustrate the key steps involved in PGD. These include examples of the micromanipulative procedures used to obtain genetic material, images of FISH–PGD, which is used in the diagnosis of numerical and structural defects of chromosomes, and some of the results using PCR–PGD for single-gene analysis.

A detailed discussion of all the possible approaches and all the complex biological issues, such as preembryo mosaicism, that may affect a diagnosis is inappropriate here. Instead, this chapter provides a general description of the basic steps involved in PGD and how diagnoses are made. For the sake of simplicity, the term 'PGD' is used even in cases where the term *preconception genetic diagnosis* may be more technically correct (see below).

Polar body and blastomere biopsy

The first critically important aspect of PGD is the collection of informative genetic material without compromising preembryo developmental potential. These efforts may include biopsy of the first polar body (or, to be more precise, *preconception genetic diagnosis*; Figure 12.2), biopsy of the second polar body, biopsy of cleavage-stage blastomeres (Figure 12.3), or biopsy of trophectoderm cells of blastocysts. In theory, trophectoderm collection represents the optimal procedure as it has the potential to harvest more cells for genetic analysis compared with the other methods[2]. Nevertheless, at present, polar body and blastomere biopsy remain the preferred approaches in most clinics[1,3–5]. Specific technical details for biopsy tend to be developed according to personal preferences and experience. Although one-step blastomere biopsy is possible, a more common and reliable method uses AT medium to open a hole in the zona pellucida (see page 195). Care must be taken in positioning the embryo and identifying a nucleus.

Fluorescent in-situ hybridization (FISH) for chromosomal analysis

As mentioned above, genetic material is generally limited to the DNA from one or two structures (polar bodies, or one or two blastomeres). Furthermore, polar-body biopsy is not applicable if the genetic disorder(s) are carried by the male. Direct chromosomal analysis is usually performed only on the first and / or second polar bodies because, at the early (six- to ten-cell) cleavage stages, metaphase chromosomes are rarely obtained. The FISH procedure, which has been developed only in the last decade, allows determination of specific chromosomal numbers by counting specific signals in interphase nuclei. The FISH procedure is very sensitive and has an acceptably high accuracy. Figures 12.4 and 12.5 demonstrate what may be expected from human blastomeres following FISH analysis. Figures 12.6–12.14 illustrate the detection of chromosomal structural abnormalities by FISH.

Polymerase chain reaction (PCR) for detection of single-gene defects

The PCR technique has revolutionized DNA analysis[6,7]. The procedure involves the repeated amplification of DNA to obtain adequate copies for analysis. Using this technique, it is now possible to detect single-gene mutations in polar bodies or blastomeres. Amplified DNA may then be subjected to mutation analysis by various methodologies, the selection of which is determined by the characteristics of the specific mutation.

Although the list of disorders for which PCR–PGD is applicable is growing rapidly, there are several problems inherent to the technique. Control of DNA contamination is of crucial importance. Even minute amounts of contaminating foreign DNA have adverse effects on the entire assay, as such material will also be amplified along with the original template of the biopsied specimen. The techniques necessary to produce a 'clean' accurate result must be stringently maintained, and an isolated working space is a prerequisite to setting up a PCR laboratory.

Other problems involve the possibility of *allele preferential amplification* or, worse, *allele drop-out (ADO)*. Recent attempts to reduce ADO have produced promising results. However, whether the complete elimination of ADO is possible remains to be seen.

In clinical PGD, cystic fibrosis and sickle cell anemia are the two major genetic disorders most commonly identified by PCR (Figures 12.15–12.17). Following PCR amplification and analysis, heteroduplex formation and restriction enzyme analysis may be carried out to obtain further information (Figure 12.18). In addition, *whole genome amplification*[8] has the potential to allow multilocus genetic analysis (Figure 12.19)[9].

Future perspectives

The application of PGD clearly involves new and challenging clinical techniques and, for this reason, is likely to remain in its research phase for several more years to come. However, in the near future, PGD will become more important and more widely used for the following reasons:

(1) The demand for PGD is continually growing. Some forms of male infertility, which may be due to genetic disorders (such as bilateral ejaculatory duct obstruction[10]), are now routinely and successfully treated with ICSI. The risk of passing on genetic disorders, which will become ever greater as the normal barriers to fertilization are bypassed by technology, may be reduced by the application of PGD. Furthermore, it is reasonable to anticipate that the Human Genome Project will be completed before the year 2010. By then, approximately 70 000 human genes will have been sequenced, and their pathogenetic relationships further clarified. This knowledge will provide more basic information for future applications of PGD;

(2) Refinement of PGD techniques will further improve the efficiency of biopsy, and thereby increase the accuracy and sensitivity of FISH and PCR while minimizing the occurrence of false-positive and / or false-negative results. With the use of laser technology, opening the zona pellucida will be a simple operation, and the risk of damage to oocytes and blastomeres will also be reduced[11]. In addition, the instrumentation for FISH and PCR continue to improve, and allow better, faster, and more accurate diagnoses[12,13]. In the future, it is anticipated that single blastomeres will first be 'fingerprinted' to exclude potential contamination[14];

(3) Improvements in the assisted reproductive technologies, particularly in the understanding of gametogenesis and embryogenesis, are likely to have direct and / or indirect effects on the future of PGD. The development and optimization of preembryo culture media, for example, will allow more days of growth for the preembryo and, thus, more time for accurate diagnosis. Furthermore, it may become possible to routinely obtain biopsies from the trophectoderm of the growing blastocyst. Improved survival rates after cryopreservation of biopsied preembryos may also allow more time in which to complete the relatively sophisticated procedures neccessary for PGD;

(4) Finally, and most important, new DNA technologies, imaging systems, and chip technology[15,16] will undoubtedly open up currently unimaginable possibilities for pinpointing single nucleotide variations within the whole of the human genome, thus allowing precise prediction of preembryo genetic makeup.

All of these foreseeable developments will have profound effects on PGD and, in turn, on us, our children, and society as a whole. Thus, the dilemma that is likely to be faced in the twenty-first century will involve the ethical barriers that are bound to be erected in the face of increasing use of PGD technology. These issues, however, are beyond the purview of this brief overview of PGD technology.

References

1. Handyside AH, Kontogianni EH, Hardy K, Winston RML. Pregnancies from biopsied human preimplantation embryos sexed by Y-specific DNA amplification. *Nature* 1990;344:768
2. Muggleton-Harris AL, Glazier AM, Pickering SJ. Biopsy of the human blastocyst and polymerase chain reaction (PCR) amplification of the β-globin gene and a dinucleotide repeat motif from 2–6 trophectoderm cells. *Hum Reprod* 1993;8:2197

3. Handyside AH, Delhanty JDA. Preimplantation genetic diagnosis: Strategies and surprises. *Trends Genet* 1997;13:270

4. Strom CM, Verlinsky Y, Milayeva S, *et al.* Preconception genetic diagnosis of cystic fibrosis. *Lancet* 1990;336:306

5. Verlinsky Y, Cieslak J, Ivakhnenko V, *et al.* Birth of healthy children after preimplantation diagnosis of common aneuploidies by polar body fluorescent in situ hybridization analysis. *Fertil Steril* 1997;66:126

6. Saiki R, Scharf S, Faloona F, *et al.* Enzymatic amplification of β-globin genomic sequences and restriction site analysis for diagnosis of sickle cell anemia. *Science* 1985;230:1350

7. Mullis KB, Faloona F. Specific synthesis of DNA in vitro via a polymerase catalyzed chain reaction. *Methods Enzymol* 1987;155:335

8. Zhang L, Cui X, Schmitt K, *et al.* Whole genome amplification from a single cell: Implications for genetic analysis. *Proc Natl Acad Sci USA* 1992;89:5847

9. Xu KP, Tang YX, Grifo JA, *et al.* Primer extension preamplification for detection of multiple genetic loci from single human blastomeres. *Hum Reprod* 1993; 8:2206

10. Meschede D, Dworniczak B, Behre HM, *et al.* CFTR gene mutations in men with bilateral ejaculatory duct obstruction and anomalies of the seminal vesicles. *Am J Hum Genet* 1997;61:1200

11. Veiga A, Sandalinas M, Benkhalifa M, *et al.* Laser blastocyst biopsy for preimplantation genetic diagnosis in the human. *J Assist Reprod Genet* 1997;14:476

12. Schrock E, Manoir SD, Veldman T, *et al.* Multicolor spectral karyotyping of human chromosomes. *Science* 1996;273:494

13. Speicher MR, Ballard SG, Ward DC. Karyotyping human chromosomes by combinatorial multifluor FISH. *Nature Med* 1996;12:368

14. Findlay I, Urquhart A, Quirke P, *et al.* Simultaneous DNA fingerprinting, diagnosis of sex and single-gene defect status from single cells. *Hum Reprod* 1995; 10:1005

15. Cronin MT, Fucini RV, Kim SM, *et al.* Cystic fibrosis mutation detection by hybridization to light-generated DNA probe arrays. *Hum Mutat* 1996;7:244

16. Castellino AM. When the chips are down. *Genome Res* 1997;7:943

The following references are referred to in the figure legends on pages 196–202.

17. Tarkowsky AK. An air drying method for chromosome preparation from mouse eggs. *Cytogenetics* 1964;5:394

18. Harper JC, Coonen E, Ramaekers FC, *et al.* Identification of the sex of human preimplantation embryos in two hours using an improved spreading method and fluorescent in-situ hybridization (FISH) using directly labeled probes. *Hum Reprod* 1994;9:721

19. Handyside AH, Lesko JG, Tarin JJ, *et al.* Birth of a normal girl after in vitro fertilization and preimplantation diagnostic testing for cystic fibrosis. *N Engl J Med* 1992;327:905

20. Sheardown SA, Findlay I, Turner A, *et al.* Preimplantation diagnosis of a human β-globin transgene in biopsied trophectoderm cells and blastomeres of the mouse embryo. *Hum Reprod* 1992;7:1297

21. Grifo JA, Tang YX, Cohen J, *et al.* Pregnancy after embryo biopsy and coamplification of DNA from X and Y chromosomes. *J Am Med Assoc* 1992;268: 727

Epilogue

Oocyte competence, sperm function and quality, culture conditions, genetic health, preembryo morphology, ovarian age, and endometrial age all emerge as factors critical for an accurate prediction of a given woman's likelihood of achieving pregnancy. Under ideal conditions, when each of these factors is optimal, pregnancy is virtually inevitable. Unfortunately, it is an extremely rare patient who presents with such model conditions. Furthermore, if the patient were to be a model case, why would she be requesting the aid of physicians and scientists? Thus, through our investigations, we continue to seek to uncover the mysteries of human reproduction.

Appendix

Glossary of terms

Activation
The process through which a secondary oocyte is stimulated to resume meiosis. This may be due to a penetrating spermatozoon or an artificial substitute

AHA
Assisted hatching; a procedure undertaken in *in vitro* fertilization (IVF) laboratories wherein a small hole is made in the zona pellucida of a preembryo to facilitate natural hatching

Aneuploidy
Any deviation, whether fewer or more, from an exact multiple of the haploid number of chromosomes

Blastocyst
The mammalian conceptus in the postmorula stage. The cells of the blastocyst form a spherical shell enclosing the blastocele, with one pole distinguished by the inner cell mass from which the embryo forms. The outer cell layer is the trophectoderm

Blastomere
One of the cells produced by cleavage of a fertilized oocyte; a cleavage cell

Conceptus
The derivatives of a fertilized oocyte at any stage of development from fertilization to birth; includes extraembryonic membranes as well as the preembryo, embryo, and fetus. The products of conception; all structures that develop from the zygote, both embryonic and extraembryonic. A term commonly used interchangeably with the term *preembryo* during IVF treatment

Compaction
A process through which a cleaving preembryo changes from a collection of individual cells into a solid mass with indistinguishable cell membranes. Compaction is the result of the formation of tight intercellular junctions which cause blastomeres to become closely apposed

Corona radiata
A closely apposed layer of follicular cells which surrounds the mature oocyte

Crossing-over
A process occurring during synapsis in which pairs of homologous chromosomes bearing linked genes mutually exchange corresponding parts

Cumulus oophorus
A multilayered mass of follicular cells surrounding the oocyte. Cells of the cumulus are instrumental, *via* gap junctions, in nurturing the oocyte during growth and possibly in passing the inhibiting factors necessary for deterring the resumption of

meiosis. The innermost layer of cells is called the *corona* or *coronal layer*. This layer expands and presents a radiant pattern as oocytes mature in response to exogenous human chorionic gonadotropin (hCG) or a midcycle surge of luteinizing hormone (LH). Near ovulation, cumulus cells loosen and expand, and are observed to retract from the zona pellucida of the oocyte, presumably cutting off previously important cellular / oocyte communication

Cytokinesis
A phase in mitosis or meiosis which involves division of the cytoplasm

Cytoplasmic fragmentation
One or more spontaneous cytoplasmic divisions, which may often superficially resemble cleavage; disorganized breakdown of the cytoplasm. Fragments may contain DNA, but are more likely to contain no nuclear material

Diandry
Triploidy in which the extra haploid set is of paternal origin

Digyny
Triploidy in which the extra haploid set is of maternal origin

Egg
A term best reserved for the nutritive object often seen on the breakfast table

Embryo
The stage of the organism after development of the primitive streak; persists until major organs are developed. Once the neural groove and first somites are present, the embryo is considered formed. In humans, the embryonic stage begins at approximately 14 days after fertilization and encompasses the period when organs and organ systems begin to develop

Fertilization
The union of male and female gametes leading to the formation of a unique zygote

Fetus
The developing conceptus after the embryonic stage; the fetal period begins at the end of the eighth postovulatory week when >90% of the >4500 named structures of the adult human body have appeared. The fetal period persists until birth

Gamete
The oocyte or the spermatozoon; a mature haploid reproductive cell; any cell which, upon union with another gametic cell, results in the development of a new individual

Haploid
Possessing half the diploid or somatic number of chromosomes

ICSI
Intracytoplasmic sperm injection; a procedure performed in IVF laboratories wherein a single sperm is injected into the cytoplasm of an oocyte to assist the fertilization process

Immature oocyte
An oocyte with chromosomes at prophase I (P I). A germinal vesicle-bearing oocyte

Intermediate oocyte
An oocyte with chromosomes at metaphase I (M I), characterized by the absence of both a first polar body and a germinal vesicle

Mature oocyte
An oocyte with chromosomes at metaphase II (M II), characterized by the presence of a first polar body

Metaphase I (M I) oocyte
An oocyte with chromosomes at metaphase I of maturation, characterized by the absence of both a first polar body and a germinal vesicle. An oocyte at an intermediate stage of maturation

Metaphase II (M II) oocyte
An oocyte with chromosomes at metaphase II of maturation, characterized by the presence of a first polar body. A fully mature oocyte. A secondary oocyte

Monosomy
A condition characterized by one less than the normal diploid number of chromosomes ($2n-1$)

Mosaicism
A condition in which a conceptus or individual possesses two or more separate and distinct cell lines

Morula
Usually, the 16-cell-stage preembryo until blastocyst formation; the stage commonly observed between 72–96 h after insemination. Some authors believe that the term is historically inappropriate for mammals

Nondisjunction
The failure of a pair of homologous chromosomes to separate during cell division

Nucleus
The spheroid mass enclosed in a thin membrane which is the center for the synthesis of specific cellular proteins and transmission of hereditary traits; contains a nucleolus or several nucleoli and a diffuse nucleoplasm

Nucleolus
A rounded, refractile structure present in the nucleus of most cells which is the site of the synthesis of ribosomal RNA; the nucleolus becomes enlarged during periods of synthesis and atrophies during quiescent periods

Oocyte
The female gamete from inception of the first meiotic division until fertilization. In oogenesis, a cell which develops from an oogonium

Oogonium
The cell that gives rise to the primary oocyte during oogenesis; oogonia proliferate by mitotic division during early fetal life

Oolemma
Plasma membrane of an oocyte

Ooplasm
Cytoplasm of the oocyte

Ooplasm / cytoplasm: Descriptive terms
Degenerative	Non-viable
Fragmented	Exhibiting extracytoplasmic fragments or blebs
Granular	Exhibiting dense granules of darkish color
Mottled	Exhibiting 'orange-peel' granularity; 'spotted'
Vacuolated	Exhibiting spaces or small cavities within the cytoplasm of an oocyte or blastomere; may be the result of an aberrant endocytosis caused by oolemma instability

Ovum
A female gamete or germ cell. An oocyte. The term is often used to refer to such disparate structures as an oocyte and a 3-week-old embryo and, thus, has little or no scientific value

Parthenogenesis
Activation and subsequent development of an oocyte without fertilization; may occur naturally or through artificial stimulation

Penetrated oocyte
An oocyte that has been penetrated by a spermatozoon; strictly speaking, an oocyte in which gamete plasma membranes have become confluent. The stage before pronuclei are formed. Penetration of the oocyte usually occurs within 3 h of sperm / oocyte exposure

Perivitelline space
Space surrounding the vitellus (in fact, the 'yolk' but, in this sense, the oocyte). The space between the oocyte and the zona pellucida. Subzonal space. This space may contain the first and second polar bodies or extracellular fragments

Polar body
First polar body: The structure extruded into the perivitelline space at the end of telophase I. Chromosomes are divided between the oocyte and first polar body (23 chromosomes, 46 chroma-

tids, 2 n DNA in each); those in the oocyte are attached to spindle microtubules. For a while after its formation, the first polar body remains connected to the oocyte by the meiotic spindle, forming a cytoplasmic bridge. Chromosomes within the first polar body may remain clumped together, may undergo a second meiotic division, or may scatter within the cytoplasm. Usually, a nucleus is not formed. The first polar body contains cortical granules because of its extrusion before sperm penetration and cortical granule release

Second polar body: The structure extruded into the perivitelline space after sperm penetration. The second polar body may be nucleated

Polyploidy
A condition in which a conceptus or individual possesses one or more sets of homologous chromosomes in excess of the normal diploid set, as in triploidy (3 n), tetraploidy (4 n), hexaploidy (6 n), or octoploidy (8 n)

Preembryo
The conceptus during early cleavage stages until development of the embryo. The preembryonic period ends at approximately 14 days after fertilization with the development of the primitive streak

Prezygote
The pronuclear oocyte. The stage of development before syngamy, when the term *zygote* becomes appropriate. Some authors refer to this stage as an *ootid*. Prezygotes are commonly observed 6–20 h after insemination or injection

Primary oocyte
The oocyte formed in the ovary before birth. Primary oocytes begin the first meiotic division before birth, but completion of prophase I does not occur until after puberty

Pronuclei
Structures formed during fertilization from sperm and oocyte chromatin. Normal pronuclei are approximately 30 μm in diameter. See *Prezygote*

Prophase I oocyte
An oocyte with chromosomes at prophase I of maturation, characterized by a germinal vesicle

Refractile body
An aggregation of lipid material and dense granules approximately 10 μm in size in the oocyte; associated with poor fertilization

Secondary oocyte
The oocyte after completion of the first meiotic division and arrest at metaphase of the second meiotic division. Also called a *mature oocyte* or *metaphase II oocyte*; the stage commonly associated with ovulated specimens or those collected from mature follicles for IVF. The secondary oocyte is characterized by a first polar body and no nucleus

Spermatogonium
A primordial germ cell that gives rise to a primary spermatocyte

Spermatozoon
A mature male germ cell, the specific output of the testes. The generative element of the semen which serves to fertilize the oocyte, it consists of a head, neck, midpiece, and tail

Spermiogenesis
The transformation of a spermatid into a mature spermatozoon

Subnuclei
Nuclear or pronuclear fragments containing scattered membrane-bound chromatin

Synapsis
The coming together in pairs of homologous chromosomes during meiosis

Syngamy
The active union of two gametes in fertilization to form a *zygote*. The process of reorganization and pairing of maternal and paternal chromosomes in the zygote after pronuclear membrane breakdown

Triploidy
A condition in which a conceptus or individual

possesses three times the haploid number of chromosomes (3 n)

Trisomy
A condition characterized by having one more than the diploid set of chromosomes (2 n+1)

Zona pellucida
The covering that surrounds the oocyte; believed to be produced largely by the surrounding follicular cells. In humans, the oocyte measures around 115 μm and the thickness of the zona is between 15–20 μm. The zona is covered externally by the corona radiata, a loose investment of granulosa cells from the ovarian follicle

Zona reaction
A process usually occurring during fertilization in which the chemistry and composition of the zona pellucida changes to render it impermeable by other spermatozoa

Zygote
The one-cell stage after pronuclear membrane breakdown and before the first cleavage. This stage is characterized by maternal and paternal chromosomes assuming positions on the first cleavage spindle and, thus, lacks a nucleus. Usually seen 18–24 h after insemination or injection

Language of human embryology: Abbreviations, symbols and terms used in the laboratory

Abbreviations and symbols used for documentation

lg, med, sm	Large, medium, small
v	Very
sl	Slightly
cent	Central
dk, dksh	Dark, darkish
oval	Oval-shaped
thk, thn	Thick, thin
m	Many
f	Faint
sl	Slow
abn	Abnormal
cont	Contracted
pb	Polar body
pn	Pronucleus / pronuclei
pvs	Perivitelline space
pvd	Perivitelline debris
fert	Fertilization
mnb	Multinucleated blastomeres
snb	Single-nucleated (mononucleated) blastomeres
subnuc	Subnuclei
clp	Clear area at periphery
zp	Zona pellucida
fz	Fractured or broken zona pellucida
zf	Zona-free
vacs	Vacuoles
rb	Refractile body
deg	Degenerative
frags	Fragments
Afrags	Large acytoplasmic fragments

÷	Cleaving (dividing)
Δ	Irregular-shaped (oocyte or blastomere)
≡	Even (equivalent)-sized blastomeres
≈	Approximately even (equal)-sized blastomeres
≢	Uneven (not equivalent)-sized blastomeres
⊜	Compacting
⊙	Large pvs
♉	Zona artifact

ô	Bilayered zona
ö	Porous zona
ō	Dark zona
Ⓜ	Mottled cytoplasm
Ⓖ	Granular cytoplasm
√	Good morphology
√ √	Excellent morphology
Ø	Poor morphology
⊗	Very poor morphology

Specific terms for ICSI

(X-o'clock) pb Position of polar body as indicated by location on a clock face

(X-o'clock) pg Cytoplasmic area of aggregated granules termed *area of polar granularity* (previously presumed to be the area of germinal vesicle breakdown and location of the meiotic spindle)

 # stabs Number of times the membrane is broken

membrane out Minimal membrane elasticity; immediate breakage of the membrane

stirring Extremely elastic membrane resulting in the need to make several attempts to break the membrane at multiple sites (with distortion of cytoplasm)

– No aspiration of cytoplasm; no mechanical activation

+/– Aspiration of cytoplasm to level of the zona

\+ Aspiration of cytoplasm beyond level of the zona

References

Dorland's Illustrated Medical Dictionary, 26th edn. Philadelphia: W.B. Saunders, 1981

Moore KL. *The Developing Human, 3rd edn.* Philadelphia: W.B. Saunders, 1982

O'Rahilly R, Muller F. *Developmental Stages in Human Embryos.* Washington, D.C.: Carnegie Institution of Washington, Publication 637,1987

Stedman's Medical Dictionary, 25th edn. Baltimore: Williams & Wilkins, 1990

Steen EB. *Dictionary of Biology.* Savage, MD: Barnes and Noble Books, 1971

Veeck LL. *Atlas of the Human Oocyte and Early Conceptus.* Baltimore: Williams & Wilkins, 1986

Section 2 Human Gametes and Conceptuses Illustrated

List of illustrations

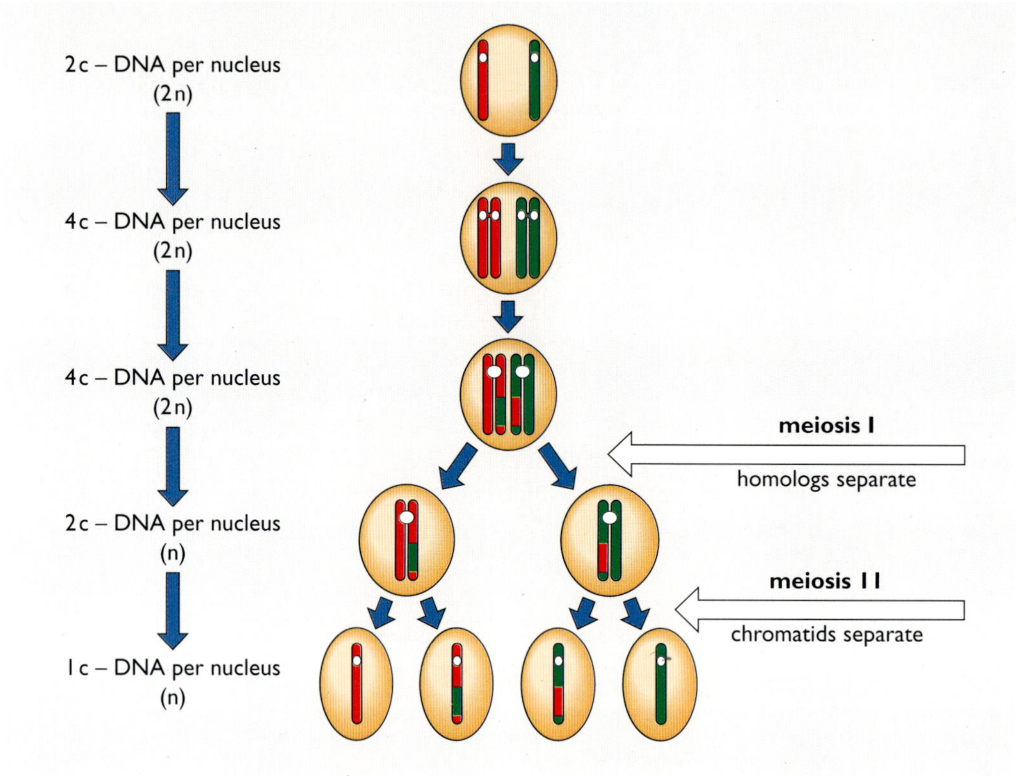

Figure 1.1 Meiosis I and meiosis II

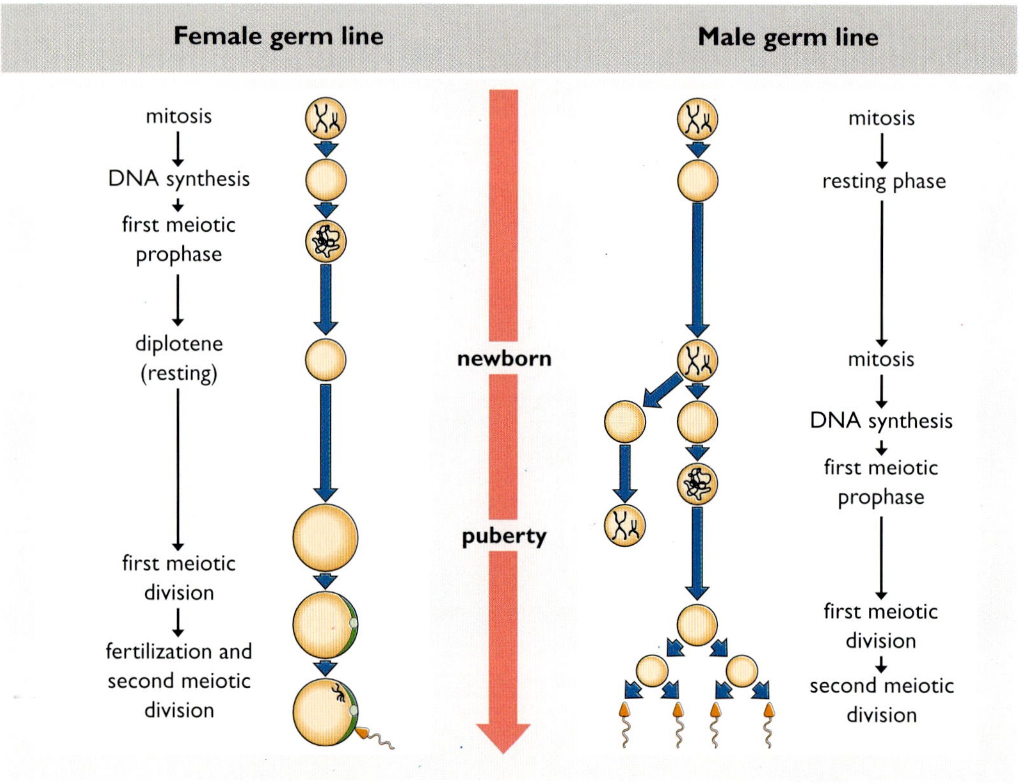

Figure 1.2 Comparison of meiosis in females and males

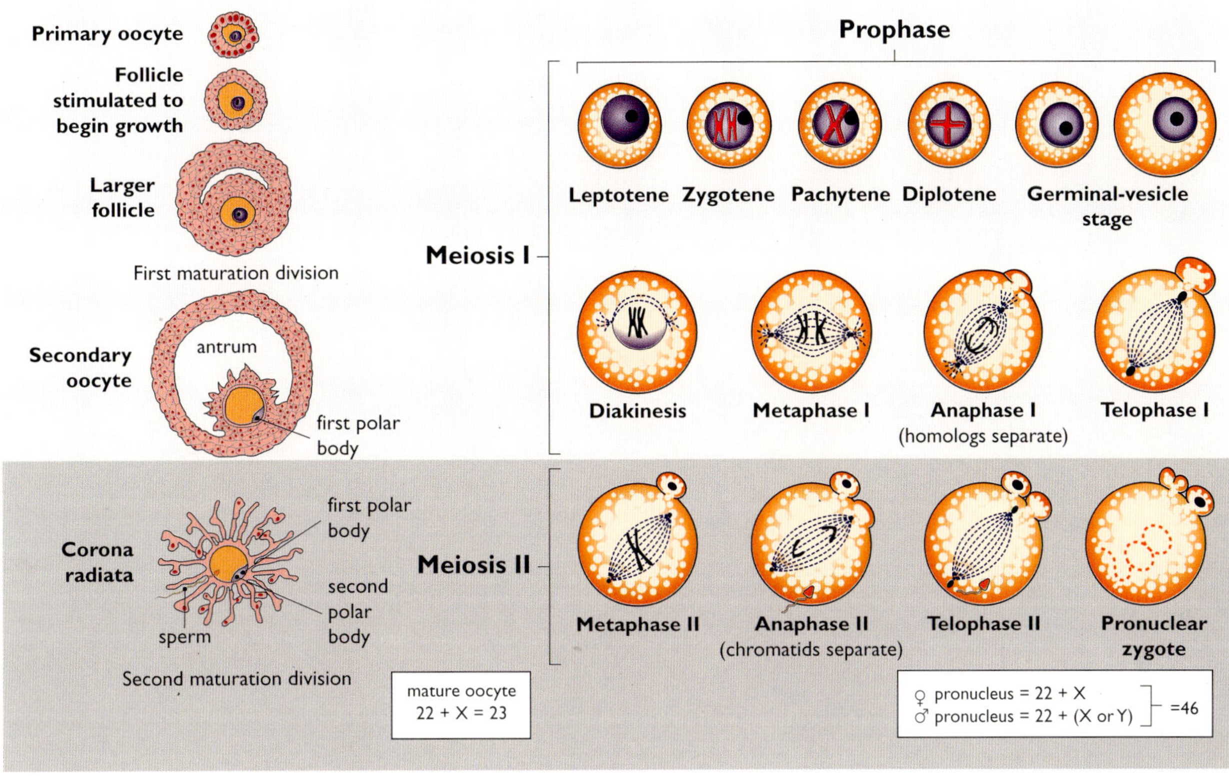

Figure 1.3 Meiosis and follicular growth in the female

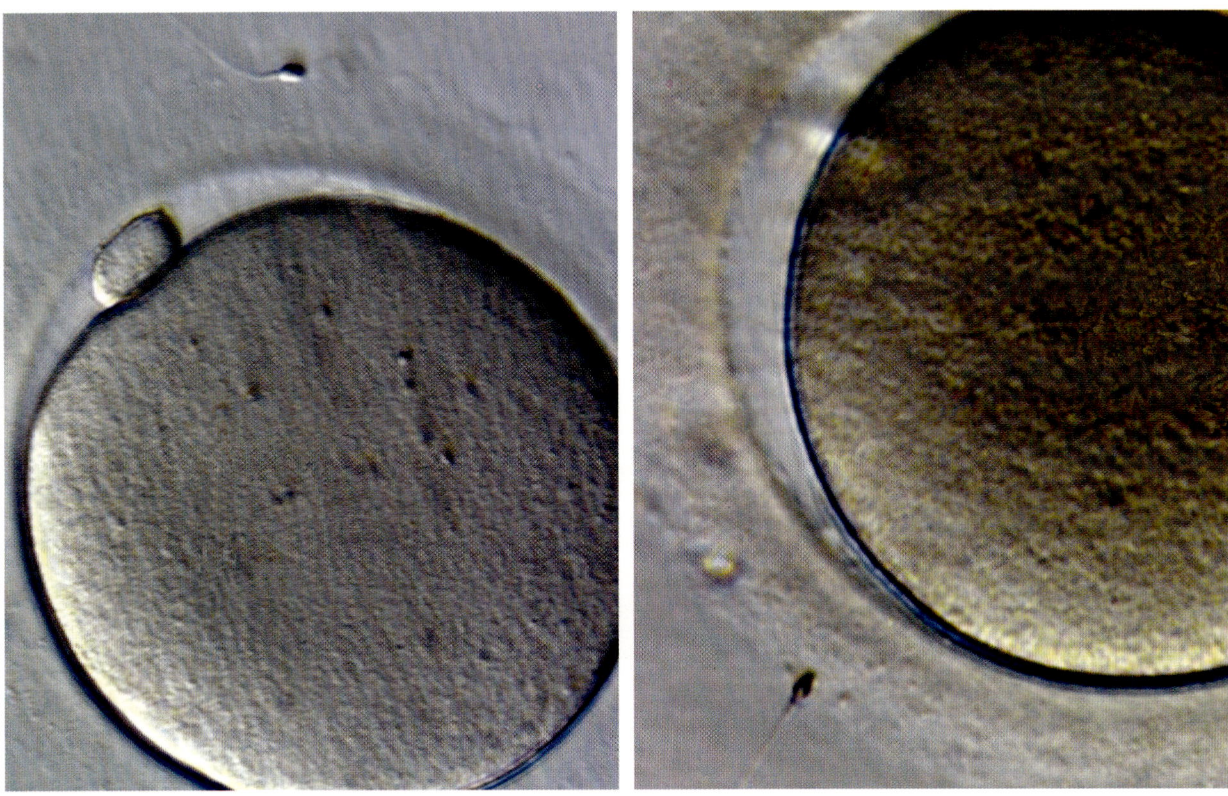

Figure 1.4 Mature oocytes and spermatozoa, the beginnings of a new life

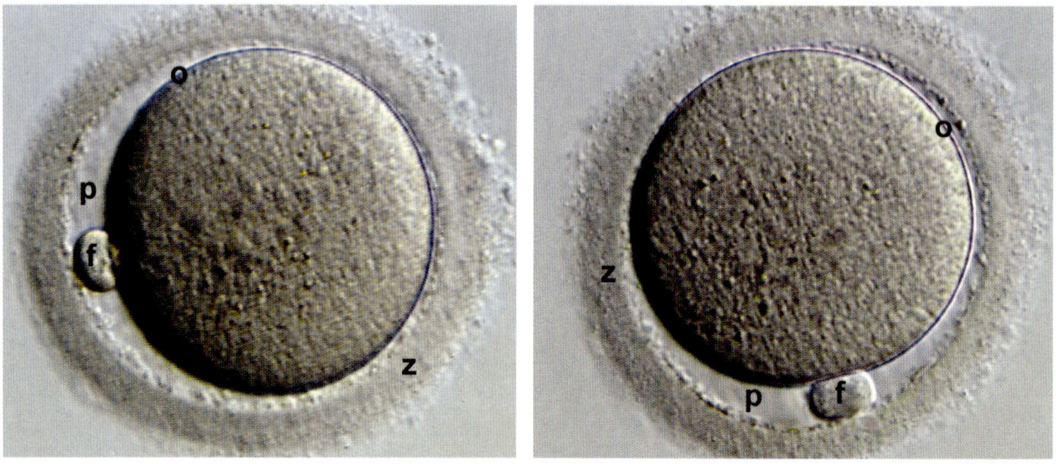

Figure 2.1 Fully mature oocytes at metaphase II (M II) of meiosis. o, oolemma; p, perivitelline space; f, first polar body; z, zona pellucida (×200)

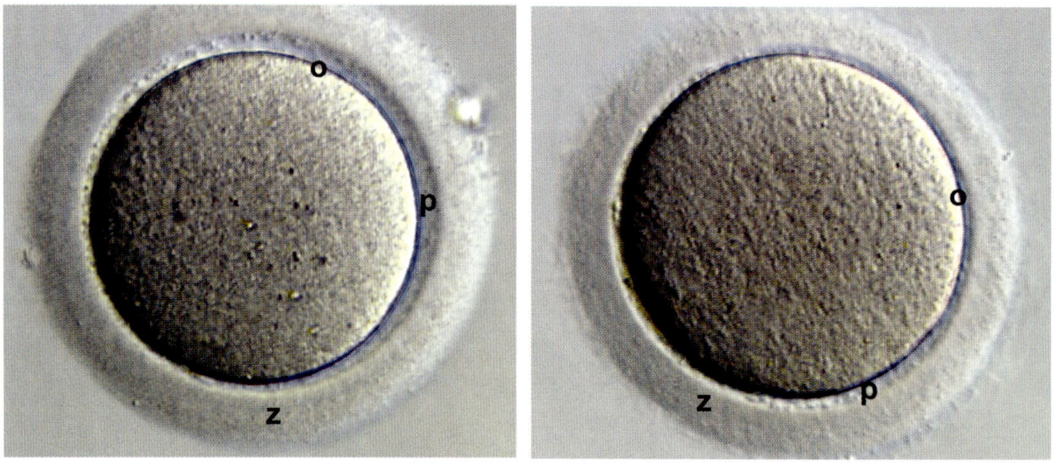

Figure 2.2 Nearly mature oocytes at metaphase I (M I) of meiosis. o, oolemma; p, perivitelline space; z, zona pellucida (no first polar body; ×200)

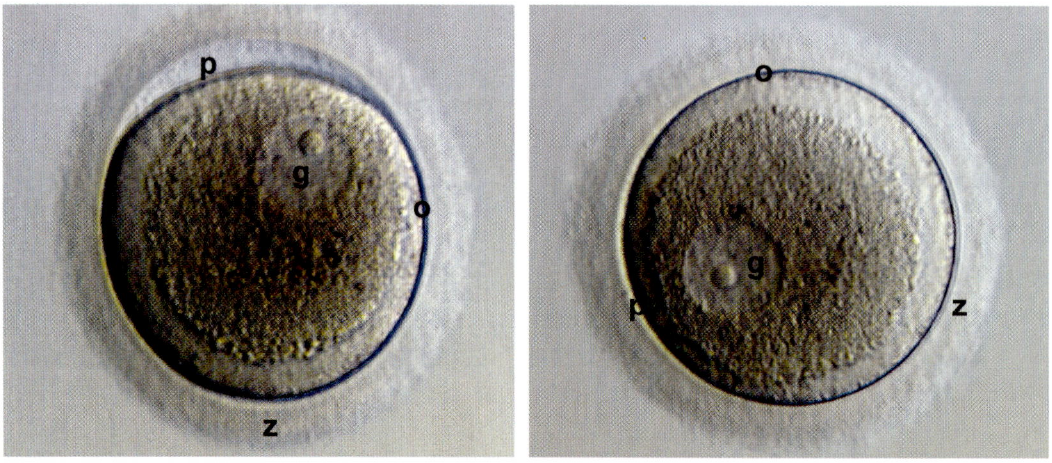

Figure 2.3 Immature oocytes at prophase I (P I) of meiosis. g, germinal vesicle; o, oolemma; p, perivitelline space; z, zona pellucida (×200)

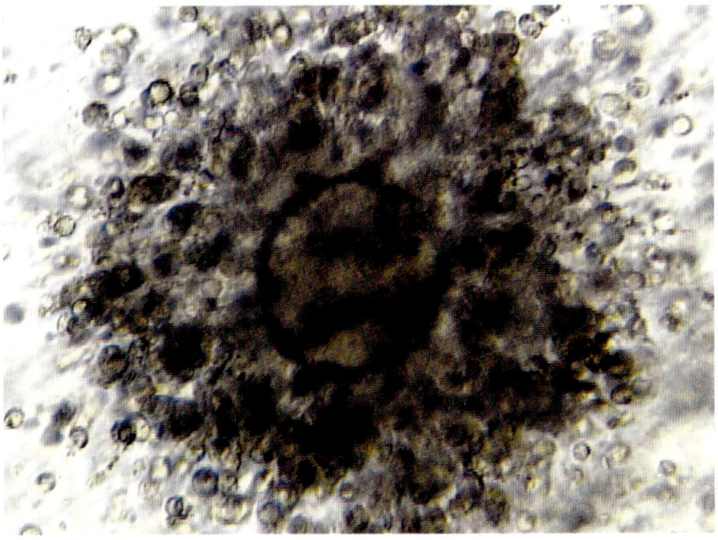

Figure 2.4 Apparently mature oocyte in its natural state near the time of ovulation. At × 100, the oocyte is seen surrounded by a radiant corona which is many layers thick, and a less dense outer cumulus oophorus. Under the cover of the obscuring cells, the oocyte itself is difficult to visualize and, therefore, its precise maturational status is uncertain

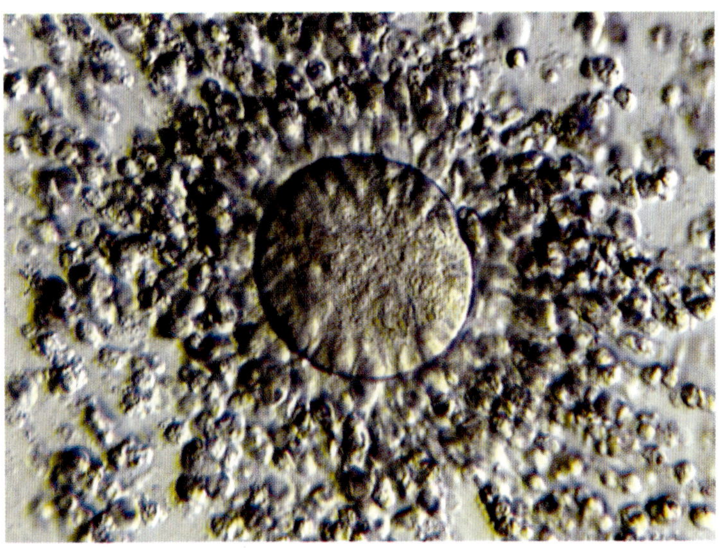

Figure 2.5 Spreading the cumulus out allows the oocyte to be visualized more clearly. This oocyte exhibits homogeneously colored ooplasm and possesses a first polar body at the two-o'clock position. The cells of the corona radiata are moderately expanded (× 100)

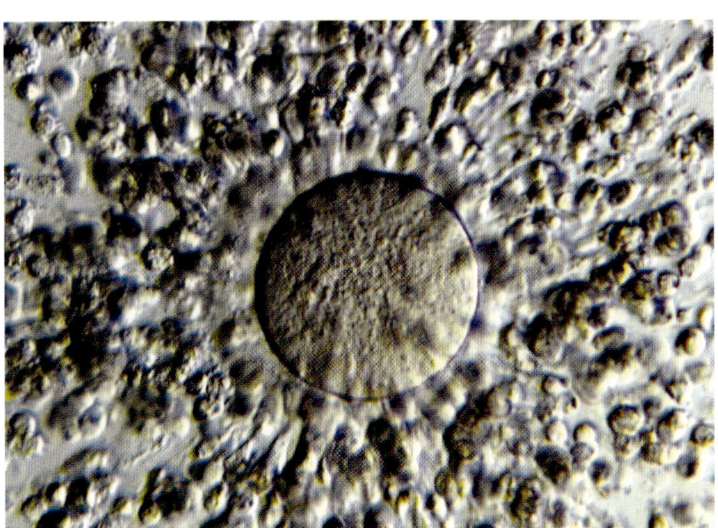

Figure 2.6 A perfectly spherical oocyte associated with a highly expanded coronal layer of cells. Although not visualized on this focal plane, a first polar body is present. Note the homogeneously colored ooplasm and the generally healthy appearance (× 100)

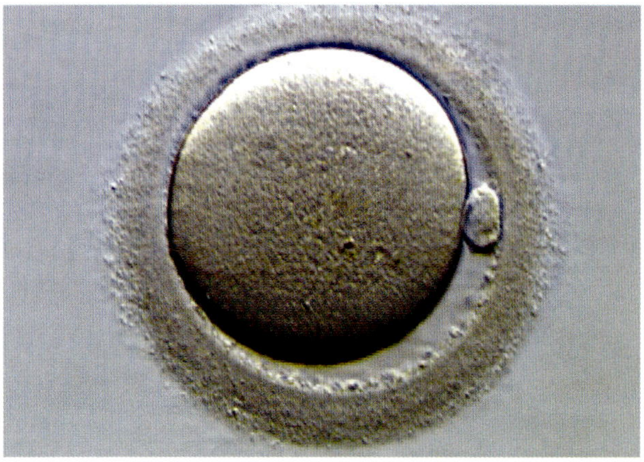

Figure 2.7 M II oocyte with a relatively large perivitelline space and a moderate amount of perivitelline debris. The ooplasm is smooth and light-colored. The zona has two distinct layers: a porous outer one and a compact inner one (×200)

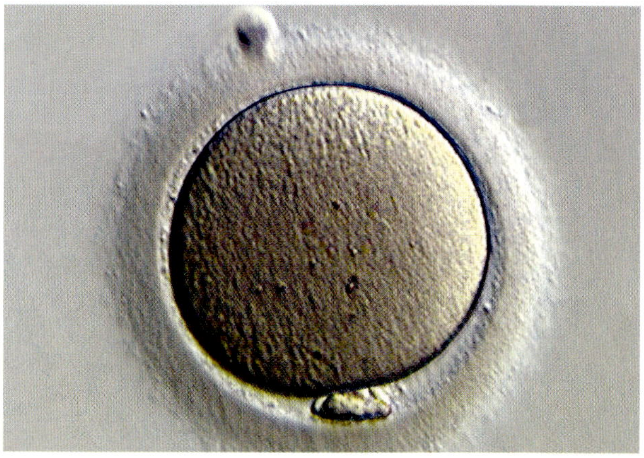

Figure 2.8 Mature oocyte with a fragmenting first polar body and cortical granularity throughout the upper and left quadrants (×200)

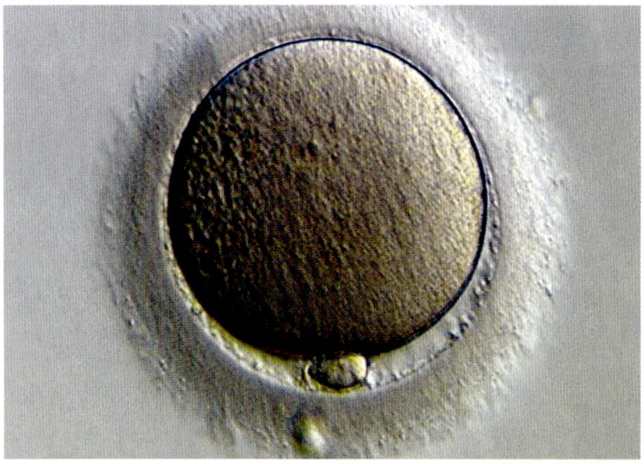

Figure 2.9 Oocyte with cortical granularity on the left. Note that the zona pellucida displays variable thickness between the upper and lower segments (×200)

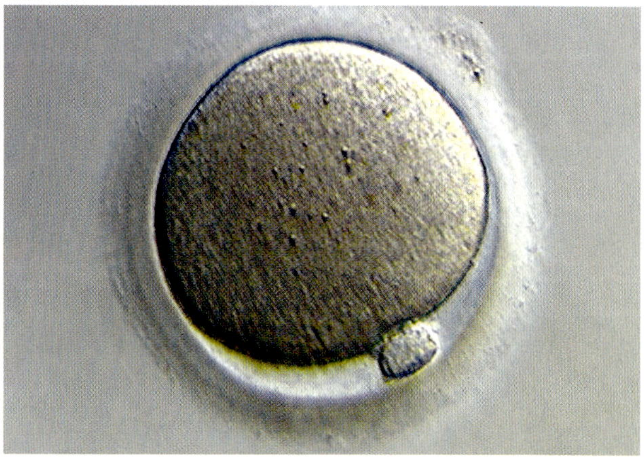

Figure 2.10 Oocyte with chromosomes at M II of maturation. Minute cytoplasmic inclusions speckle the oocyte surface. Minor defects are apparent in the zona at the one- and six-o'clock positions. The zona is relatively thin and compact (×200)

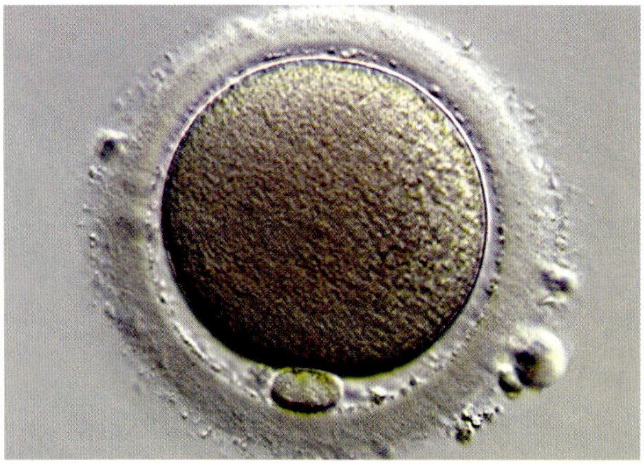

Figure 2.11 Oocyte from a woman undergoing natural-cycle IVF. Cortical granularity is evident along the right. Moderate perivitelline debris lines the inside of the thin zona pellucida (×200)

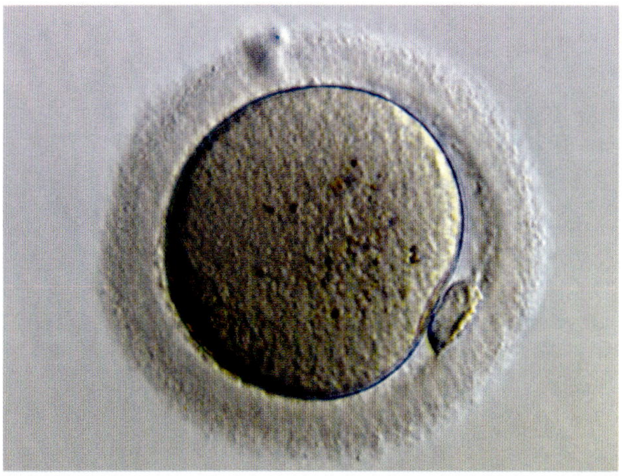

Figure 2.12 MII oocyte after maturation *in vitro* from PI of meiosis. The relatively thick zona displays little or no variation in diameter throughout its circumference (×200)

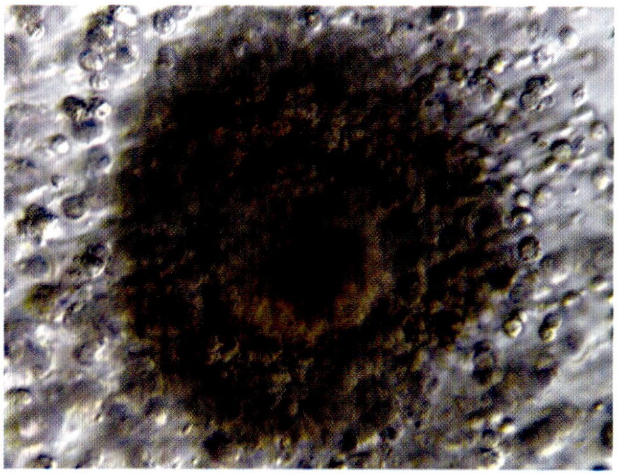

Figure 2.13 Apparently immature oocyte by cumulus and corona cell morphology. The coronal layer, at least five cells deep, is compact rather than radiant and completely obscures the oocyte. The oocyte itself appears dark centrally, a frequent observation in PI oocytes, but proved to be at MI of maturation after removal of cumulus cells with hyaluronidase (×100)

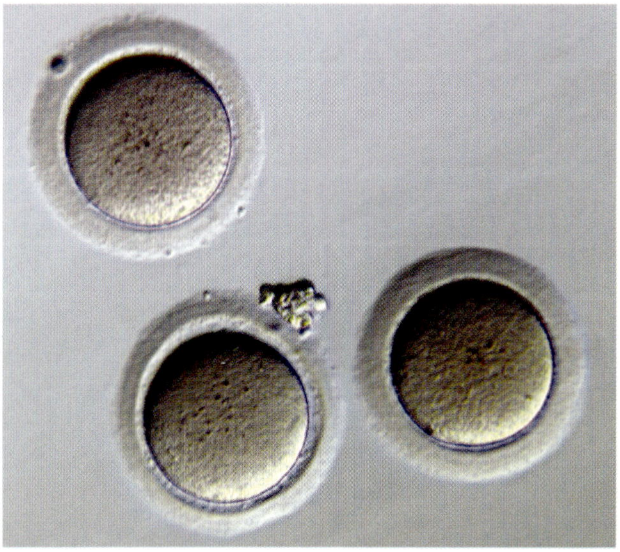

Figure 2.14 Three MI oocytes presumed to be near maturity because of their spherical shapes and homogeneously colored ooplasm. The zona varies in diameter among sibling oocytes, the thinnest associated with the largest perivitelline space (×100)

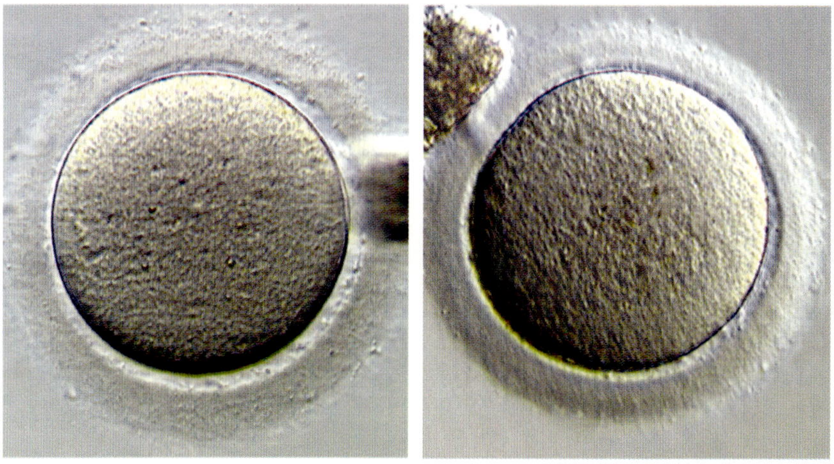

Figure 2.15 Late MI oocytes: (left) spherical with clear ooplasm and a porous outer zona; (right) thin zona pellucida is distinguished by two distinct layers (×200)

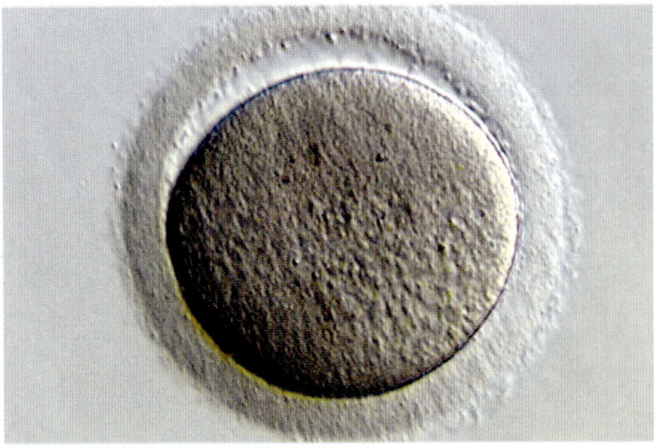

Figure 2.16 Early MI oocyte with somewhat coarse ooplasmic granularity and a slightly irregular shape. This appearance suggests that several hours of culture are required before first polar-body extrusion occurs (×200)

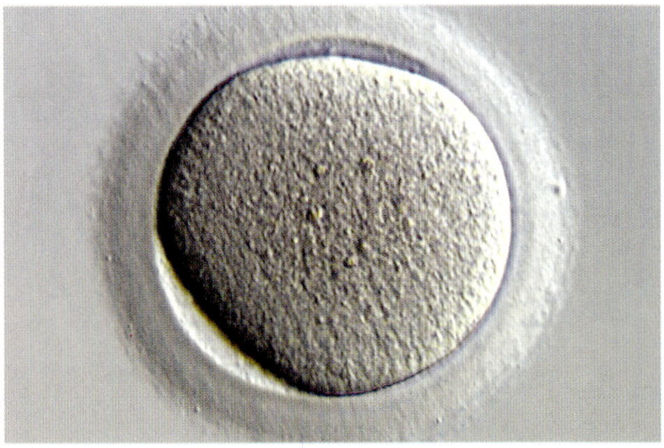

Figure 2.17 Early MI oocyte with a slightly darkened, coarse ooplasm and an irregular shape at two poles. Such an oocyte has most likely undergone fairly recent germinal-vesicle breakdown (GVBD) (×200)

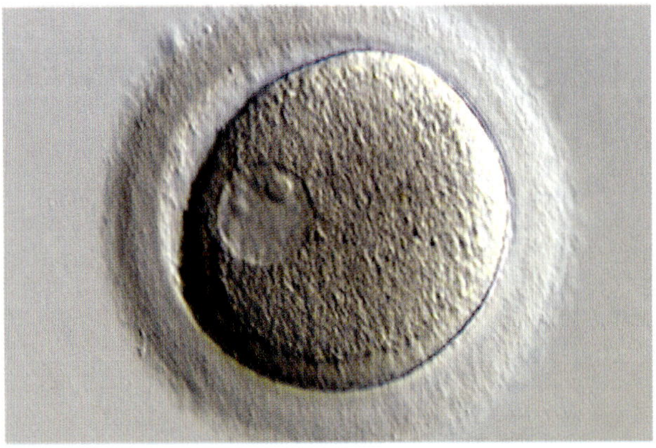

Figure 2.18 Typical germinal vesicle (GV)-bearing oocyte shows coarse central granularity, a clear peripheral zone, and an irregular shape. The GV has a large exocentric nucleolus and two smaller indistinct bodies and, as it lies peripherally, GVBD is probably imminent (×200)

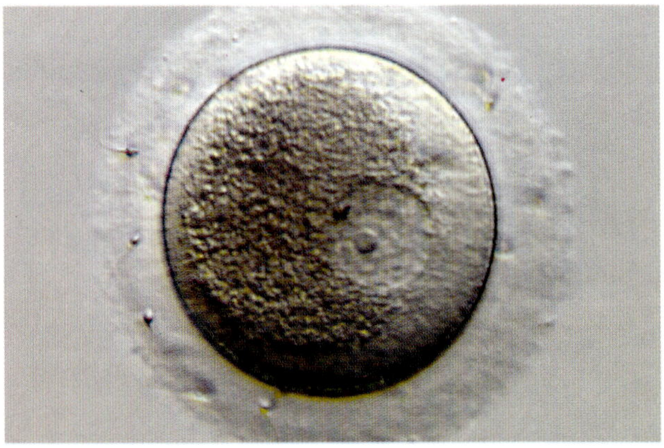

Figure 2.19 PI oocyte showing the typical thickened zona, a barely off-center GV, and an extremely clear right-sided cortical zone. This oocyte failed to undergo GVBD 22 h after harvest. After mechanical removal of obscuring cells, spermatozoa can be seen bound to the zona after insemination (×200)

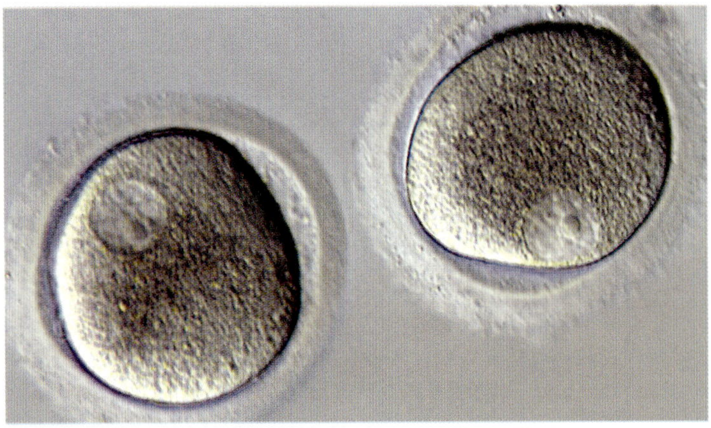

Figure 2.20 Sibling PI oocytes shown just before GVBD. Note the exocentric germinal vesicles and perinuclear aggregation of dark-colored granules. When observed again after 4 h of culture, both oocytes had proceeded to MI of maturation (×200)

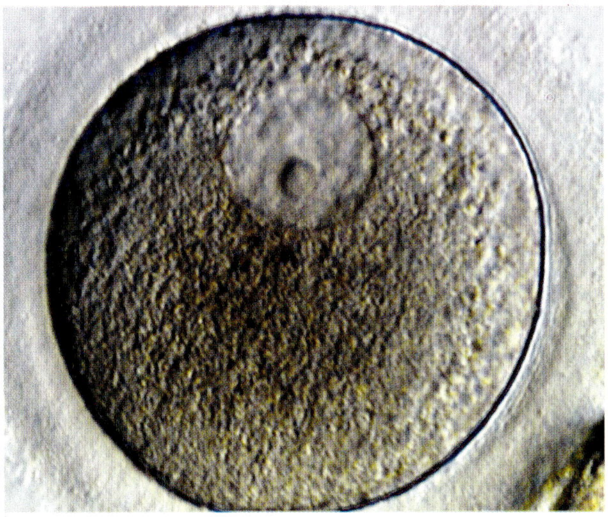

Figure 2.21 Germinal vesicle-bearing oocyte showing coarse granularity in the ooplasm, especially in perinuclear regions. A thin and discontinuous clear cortical zone is seen. Both the GV and its nucleolus are positioned off-center, typical of immature oocytes (×400)

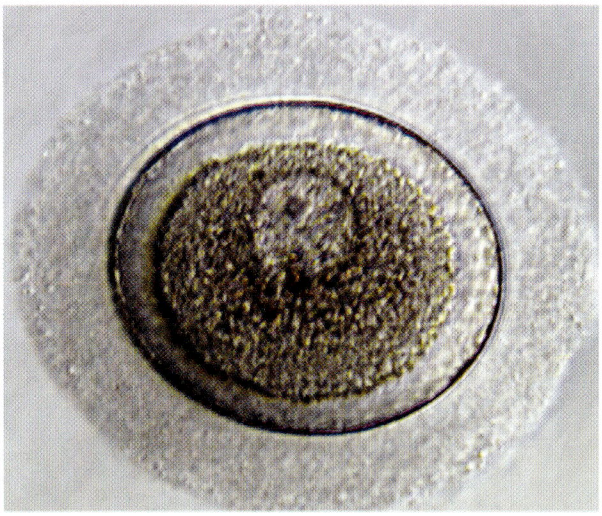

Figure 2.22 Typical appearances of an oocyte arrested at PI of maturation. Note the nearly central nucleus, the continuously wide and vacant cortical zone, irregular shape, and extremely thickened zona (diameter almost double that of healthy oocytes). Such an oocyte is not expected to complete meiotic maturation *in vitro* (×200)

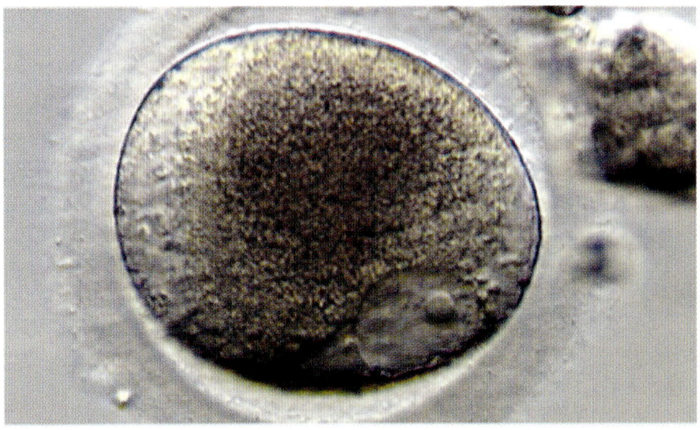

Figure 2.23 PI oocyte with ooplasm showing an extremely dark-colored area that is not associated with the peripheral germinal vesicle. It was thought that the oocyte had sustained damage during enzymatic and mechanical removal of cumulus cells for intracytoplasmic sperm injection (ICSI). Nevertheless, the oocyte retained the capacity for maturation *in vitro*, and proceeded to MII within 24 h of culture (×200)

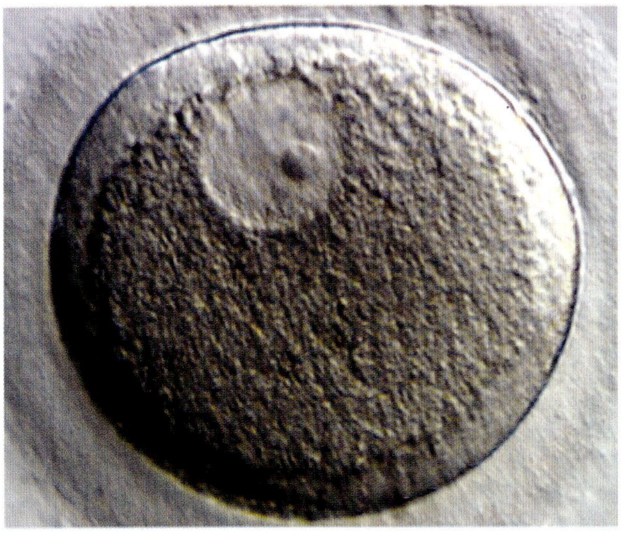

Figure 2.24 PI oocyte showing an exocentric germinal vesicle, a large and distinct nucleolus, and a thin and continuous clear cortical zone (×400)

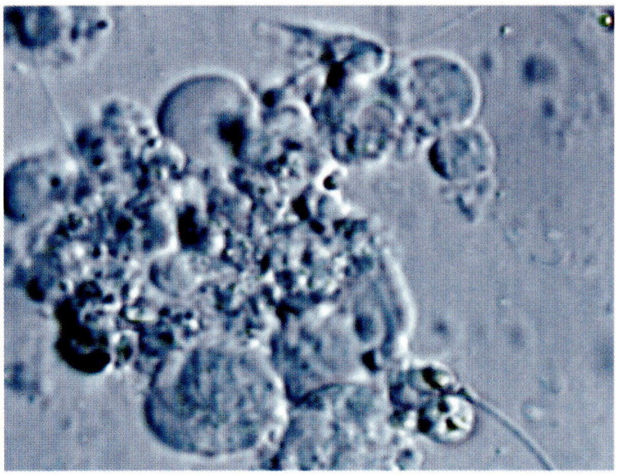

Figure 3.1 Testicular tissue sample with spermatogenetic cells. The gametes are spermatids, not spermatozoa, as they are attached to Sertoli cells. Their morphology is indistinguishable from spermatozoa in the ejaculate. As testicular spermatozoa are immature, cytoplasmic droplets are often seen

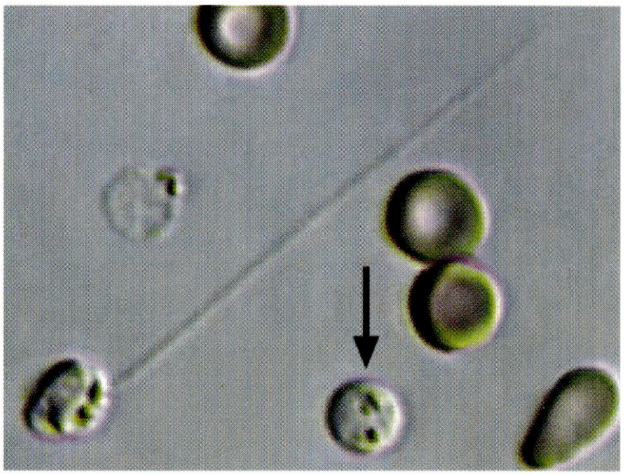

Figure 3.2 Round spermatid (arrowed), from a testicular biopsy, in the early (acrosome) phase before development of a tail. Two to four proacrosome granules are seen in the cytoplasm

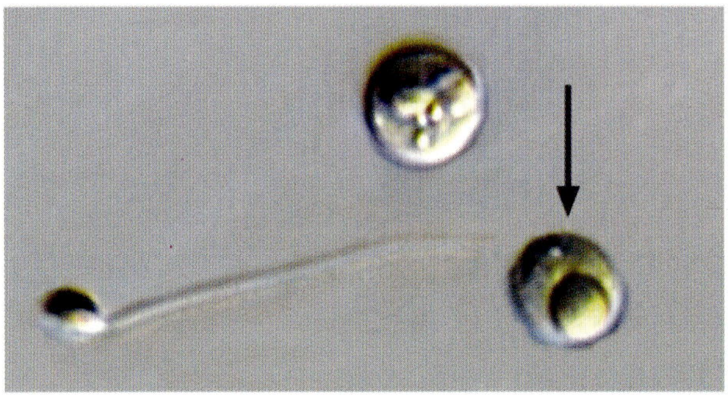

Figure 3.3 Round spermatid (arrowed), from a testicular biopsy, in the Golgi cap phase, the first stage after secondary spermatocyte division. Its size (7–8 μ) is similar to that of red blood cells and small lymphocytes. There is a central rounded thickened nucleus. The developing acrosome, seen as a small protrusion to one side, aids identification

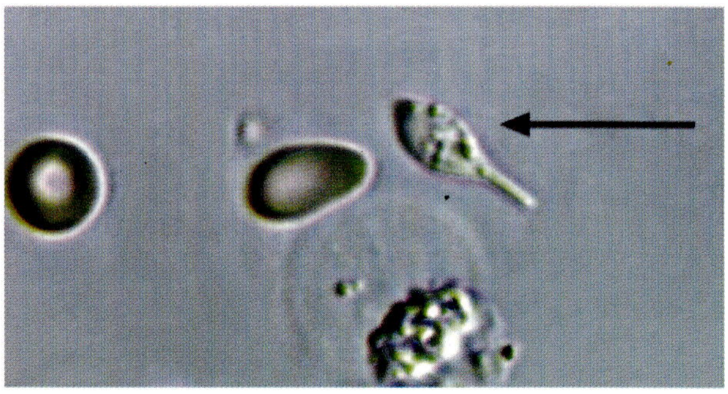

Figure 3.4 Elongating spermatid (arrowed), from a testicular biopsy, shows proacrosome granules in the cytoplasm. The head is oval-shaped, but the tail is still not completely developed

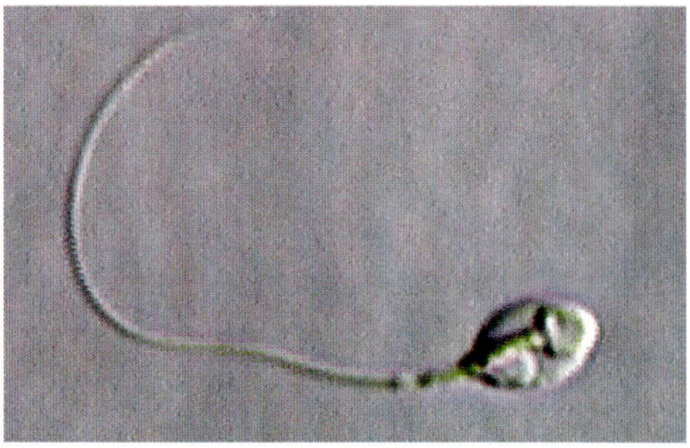

Figure 3.5 Elongated spermatid from a testicular biopsy. The only step remaining to the spermatozoon stage is extrusion of the residual body and delivery to the lumen of the seminiferous tubule

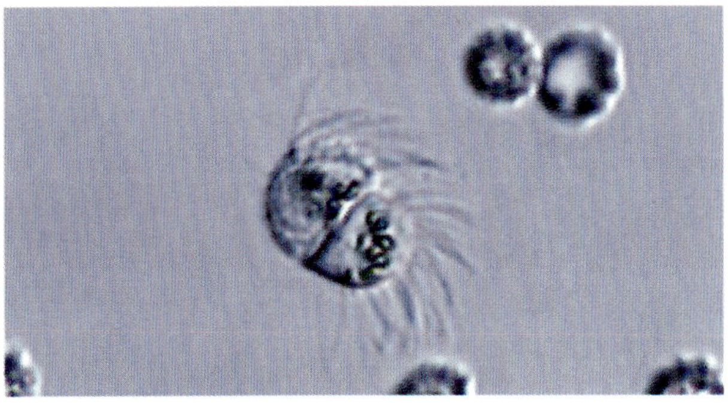

Figure 3.6 Ciliated epithelial cells from an epididymal aspiration sample. These cells have two functions: reabsorption of fluid from the testicles; and release of various secretions to the epididymal lumen. Transport of spermatozoa through the epididymal duct apparently does not involve the cilia (specifically, stereocilia) of these cells, but is promoted by epididymal contractions and testicular fluid pressure

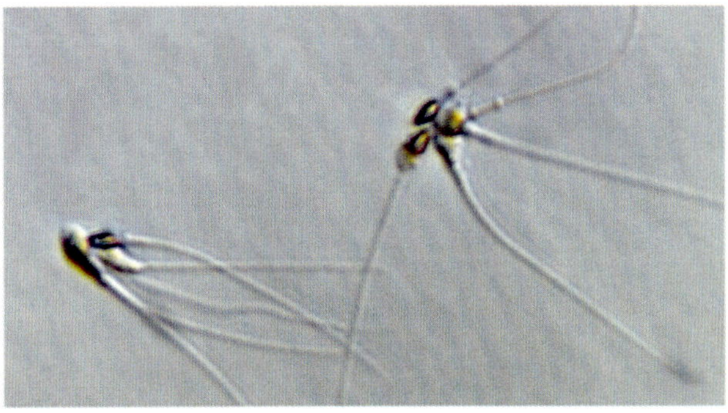

Figure 3.7 Agglutinated spermatozoa, from an epididymal aspiration sample. Agglutination may be the result of an immunological factor

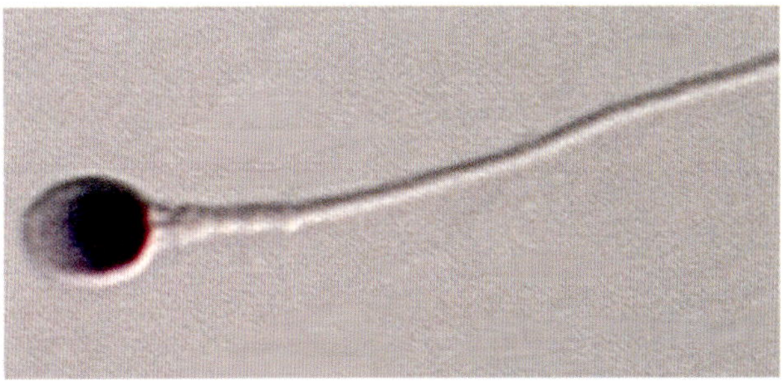

Figure 3.8 Normal spermatozoon has an elliptical head, and the head and tail share the same long axis. The acrosome and midpiece appear normal and no duplicate structures are seen. The different structures are normal-sized

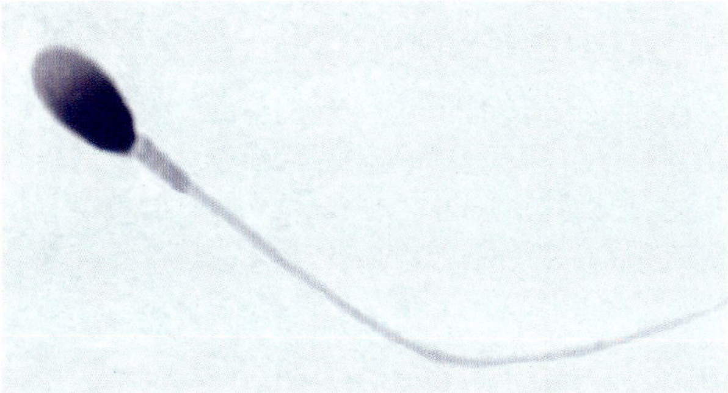

Figure 3.9 Slightly amorphous (borderline) spermatozoon has a narrow postacrosomal region. Such forms are found in the upper endocervical canal mucus after coitus

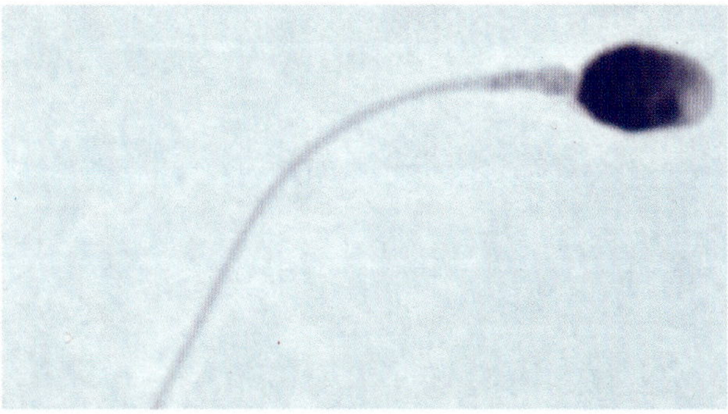

Figure 3.10 Spermatozoon with a small acrosome, which decreases its ability to penetrate the oocyte. This is an indication for ICSI

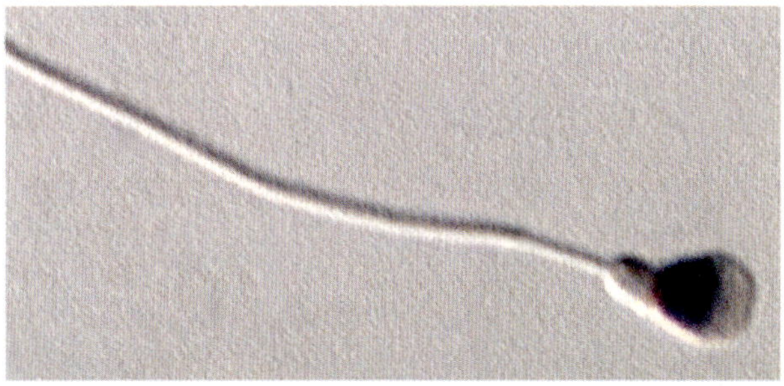

Figure 3.11 Pyriform spermatozoon with a narrow postacrosomal region. This defect is considered a mildly tapered form

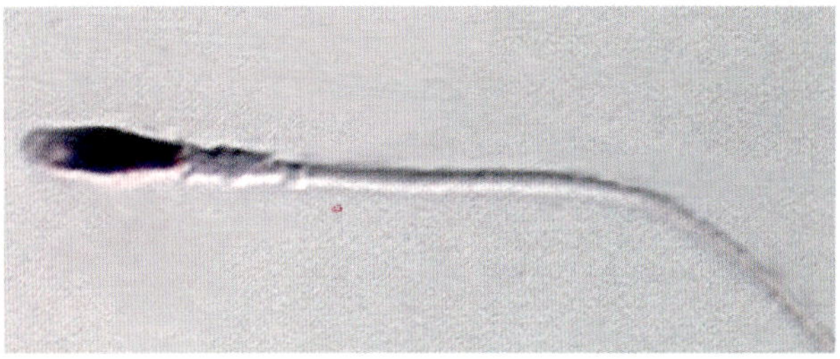

Figure 3.12 Tapered spermatozoon with a very elongated head, an anomaly often seen in patients with varicocele

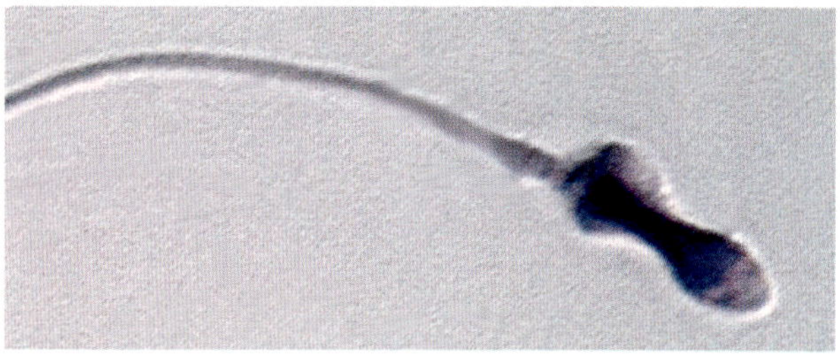

Figure 3.13 Spermatozoon with a dumb-bell-shaped head. This defect is usually described as 'amorphous'

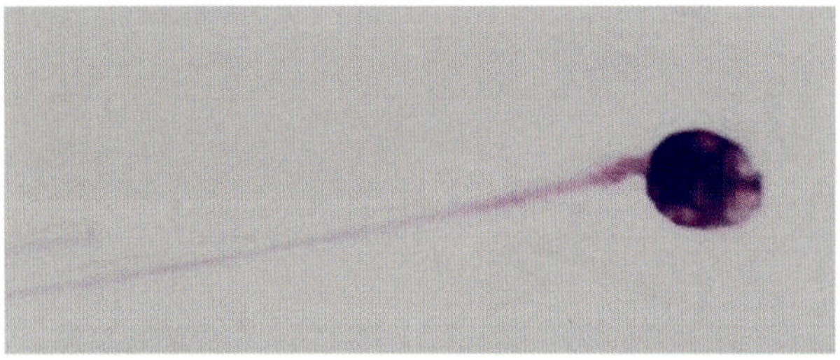

Figure 3.14 Vacuolated spermatozoon. It is not known whether this anomaly affects fertilization

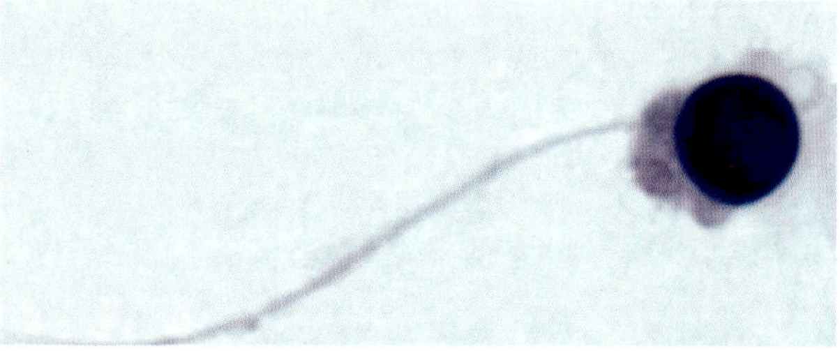

Figure 3.15 Round-headed spermatozoa lack an acrosome, as revealed by TEM studies

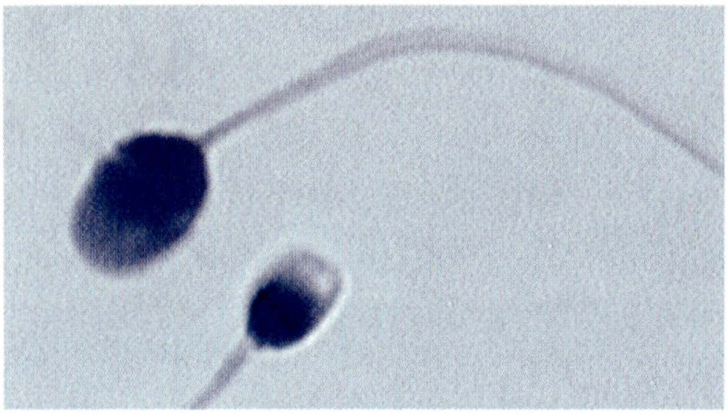

Figure 3.16 Large-headed spermatozoon. This anomaly is correlated with diploid spermatozoa

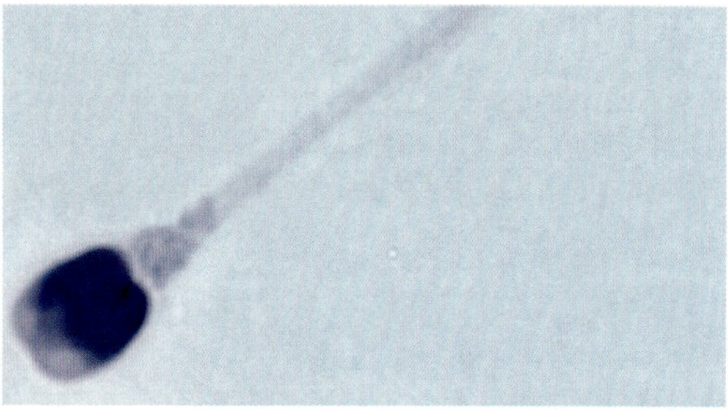

Figure 3.17 Double-headed spermatozoon. Each head has its own membrane

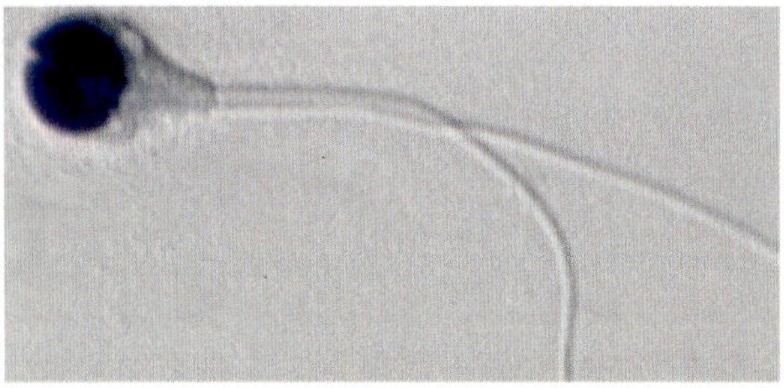

Figure 3.18 Spermatozoon with a binucleated head. In this case, the head contains two nuclei surrounded by only one membrane

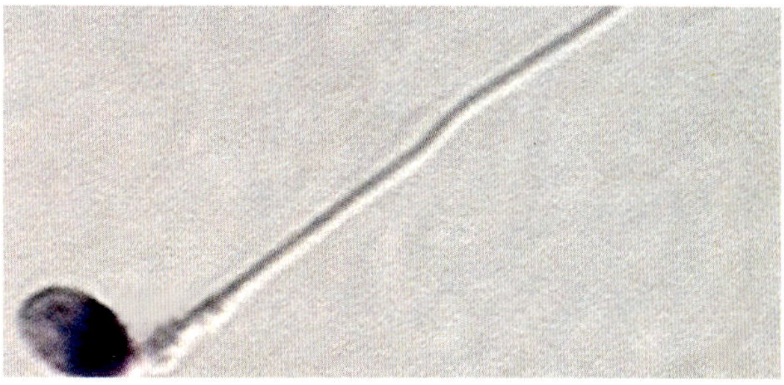

Figure 3.19 Spermatozoon with a bent neck, a defect causing motility, if present, to be very poor

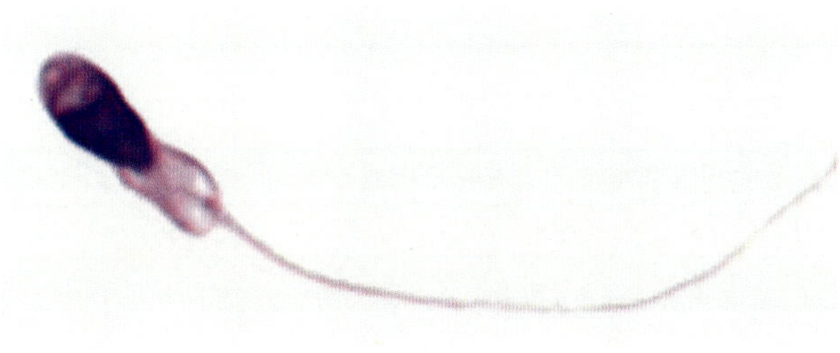

Figure 3.20 Spermatozoon containing a cytoplasmic droplet, a sign of immaturity or incomplete spermiogenesis

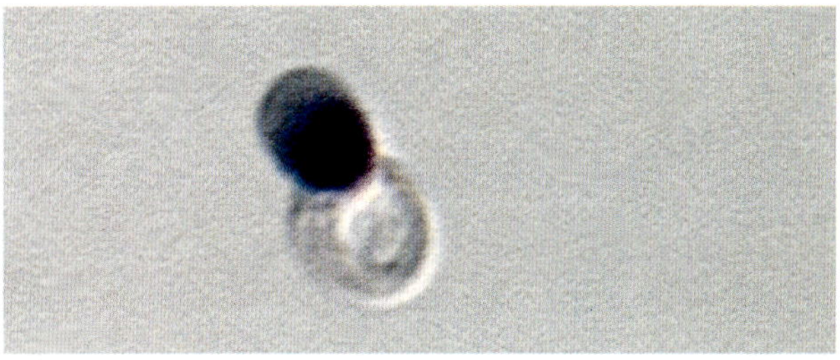

Figure 3.21 Spermatozoon with a coiled tail, an anomaly associated with epididymal infection

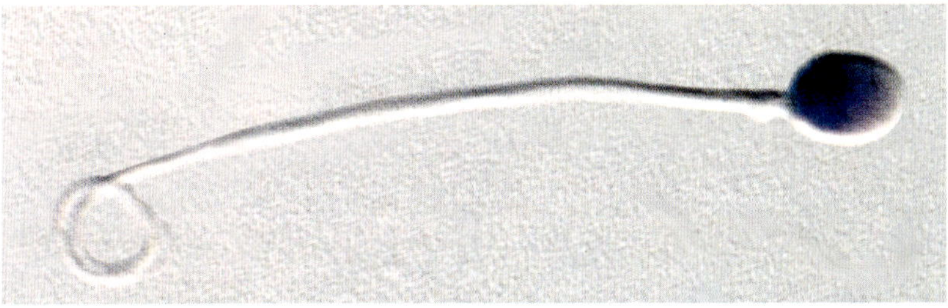

Figure 3.22 Spermatozoon with a partially coiled tail, which may be due to osmotic stress

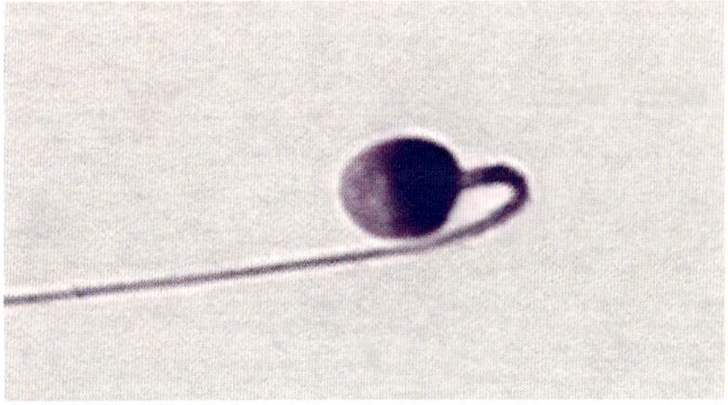

Figure 3.23 Spermatozoon with a bent tail, which confers poor motility

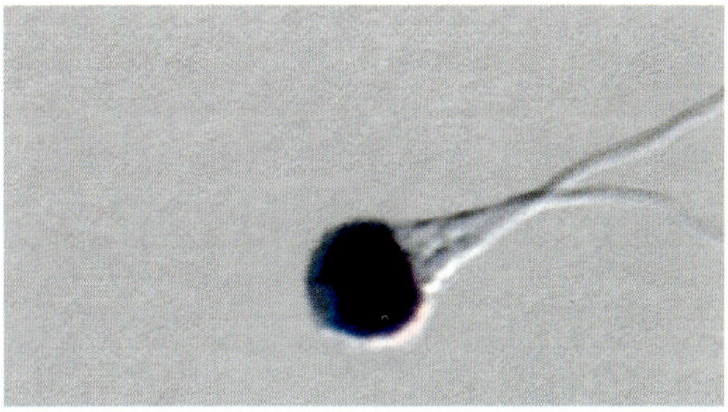

Figure 3.24 Spermatozoon with a double tail, the result of a centriole anomaly

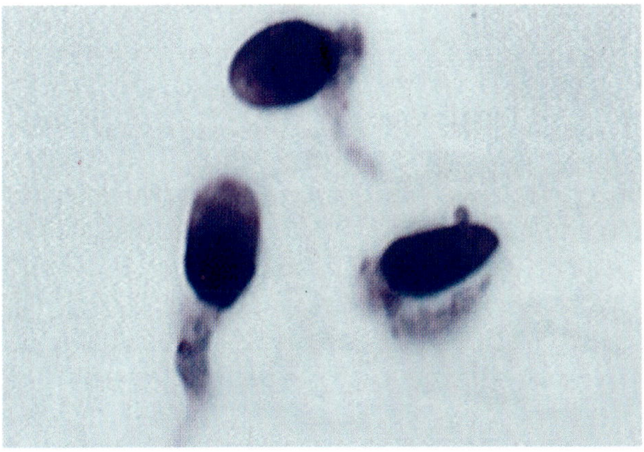

Figure 3.25 Spermatozoa with short tails due to an anomaly in axoneme development. All of the patient's spermatozoa (ejaculated and testicular) showed this defect

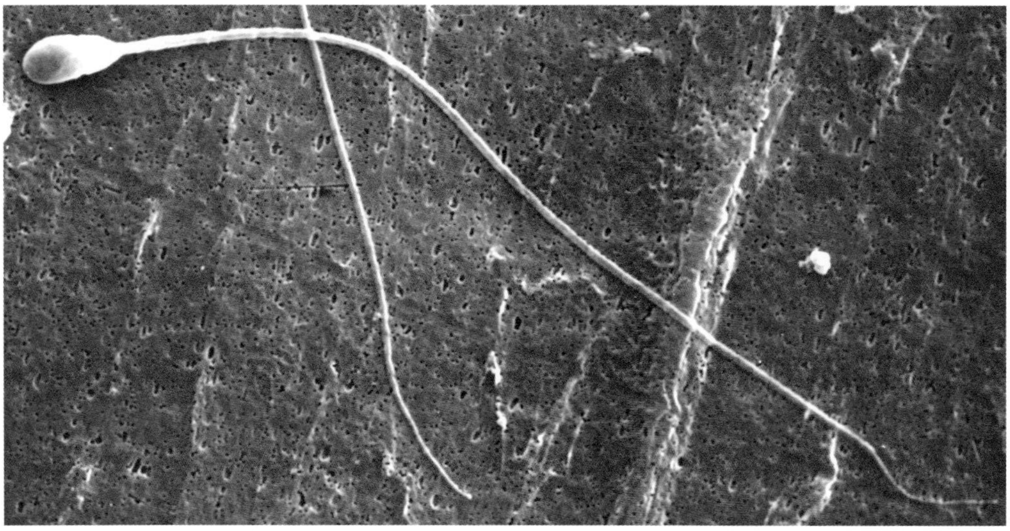

Figure 3.26 SEM (× 1800) of a normal spermatozoon, which has an acorn-shaped head of normal size, a well-defined midpiece, and a normal tail; the terminal piece is thin because the axoneme is covered only by cytoplasmatic membrane

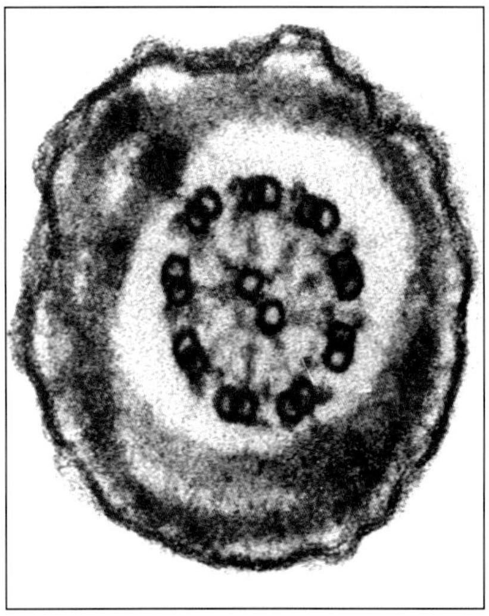

Figure 3.27 TEM (× 150 000) of a normal spermatozoon, seen in transverse section at the level of the principal piece (tail), shows nine pairs of peripheral microtubules and one pair of central microtubules surrounded by a coarse fibrous sheath. Each doublet consists of an A subunit, circular in cross-section, and a B subunit (C-shaped and attached to the wall of subunit A). A subunits join the coarse sheath surrounding the central pair by the radial spokes. Each A subunit has two dynein arms, an outer and an inner, following slightly diverging courses towards the B subunits of the next doublet. The nexin links, a system of long thin filaments, traverse the interdoublet space and connect subunit A of each doublet to subunit B of the adjacent one. Dynein is a heterogeneous protein possessing ATPase activity. In the dynein arms, ATP synthesized in the mitochondria is hydrolyzed to ADP, phosphate, and energy. The radial spokes regulate the relative sliding of the peripheral tubules alongside one another[18]

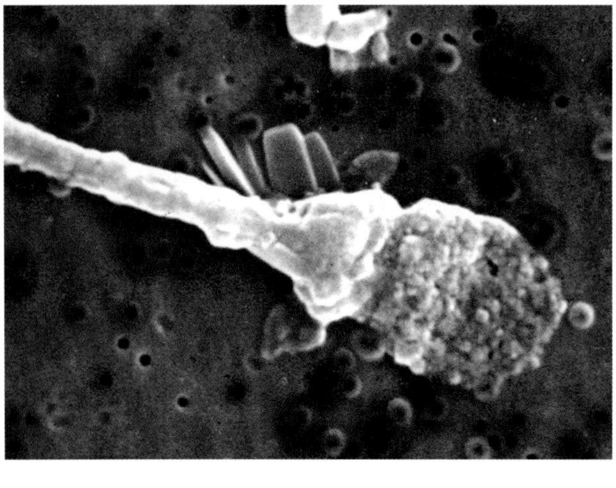

Figure 3.28 SEM of necrozoospermia (× 9275), an infrequently observed pathology. In this case, 100% of the spermatozoa were dead (eosin–nigrosin stain). With the absence or diminution of the enzyme carboxyl-o-methyltransferase, spermatozoa do not produce lactic acid from fructose[19]. The genetic basis of this abnormality is not confirmed; it may be an acquired pathology[20]. Fertilization may be achieved using ICSI with testicular sperm[21]

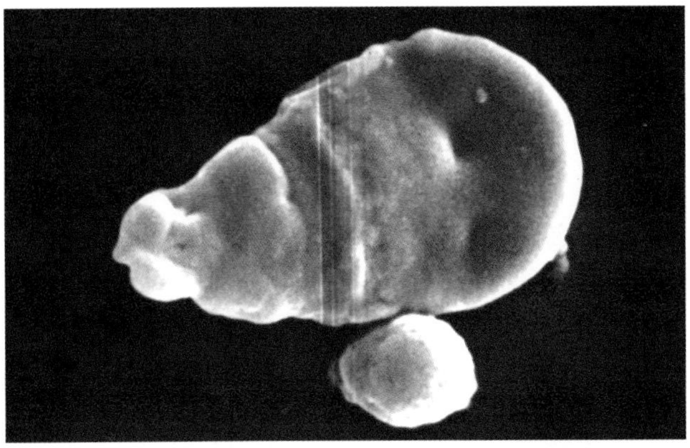

Figure 3.29 SEM of decapitation defect (×9300), first described by Lüders[22], due to a severe abnormality of the connecting piece. The semen showed moving tails. Dissociation of the head and tail occurred in either the testis or epididymis. On LM, these may be confused with pinhead defects. On SEM, a normal flagellum is seen with a cytoplasmic droplet at the proximal end. This pathological condition is considered a congenital defect due to either failure of connection[23] or alteration of the proximal centriole[24]

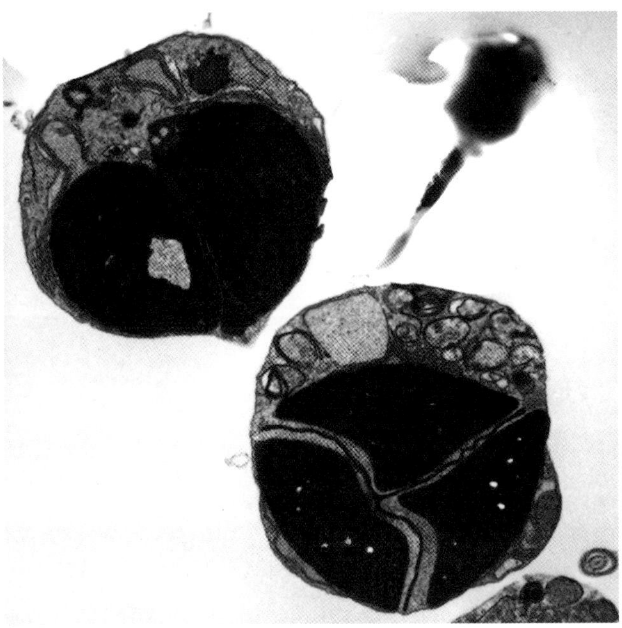

Figure 3.30 TEM (×13 000) of polynucleated spermatozoa, which have two or more nuclei and one shared acrosome, and originate from polynucleated spermatids. If binucleated, more than one tail is usually present; if polynucleated, the tail is usually absent

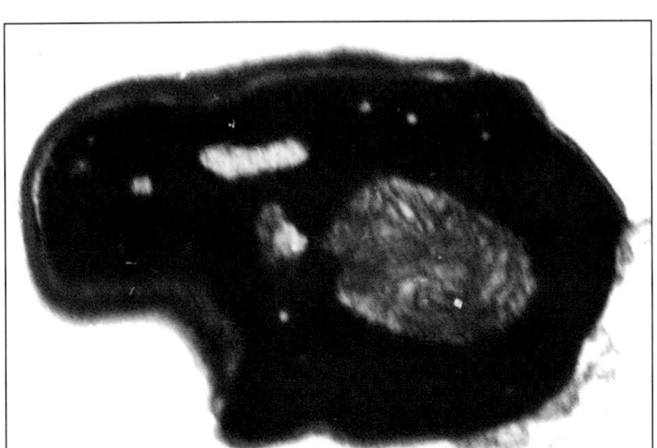

Figure 3.31 TEM (×25 200) of nuclear vacuoles, which are seen in almost all semen samples from infertile patients, but also commonly observed in normal ejaculates. These vacuoles do not possess membranes

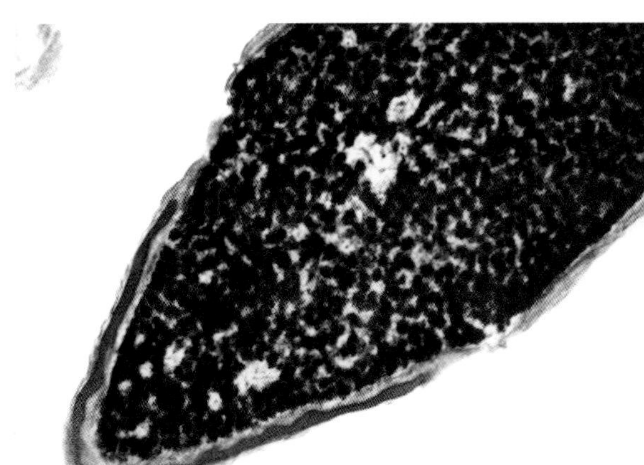

Figure 3.32 TEM (×30 000) of chromatin subcondensation, a frequent alteration seen in infertile patients and associated with chromosomal abnormalities[25]. One causal theory is that histones have failed to become substituted by protamines[26]

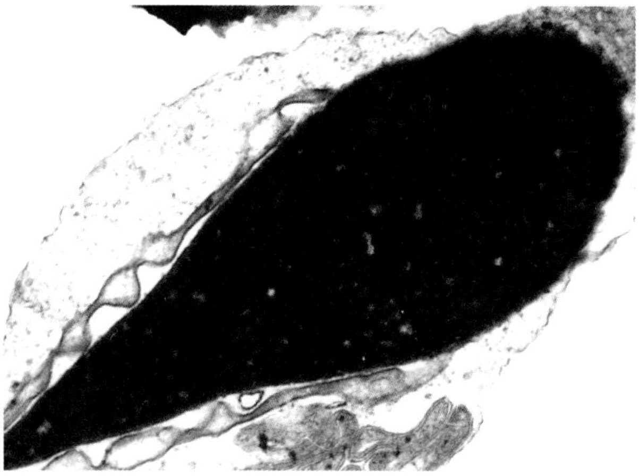

Figure 3.33 TEM (×28 900) of cephalic cytoplasm, seen between the membrane of the sperm and that of the external acrosome. This is considered to be a sign of sperm immaturity

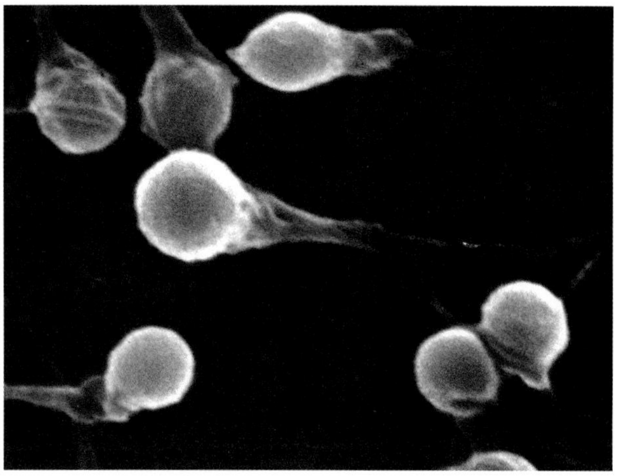

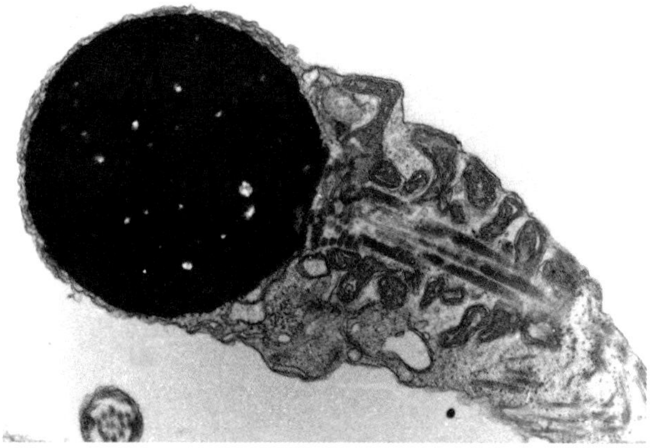

Figure 3.34 SEM (upper; ×4000) and TEM (lower; ×20 000) of absent acrosome defect. The sperm are round-headed (globozoospermia) and the chromatin is decondensed[27,28]. It has been suggested that the pathology is due to a polygenic hereditary condition[29]. Spermatozoa with this defect cannot pass the zona pellucida, although pregnancies have been achieved with ICSI[30]. Hypoplasic acrosome defect also affects fertility

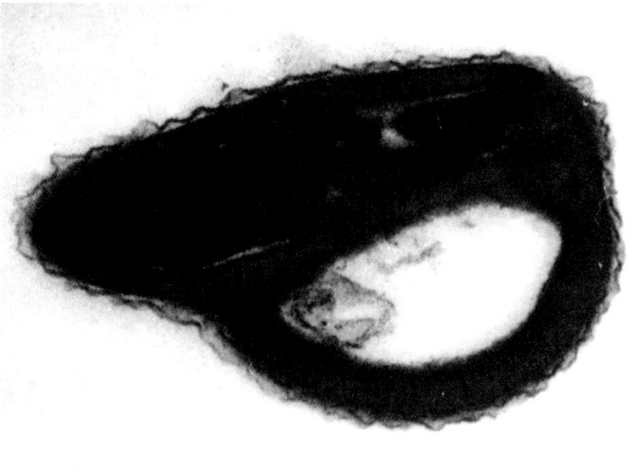

Figure 3.35 TEM (×45 000) of a deformed acrosome, usually associated with nuclear alterations

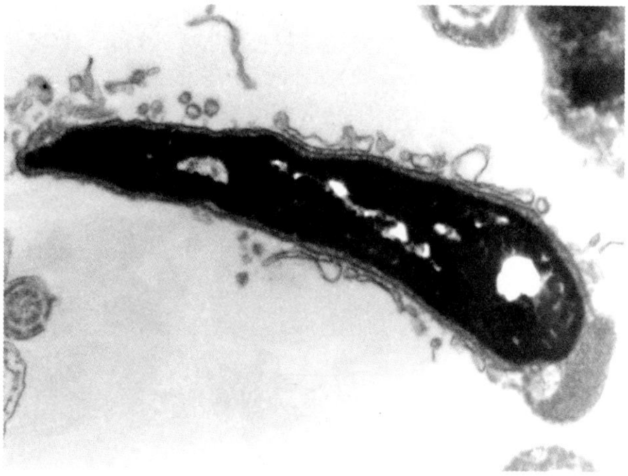

Figure 3.36 TEM (×25 000) of a reacted acrosome. If the acrosome reaction takes place in the ejaculate before the spermatozoon contacts the oocyte, it is not likely to be able to traverse the zona pellucida

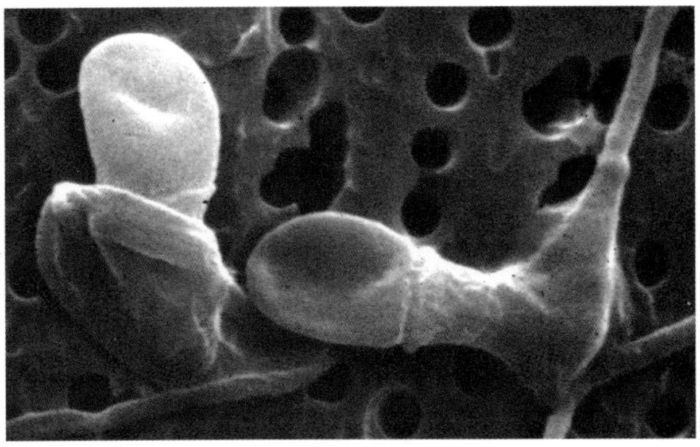

Figure 3.37 SEM (× 13 400) of angulation and coiled-tail defects, which can also be seen by LM. Spermatozoa with these defects cannot acquire hyperactive motility, or may be immotile

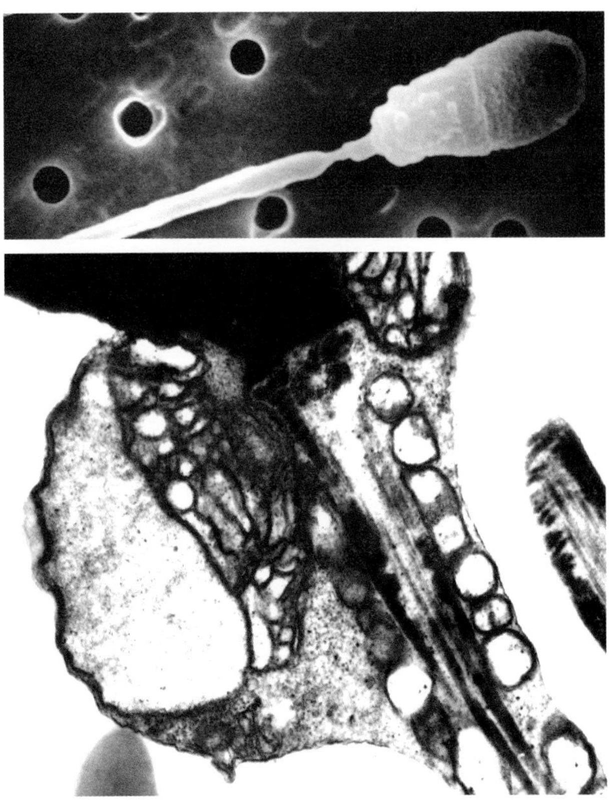

Figure 3.38 SEM (upper; × 9600) and TEM (lower; × 26 500) of mitochondrial sheath alteration. The midpiece is the part of the flagellum that contains the mitochondria, which are distributed in a helicoidal pattern of 12–15 gyres, each containing two mitochondria[31]. The ATP produced in the mitochondria is transformed into mechanical energy in the dynein arms. Mitochondrial absence results in a lack of motility

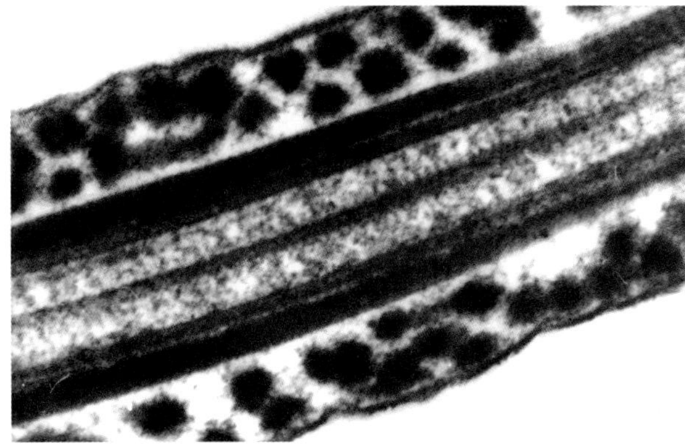

Figure 3.39 TEM (× 100 000) of fibrous sheath defect. The fibrous sheath begins just below the last mitochondrial gyre, and surrounds the outer dense fiber and the axonemal microtubules over the principal piece. It consists of two longitudinal columns positioned 180° to each other, and a regular series of transversal ribs. Defects of the fibrous sheath result in sperm immotility[32] or severe asthenozoospermia, and affected patients may have respiratory cilia pathology. Fibrous sheath defects have been described in brothers[33]. A system of nine outer dense fibers wraps the axoneme along the whole of the midpiece and principal piece. Cranially, each fiber fuses with a segmented column of the connecting piece whereas, caudally, the fibers terminate by fusing to the wall of its corresponding doublet. Not considered to be contractile elements, defects of the outer dense fibers are not frequently observed

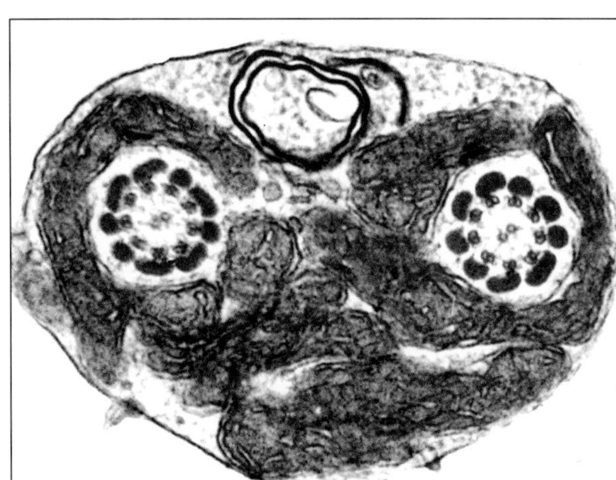

Figure 3.40 TEM (× 4000) of polyaxoneme defect. This alteration may be related to centriole abnormalities

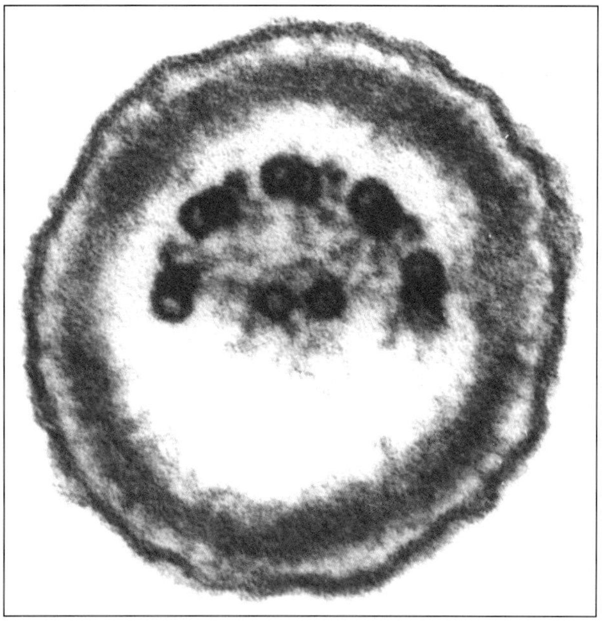

Figure 3.41 TEM (× 173 400) of axonemal peripheral doublet alteration. This abnormality is usually observed together with other defects; changes in the number of doublets or doublet disorganization may be present. The microtubules derive from the centriole during spermiogenesis[34]

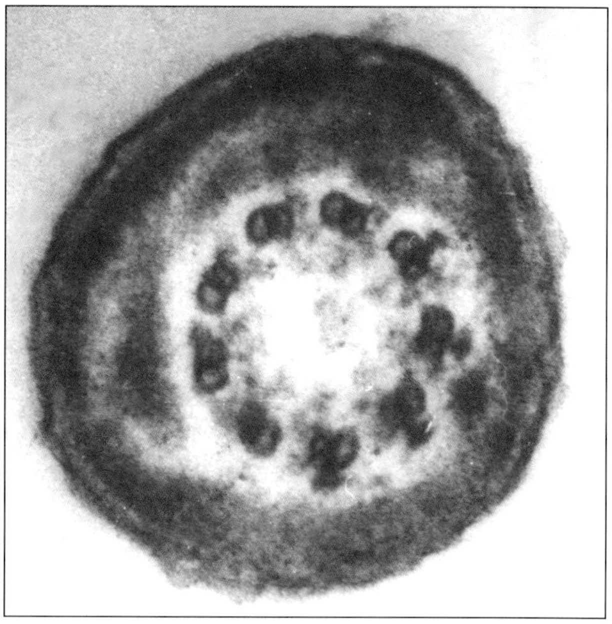

Figure 3.42 TEM of central axonemal pair alteration, 9 + 0 formula (× 132 600), which does not occur frequently, but is the most common central-pair abnormality observed. Spermatozoa with this abnormality are immotile. The fibrous sheath is also defective. Formula 9 + 1 or 9 + 3 may also be found, but is rare[17]

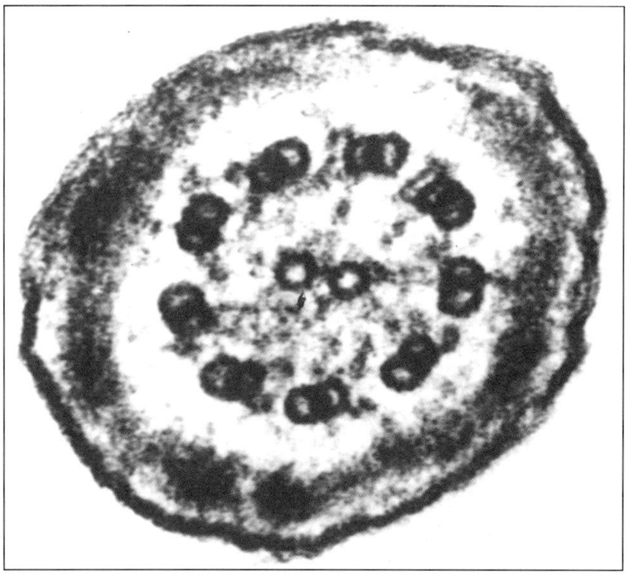

Figure 3.43 TEM of absence of dynein arms (× 132 600). As dynein is essential for flagellar and ciliar movement, its absence provokes asthenozoospermia, sinopulmonary infections, and bronchiectasis. Dynein absence can only affect either the spermatozoon[35] or cilia[36]. If bronchiectasis and situs viscerum inversus are also present, it is referred to as Kartagener's syndrome. Such patients may have normal ciliar ultrastructure and motile sperm[36]. Fertility has also been reported[37]. It is concluded that the genes regulating dynein synthesis for spermatozoa and for bronchial cilia are different[38]. Less frequently, the absence of only either external or internal dynein arms is observed. Spermatozoa lacking external dynein arms may demonstrate some type of movement[39]

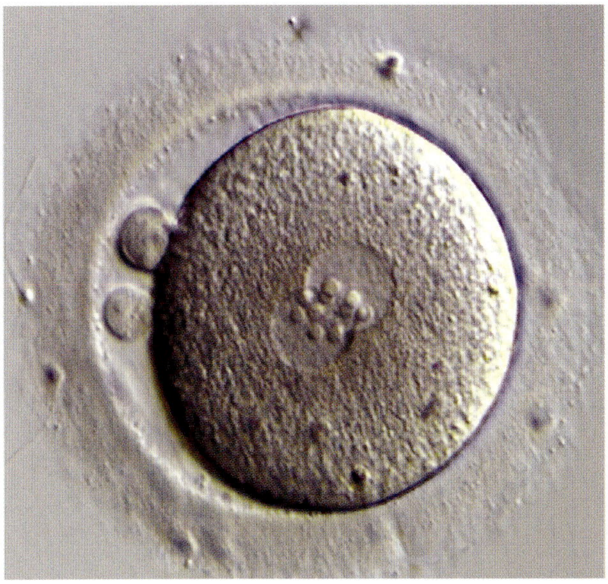

Figure 4.1 Typical appearance of an oocyte with two pronuclei and two polar bodies. The upper pronucleus is slightly larger than the lower one, and its position in relation to the polar bodies provides little information for predicting its origin. Nucleoli within the pronuclei are beginning to migrate to the area of juxtaposition

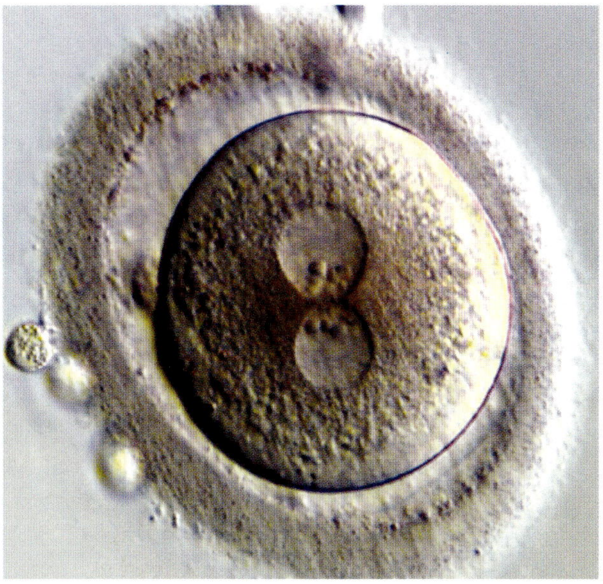

Figure 4.2 Double-pronucleate oocyte with a large perivitelline space and clear cortical zone. The aggregation of cytoplasmic organelles causes a deepening of color in the area adjacent to the pronuclei. The upper pronucleus is somewhat larger than the lower one; nucleoli in each are migrating to the area of pronuclear juxtaposition

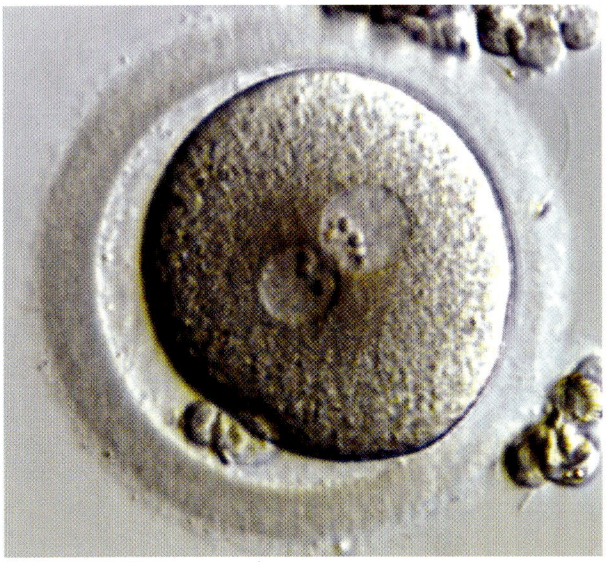

Figure 4.3 Fertilized oocyte with two pronuclei, two polar bodies, and a single spermatozoon bound to the zona. One pronucleus is larger than the other, and nucleoli within both are aligning at adjacent poles. Accumulation of organelles causes a discoloration in the area surrounding the pronuclear structures

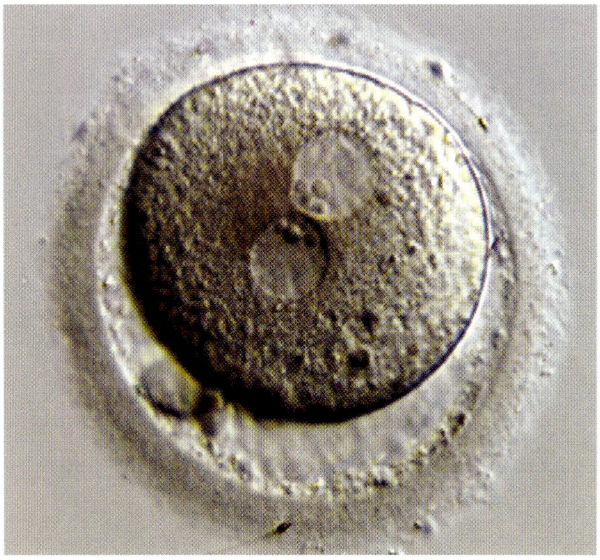

Figure 4.4 Granular oocyte displaying an extremely large, debris-filled, perivitelline space. The slightly smaller lower pronucleus with completely aligned nucleoli is nearest the site of polar body extrusion. Two spermatozoa can be seen bound to the thin zona pellucida

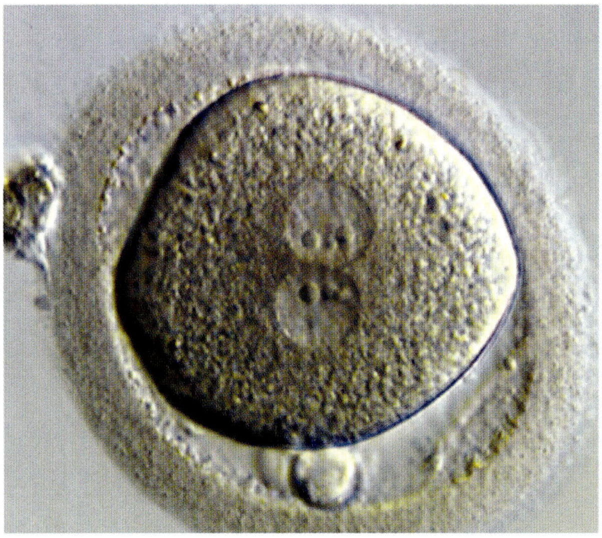

Figure 4.5 The slightly darkened zona of this pronuclear oocyte is thickened (typically called 'bilayered') in the lower right and upper left quadrants. Two closely apposed polar bodies can be seen at a six-o'clock position. The oocyte exhibits granular ooplasm and discoloration in the area surrounding the similarly sized pronuclei. Nucleoli within each pronucleus are lined up at adjacent borders

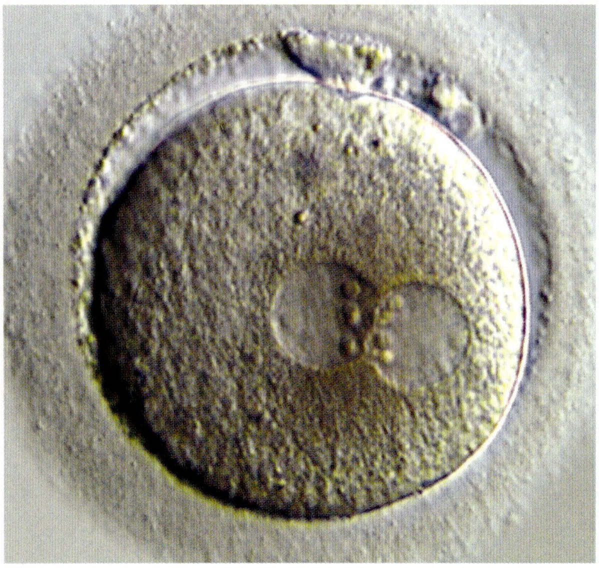

Figure 4.7 Two pronuclei of equal size are positioned off-center in this oocyte. Two polar bodies are located at twelve- and one-o'clock. At 20 h post-ICSI, this oocyte is close to entering syngamy as evidenced by the large pronuclear size and the precise alignment of nucleoli at opposing borders

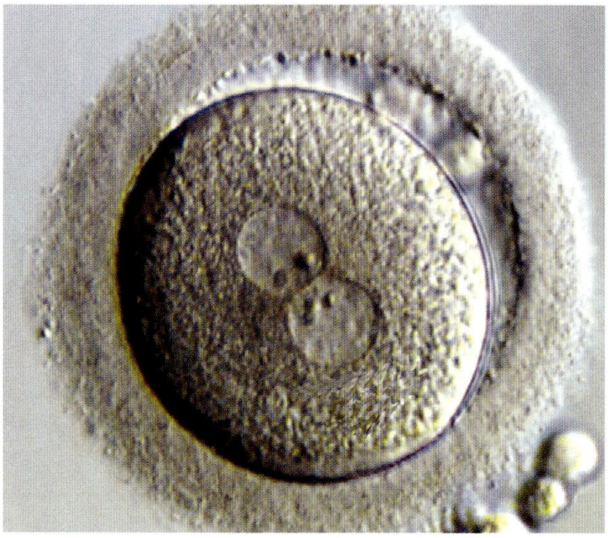

Figure 4.6 Two pronuclei, two polar bodies, and a thick and darkened zona are seen in this example of an oocyte 18 h after ICSI. The two pronuclei are of similar size and contain few nuceloli

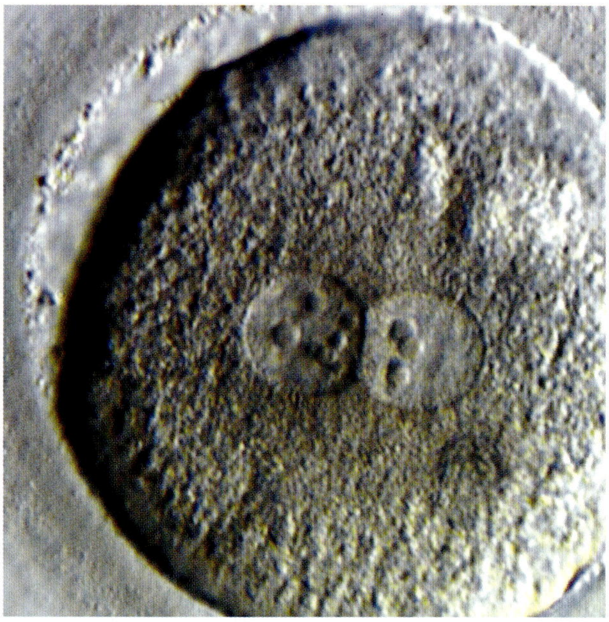

Figure 4.8 High-power view shows two small pronuclei of equal size at 9 h postinsemination. Nucleoli are scattered within, and differ in number between, the pronuclear structures. Polar bodies can be seen (out of focus) above the pronucleus on the right. The ooplasm is granular and exhibits darkening in the area surrounding the pronuclei. Moderate perivitelline debris is evident in the upper left perivitelline space

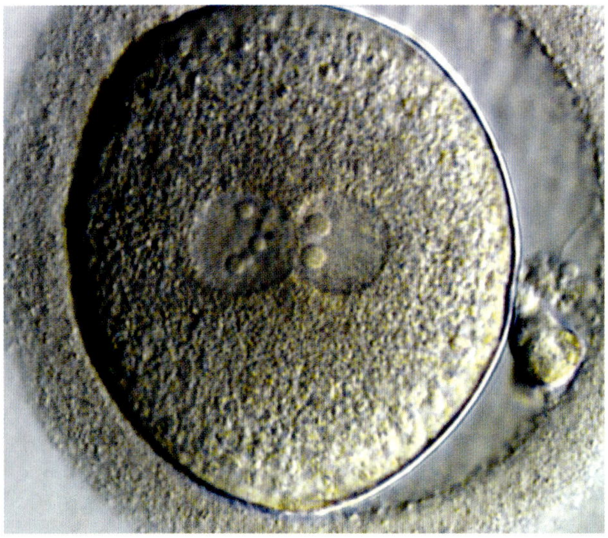

Figure 4.9 Extremely large perivitelline space surrounds this fertilizing oocyte at 18 h post-ICSI. One of the polar bodies has fragmented within the perivitelline space to the right. The zona appears slightly darkened and very speckled. The pronucleus on the left has six or seven small nucleoli whereas the slightly smaller pronucleus on the right has only two or three, but much larger, nucleoli

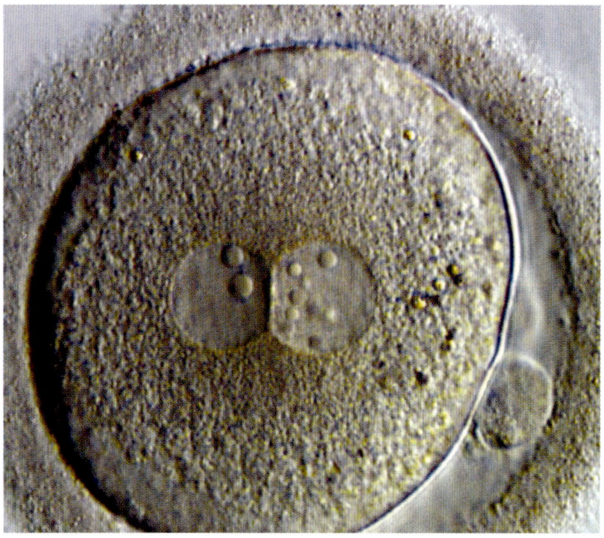

Figure 4.10 The larger pronucleus on the right shows 10 small, randomly positioned, nucleoli. The second pronucleus has only two nucleoli, which are considerably larger than any in the other pronucleus. If it is true that the smaller pronucleus with fewer nucleoli is most likely of maternal origin, then its location furthest away from the two polar bodies is contrary to typical development

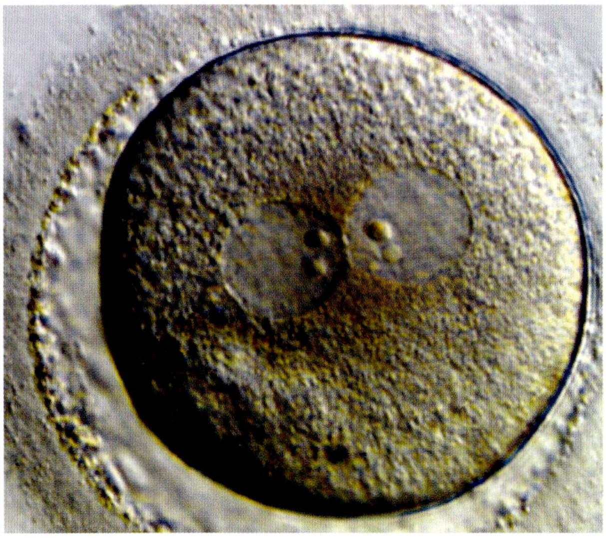

Figure 4.11 Two pronuclei of similar size are centrally located within this slightly granular oocyte. Few nucleoli can be seen in either structure, an observation considered by some to be a negative finding. Significant perivitelline debris covers the inner layer of the thin zona. The preembryo developing from this prezygote was transferred and resulted in a pregnancy

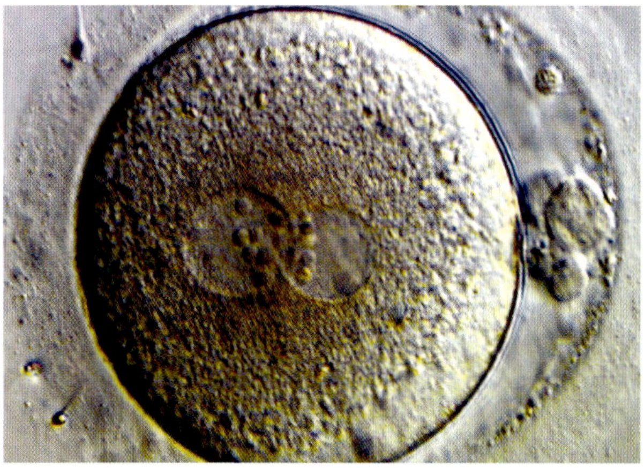

Figure 4.12 At 15 h postinsemination, this oocyte has two pronuclei and two polar bodies, one of which is fragmenting. Two-thirds of the cortical area is a clear organelle-free zone. The area surrounding the pronuclei is darkened. The pronucleus on the left has eight or nine migrating nucleoli; that on the right has six or seven, five of which are aligned to the inside and one, or possibly two, are separated on the opposite side. Here, the smaller pronucleus with the fewest nucleoli is indeed nearest the polar bodies

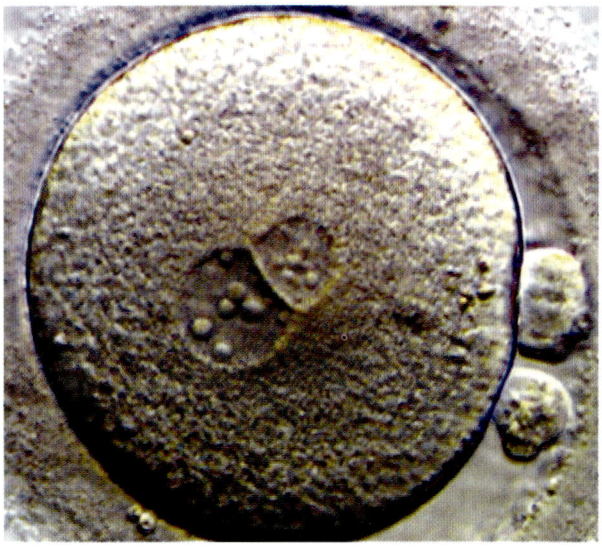

Figure 4.13 At 15 h post-ICSI, this oocyte had a single pronucleus. At 21 h, these two atypical pronuclei were seen. The one on the left is larger and contains larger nucleoli, none of which has migrated to the area of pronuclear juxtaposition. This is an irregular finding so many hours after oocyte activation. The smaller pronucleus is late-developing, has smaller nucleoli, and sits closer to the two clearly visualized polar bodies

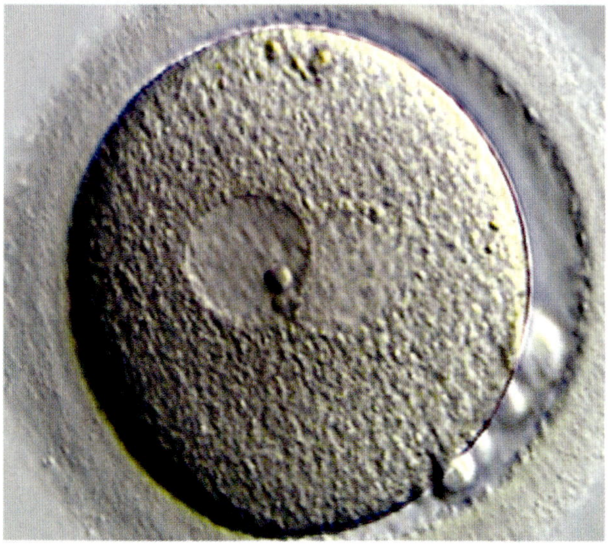

Figure 4.14 At 19 h post-ICSI, this oocyte is undergoing pronuclear breakdown. The pronucleus on the right is dismantling its membrane ahead of the one on the left and presents only a ghost of its previous form. Fragmented polar bodies are seen to the lower right. Less discoloration is noted in the pronuclear area compared with earlier observations

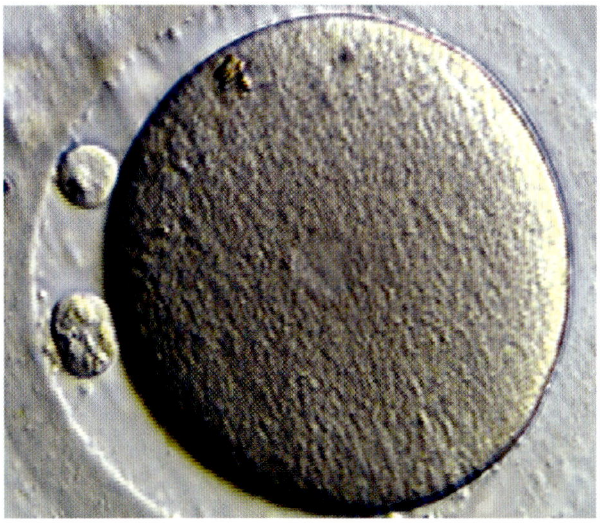

Figure 4.15 At 22 h postinsemination, pronuclear membranes have all but disappeared in this oocyte. Only a faint outline indicates the location of one of the original two pronuclei. First and second polar bodies can be seen a slight distance apart within the perivitelline space to the left. The ooplasm is homogeneously light-colored and agranular

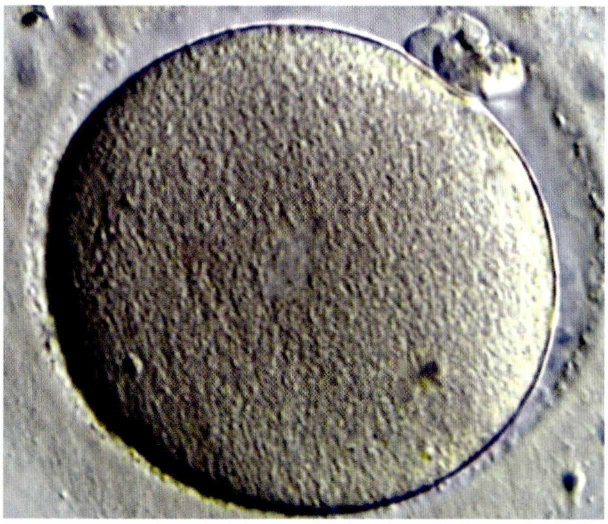

Figure 4.16 Pronuclear membranes have faded almost to extinction in this syngamous oocyte. The ooplasm has regained a homogeneous color and granularity. The polar bodies are fragmenting

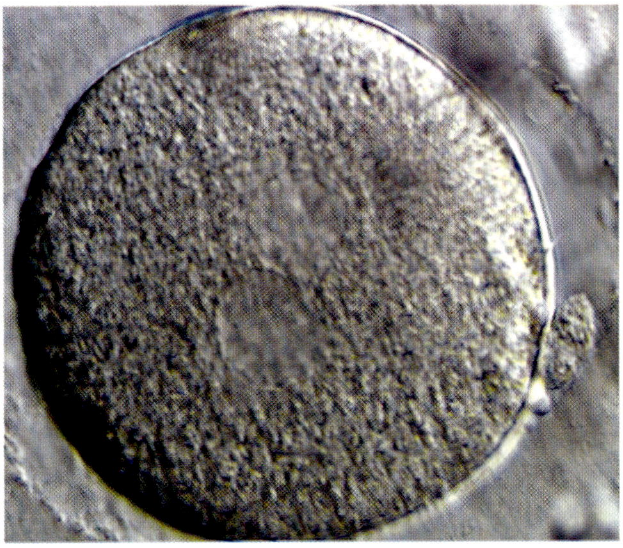

Figure 4.17 Two fading pronuclei are disappearing asynchronously in this granular, unhealthy-looking oocyte. A polar body, also granular and perhaps degenerating, is located at a four-o'clock position

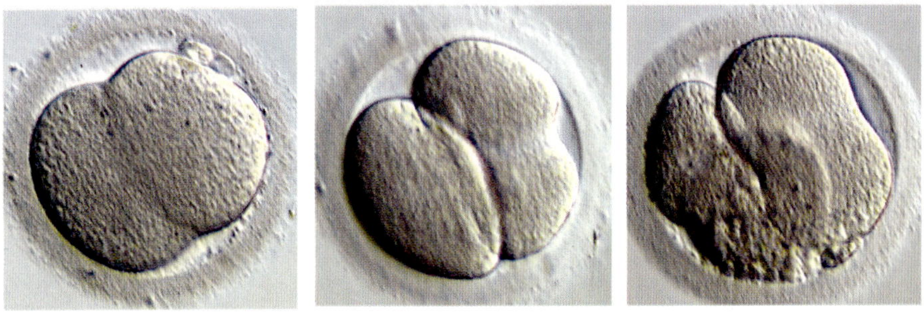

Figure 5.1 Cytoplasmic division: (left) One-cell zygote dividing into two blastomeres during the first cleavage. As the first cleavage mitosis reaches telophase, the cytoplasm elongates and the surface contracts around the lesser circumference; (middle) Two-cell conceptus cleaving to three cells; (right) Three-cell preembryo just before division into four blastomeres

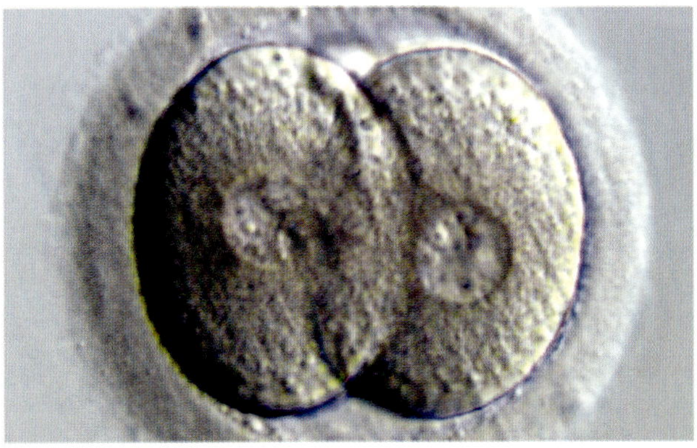

Figure 5.2 Two-cell conceptus. Despite the presence of distinct nuclei, the cleavage process does not appear to have been fully completed

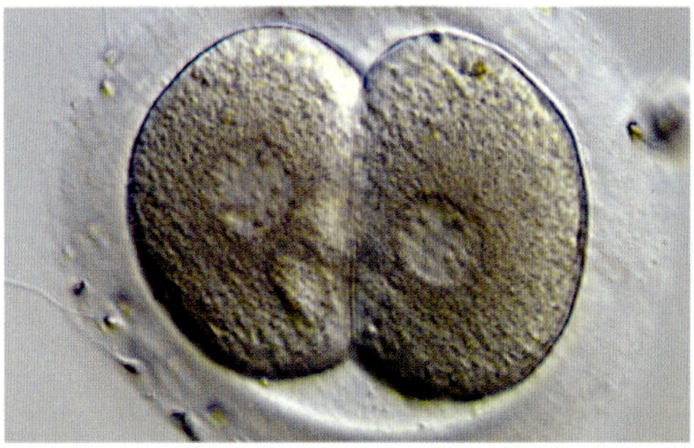

Figure 5.3 Two-cell conceptus with closely apposed blastomeres and distinct nuclei. Two polar bodies are faintly visualized on a separate plane of focus above the left blastomere. Several spermatozoa are bound to the zona pellucida

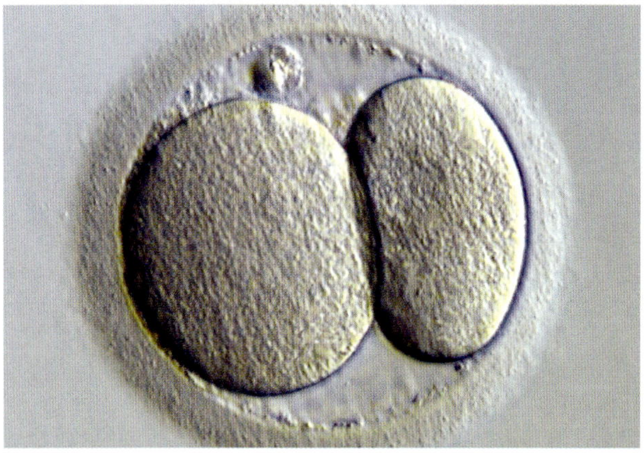

Figure 5.4 Two-cell conceptus with asymmetrical division. One blastomere is larger than the other, very likely the result of recent or impending cleavage. Faint nuclei can be visualized in each blastomere, particularly in the blastomere on the right

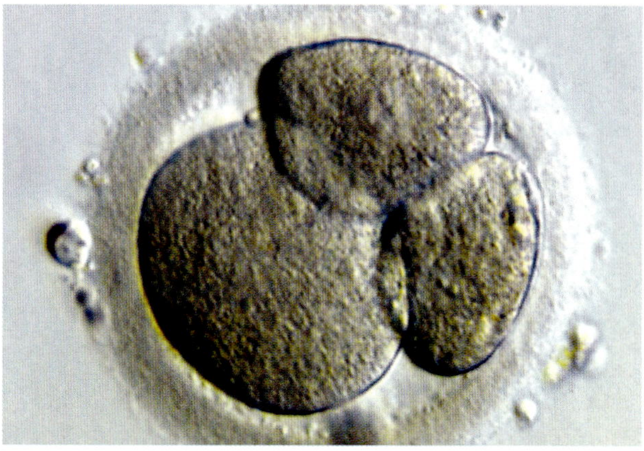

Figure 5.5 Three-cell conceptus with one larger and two smaller blastomeres. Both smaller blastomeres have nuclei whereas the larger blastomere displays only a faint central nuclear remnant

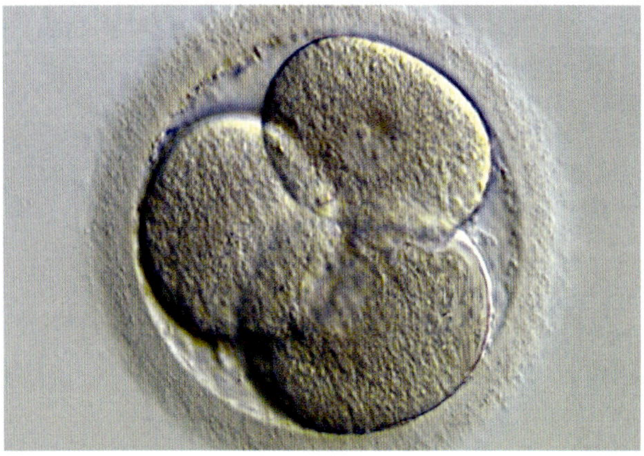

Figure 5.6 Three-cell conceptus with blastomeres that are more equal in size compared with those in Figure 5.5. Two upper blastomeres are the result of division of a single superior blastomere

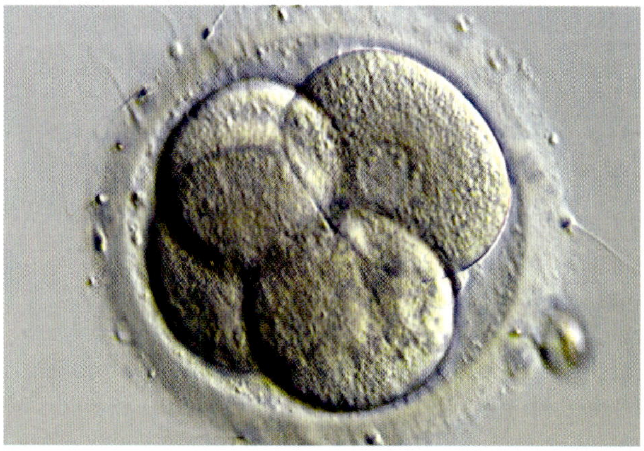

Figure 5.7 Typical four-cell conceptus showing two blastomeres on one plane of focus and a further two in alternate apposition on another plane

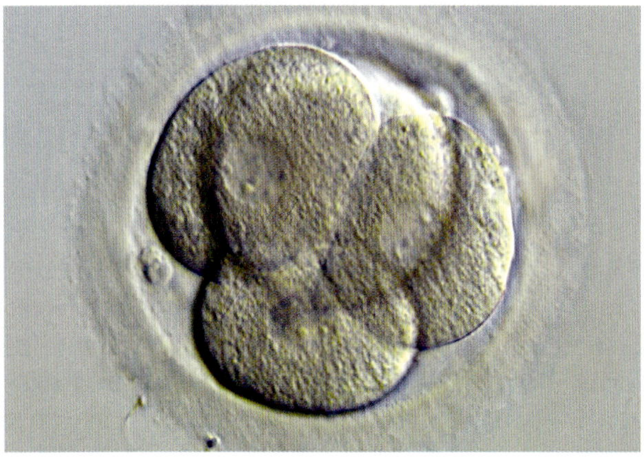

Figure 5.8 Four-cell conceptus showing nucleation of all blastomeres, including the uppermost which is out of focus

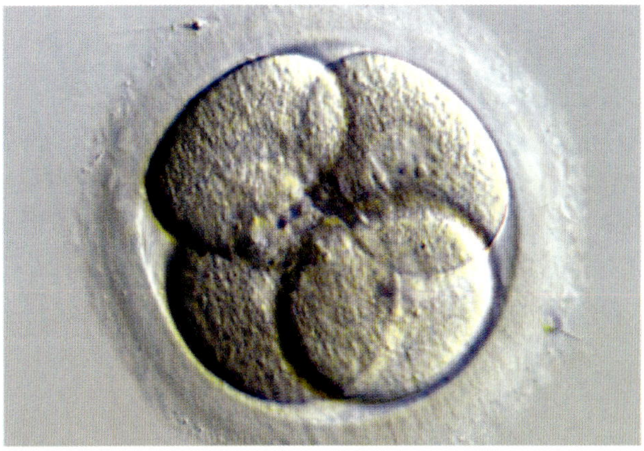

Figure 5.9 Typical healthy-looking four-cell preembryo showing two distinct zona pellucida layers

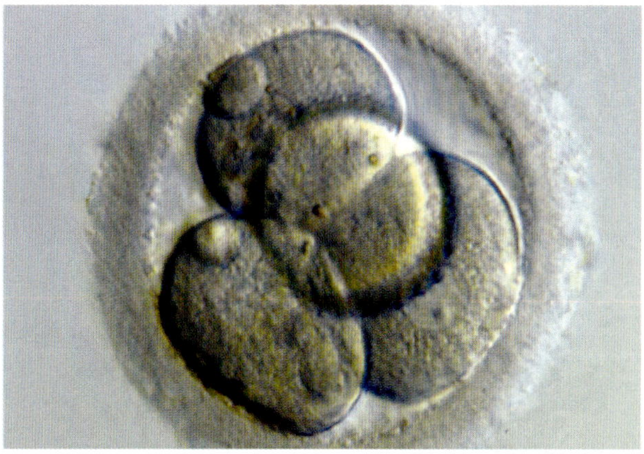

Figure 5.10 Four-cell conceptus with slightly irregular blastomeres. The two polar bodies are associated with two blastomeres to the left

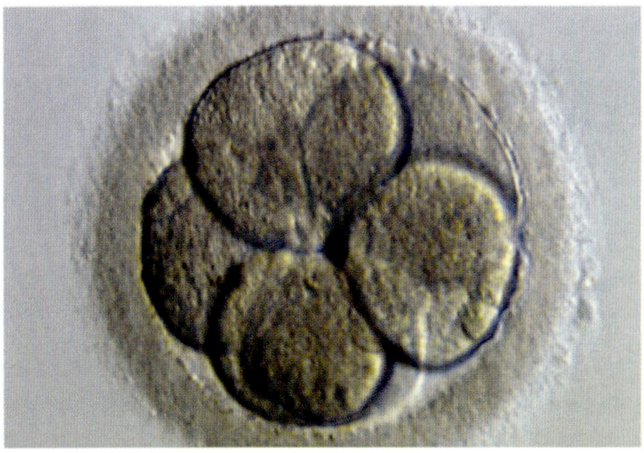

Figure 5.11 Six-cell conceptus with blastomeres of roughly equal size, two of which can be seen faintly above the plane of focus. The zona is rather porous throughout its circumference

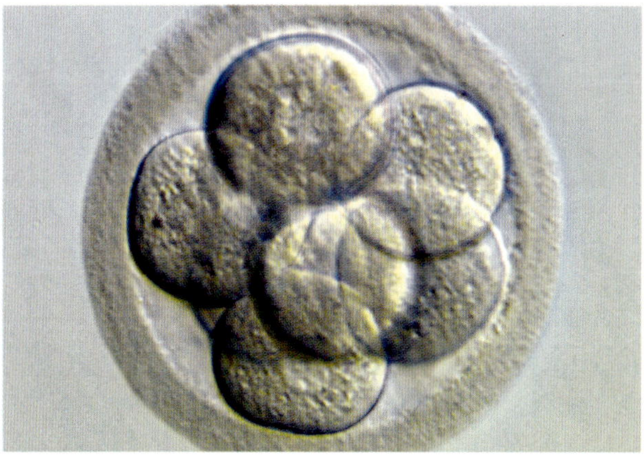

Figure 5.12 Seven-cell conceptus with equal-sized blastomeres, many of which are nucleated, and a rather condensed zona. Minor cytoplasmic vacuolization is present in most of the blastomeres

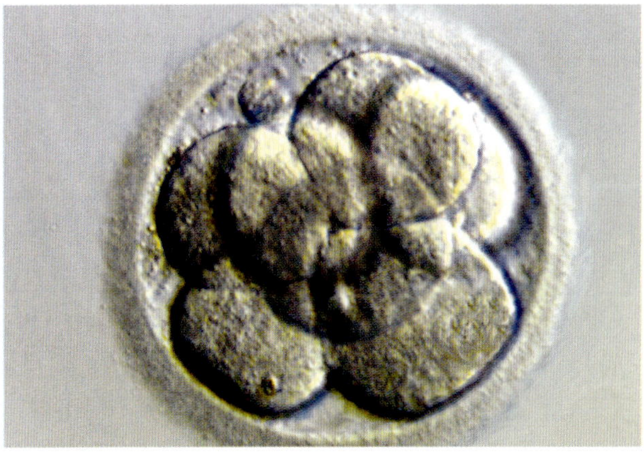

Figure 5.13 Seven-cell conceptus with six equal-sized blastomeres to the center and left, and one slightly larger blastomere to the lower right. The zona is rather thin and condensed. Large inclusions can be seen in the lower left and right blastomeres

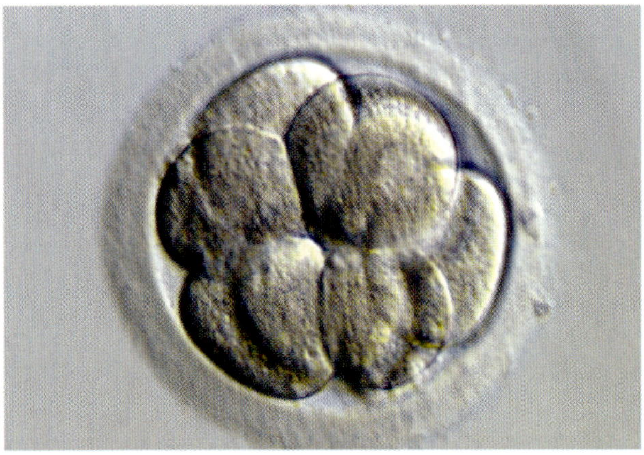

Figure 5.14 Eight-cell conceptus showing minor, but normal, variation in blastomere size

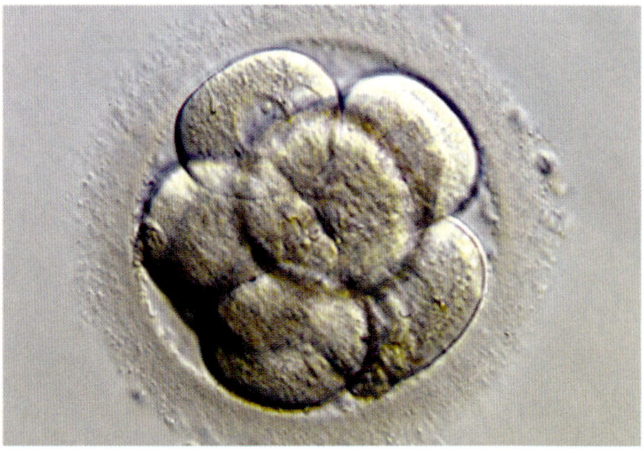

Figure 5.15 Eight-cell conceptus possessing a very porous and slightly thickened zona pellucida

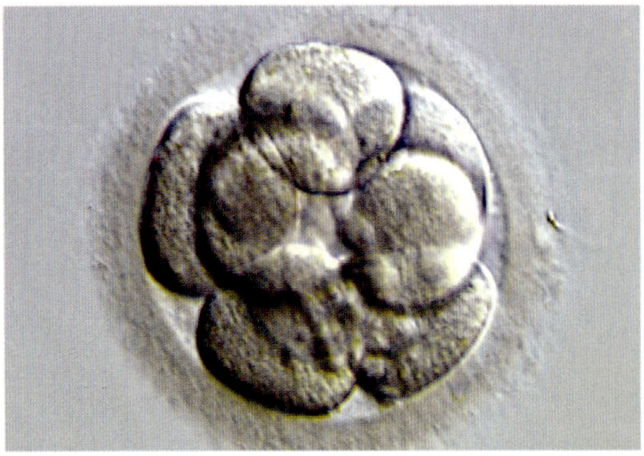

Figure 5.16 Eight-cell conceptus with porous and thin zona pellucida

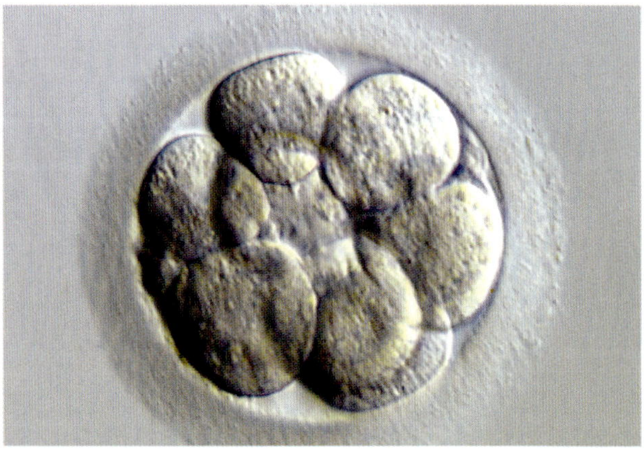

Figure 5.17 Ten-cell conceptus with four blastomeres faintly discernible above the plane of focus. Typical of cleaved conceptuses beyond the four-cell stage, the blastomeres are slightly wider and flatter in areas apposed to the zona compared with inner areas where triangular shapes can be seen

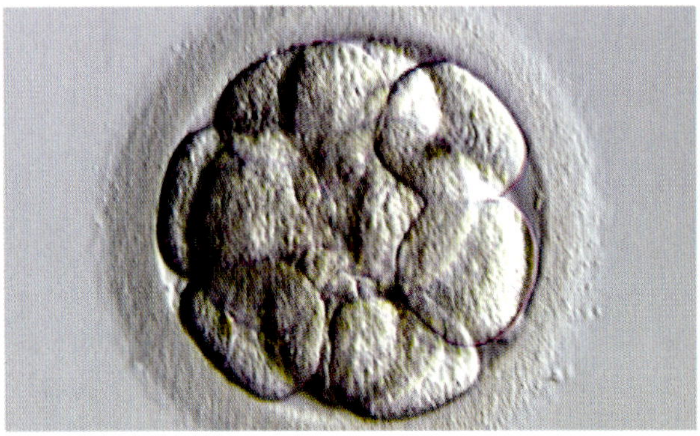

Figure 5.18 Healthy-looking 10-cell conceptus showing little variation in zona pellucida thickness

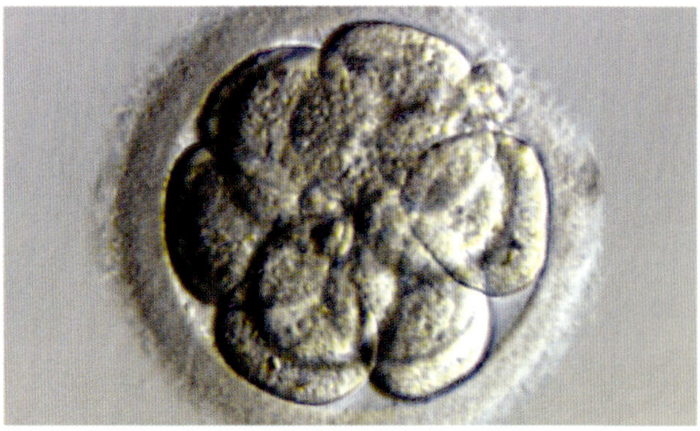

Figure 5.19 Twelve-cell conceptus with a flattened zona (upper right) due to the application of AHA

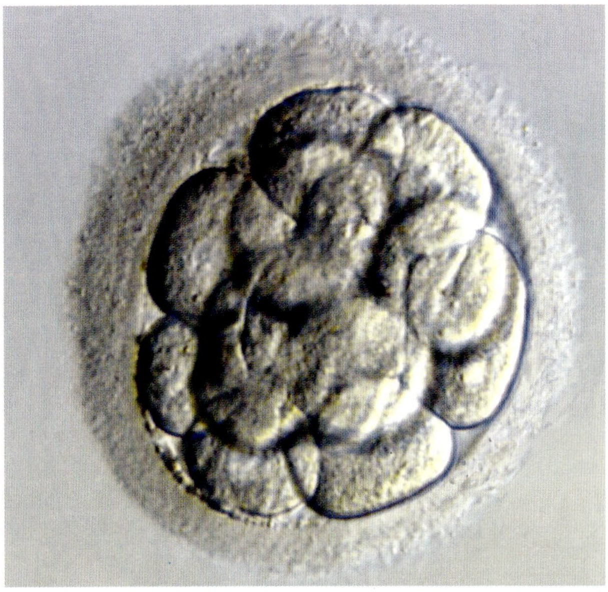

Figure 5.20 Fourteen-cell conceptus with blastomeres of varying sizes and shapes. The zona is alternately thick and thin. The blastomeres remain distinct and separate despite the advanced cleavage status of the preembryo

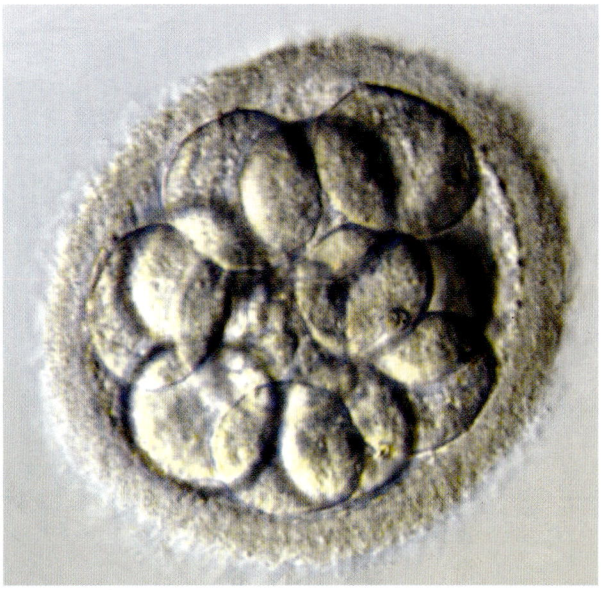

Figure 5.21 Fourteen-cell conceptus with a thin and darkened porous zona, and no evidence of impending compaction

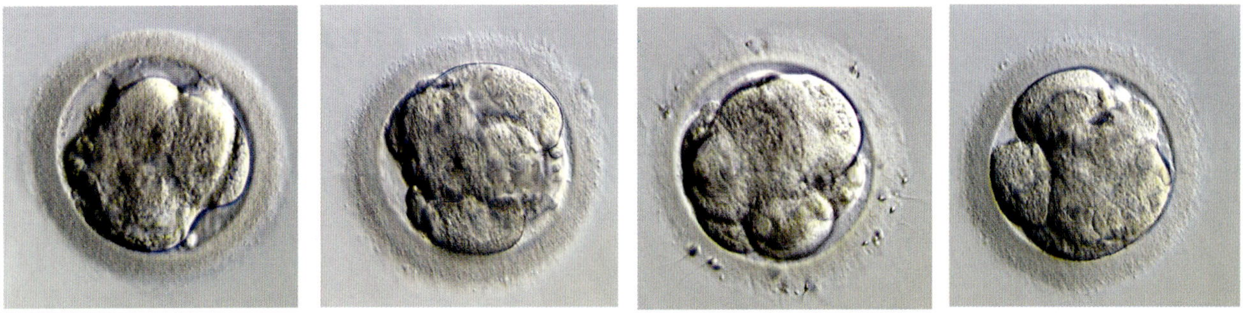

Figure 5.22 Compacting preembryos: These eight-cell conceptuses are losing their cellular distinction as the blastomeres form tight intercellular junctions, thus becoming closely apposed

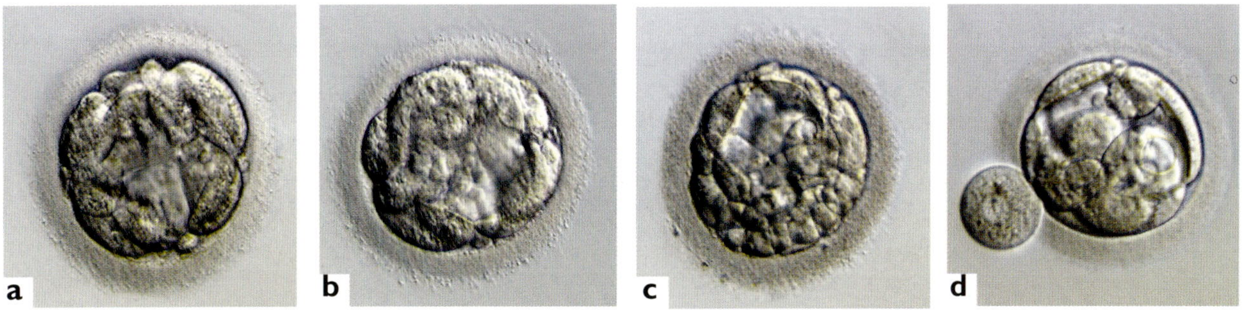

Figure 5.23 Vacuolating (a & b) and cavitating (c) morulae, and cavitating morula with one large nucleated blastomere extruding through an artificial opening created after AHA (d; note the thick zona)

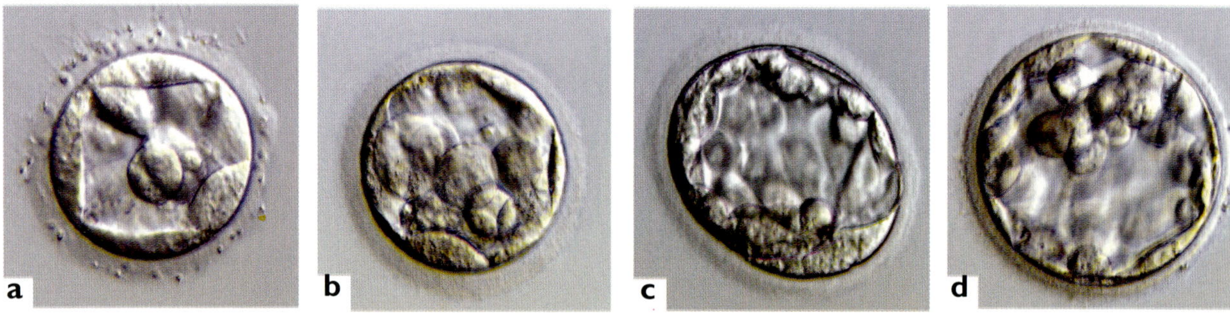

Figure 5.24 Late cavitating morulae (early blastocysts), composed of rather large cells, showing formation of early blastoceles and zona thinning (a & b). Early blastocysts with thinning zonae and accumulation of cells to one pole (c & d)

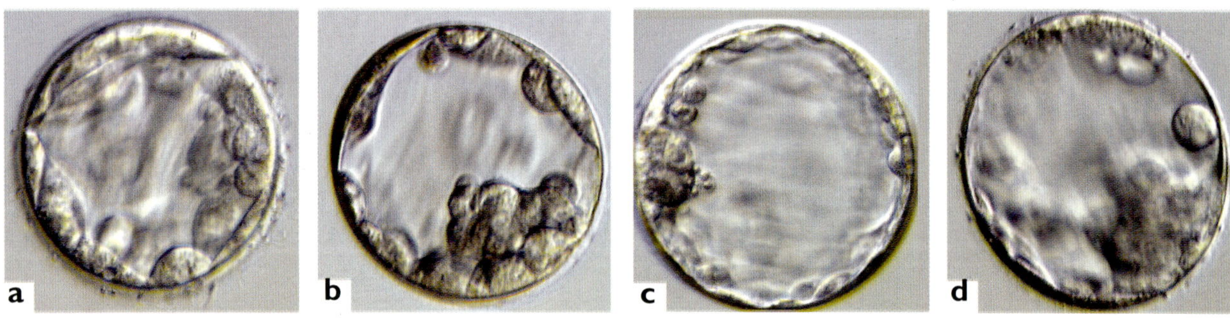

Figure 5.25 Blastocyst formation and zona thinning: As the blastocyst forms, the zona becomes thin in response to the increasing pressure of accumulating fluid within the blastocele. Cells accumulate at one pole to give rise to the inner cell mass. As development proceeds, the conceptus enlarges overall. (a) Early blastocyst with relatively large cells and delineation of trophoblastic and inner cell lines. The conceptus is slightly enlarged due to fluid accumulation, and the zona has thinned. (b) The inner cell mass (on the lower right) is clearly distinguishable and the zona is very thin. (c) The inner cell mass is out of focus (on the lower left) and trophoblastic cells have segregated into a single ring at the conceptus periphery. (d) The inner cell mass is forming (on the lower right) and a single large cell persists above it

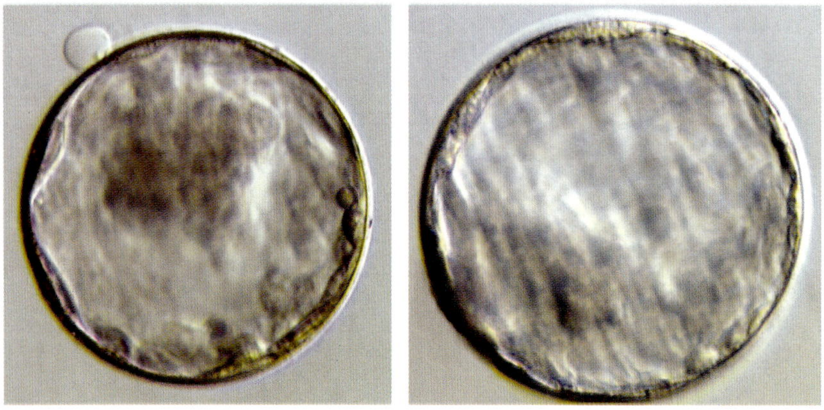

Figure 5.26 Enlarging blastocysts: (left) As fluid volume increases, the zona thins to the point where it is difficult to visualize; membranous material is escaping through a thinned section of the shell. The inner cell mass is evident behind the plane of focus as a darkened area of accumulating cells; (right) Fully expanded blastocyst with an almost non-existent zona, single-layered trophoblastic cells, and an inner cell mass (on the lower left) which is out of focus, but identifiable

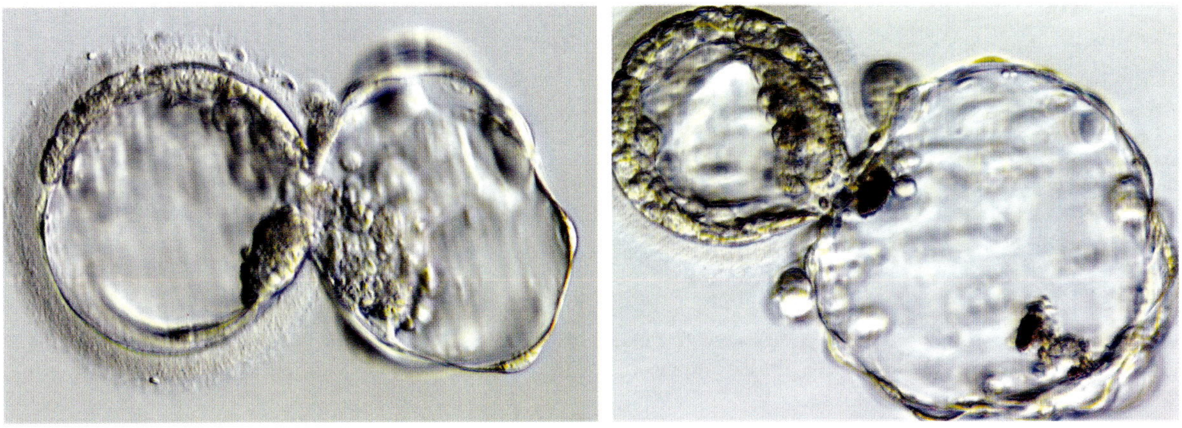

Figure 5.27 Hatching blastocysts seen after a hole has been made in the zona by an AHA procedure. When a hole is made in the zona (see Chapter 11), it fails to thin normally and the blastocysts generally hatch earlier. In these examples, abundant cellular material has been left behind in the zona shell

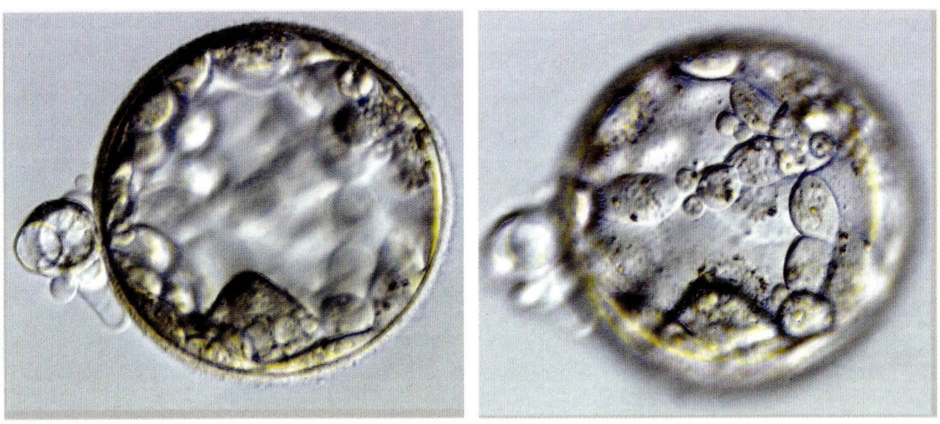

Figure 5.28 Initial stages of the hatching process: The zona is rather thin; membranous material has escaped ahead of the trophoblast. Focusing on the zona (left), large cells can be seen along the rim of the blastocyst and relatively few cells have accumulated at a six-o'clock position; focusing above the plane of the zona (right), large non-conjoined cells can be seen. Whether such a blastocyst has the potential to develop normally is not known

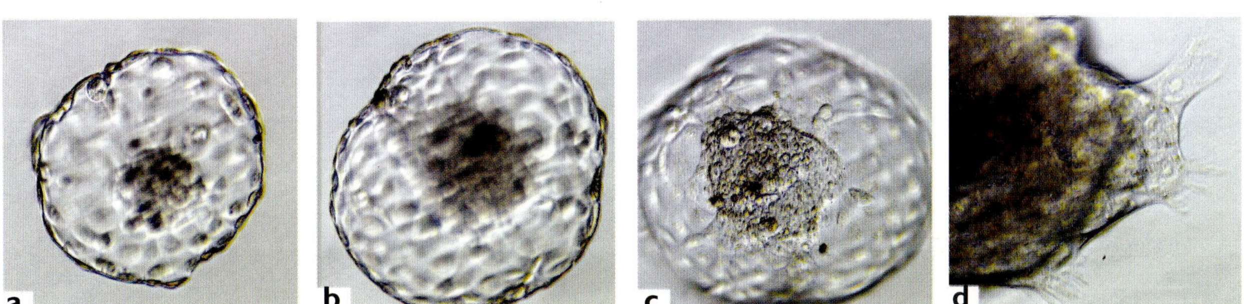

Figure 5.29 Hatched blastocyst enlarging in culture. The heavier inner cell mass routinely positions itself towards the bottom of the culturing vessel: (a–c) On day 6 after harvest, the blastocyst and its inner cell mass enlarge after normal hatching; (d) on day 7, the blastocyst has become attached to the plastic surface of the culturing vessel

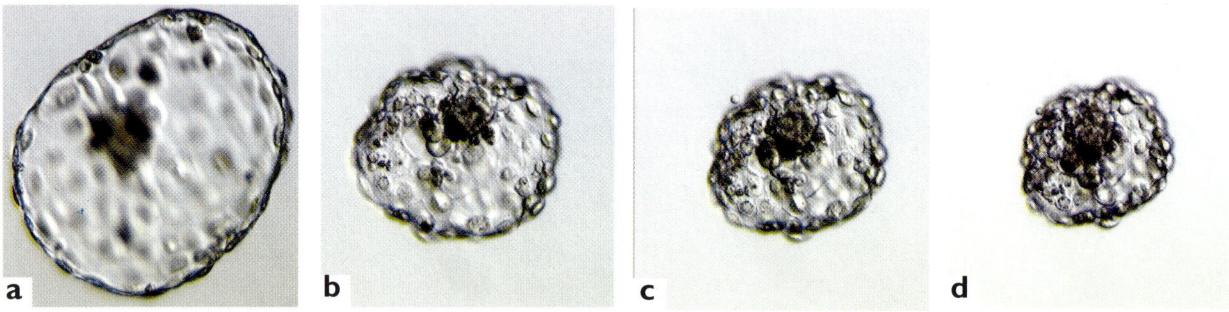

Figure 5.30 Blastocyst collapse: (a–d) On day 7, a blastocyst is observed over a 5-min period after disturbance of its preliminary attachment to the culturing vessel. The result is rapid collapse and loss of fluid

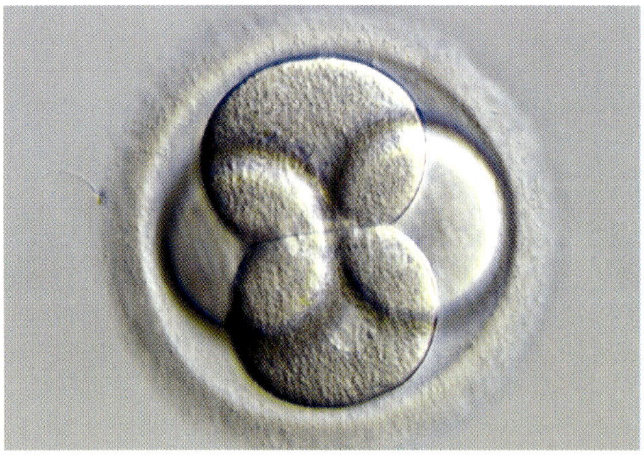

Figure 6.1 Four-cell conceptus with perfect morphology. The blastomeres are symmetrical and of equal size; two lie in one plane of focus and two others, with opposing polarity, lie in another. No cytoplasmic fragments are observed. The cytoplasm is clear and homogeneous. The zona shows normal morphology and is relatively thin

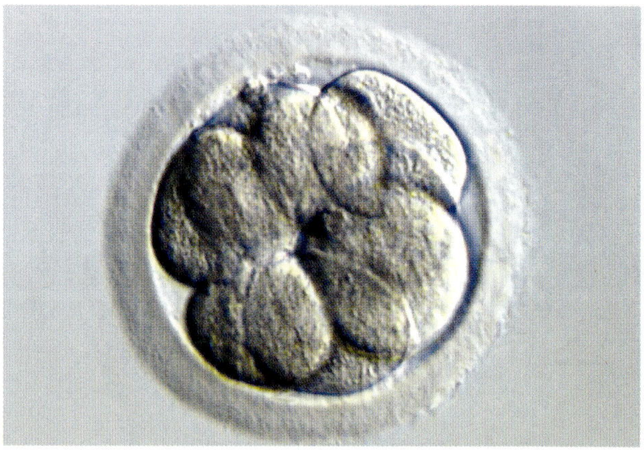

Figure 6.3 Eight-cell conceptus has a grading of I on the basis of its healthy appearance, equal size of blastomeres, and lack of cytoplasmic fragments. Polar bodies are located at a twelve-o'clock position

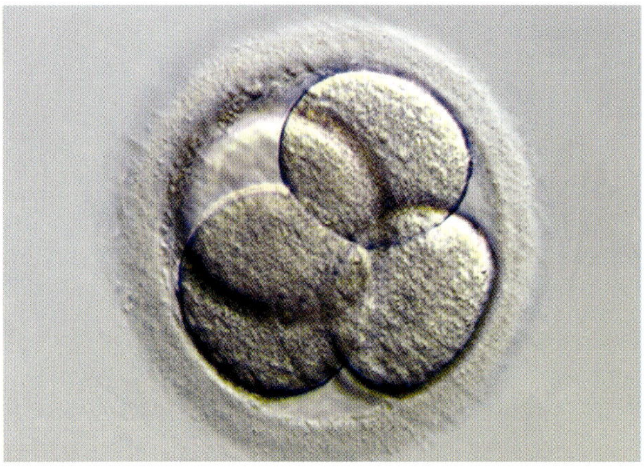

Figure 6.2 Slightly granular grade I conceptus

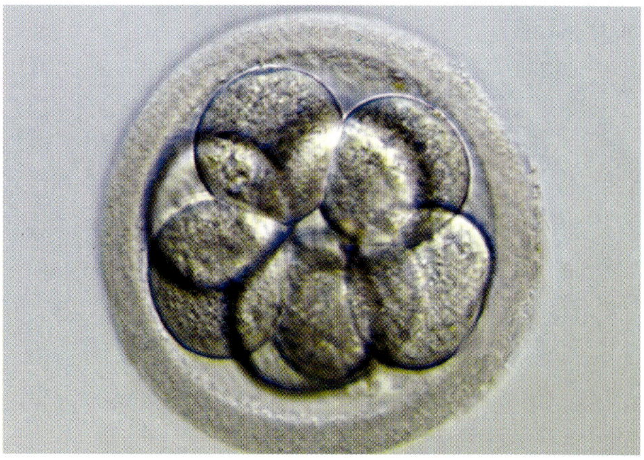

Figure 6.4 Eight-cell conceptus with a near-perfect morphology. The zona is relatively compact and exhibits almost uniform thickness

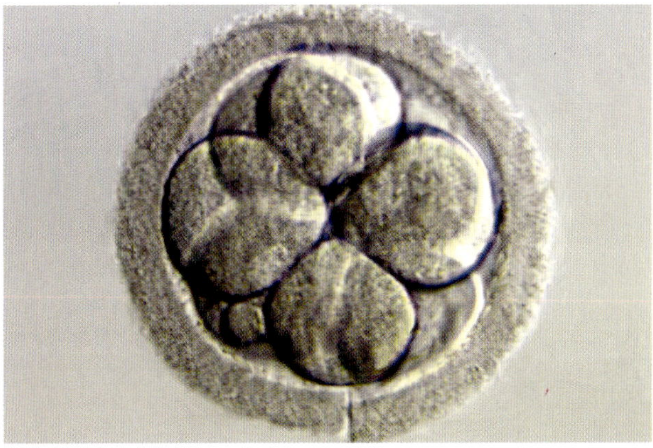

Figure 6.5 Eight-cell conceptus with excellent morphology except for a dark zona. The breach in the zona at six-o'clock is probably the result of too much pressure during removal of cumulus cells

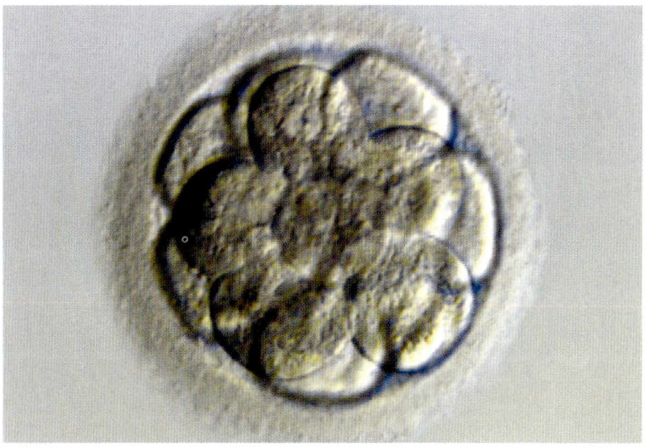

Figure 6.6 Fourteen- to sixteen-cell conceptus with grade I morphology

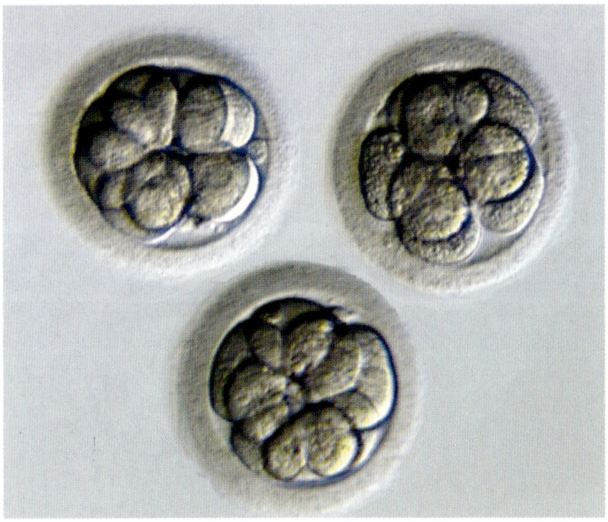

Figure 6.7 Intrauterine transfer of three grade I preembryos. The result was the delivery of one healthy child

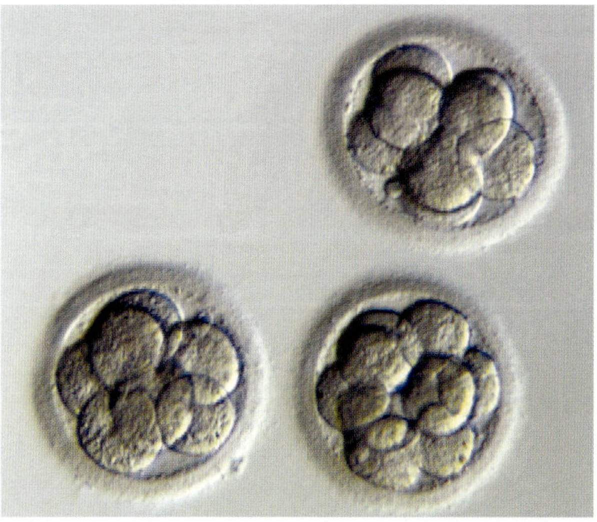

Figure 6.8 These grade I preembryos were transferred to a 41-year-old woman after each had been subjected to AHA. No pregnancy was established

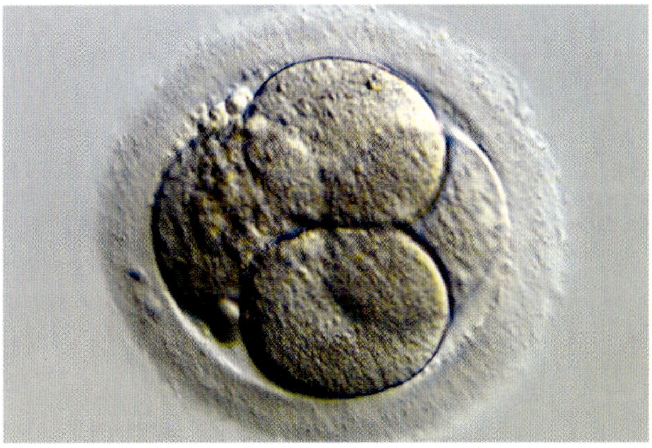

Figure 6.9 Four-cell grade 2 preembryo with symmetrical blastomeres. Minor cytoplasmic fragmentation is noted between nine- and eleven-o'clock, presumably as a result of blastomere cleavage in the upper plane of focus. One polar body is situated between the left and lower blastomeres

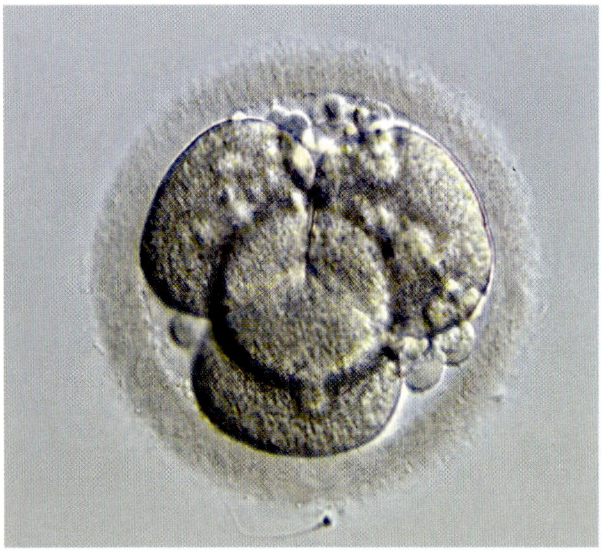

Figure 6.10 Grade 2 conceptus with minor to moderate cytoplasmic fragmentation, but in association with four equal-sized blastomeres. Fragments are scattered throughout the upper and right-sided poles. These fragments are easily removed during AHA procedures

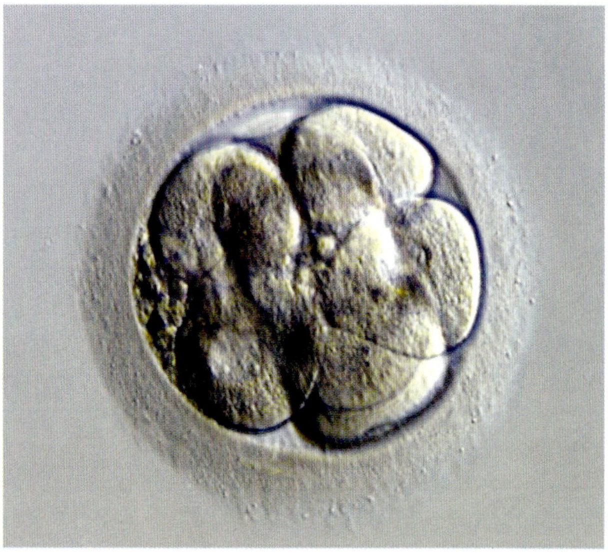

Figure 6.11 Minor localized cytoplasmic fragmentation at a nine-o'clock position in this eight-cell conceptus. A few centralized fragments are also seen in another focal plane

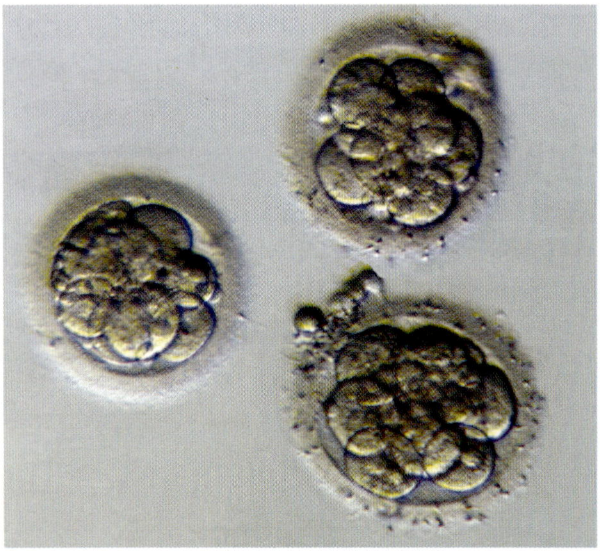

Figure 6.12 Three grade 2 preembryos with minor cytoplasmic fragmentation associated with otherwise healthy appearances. Each contains fragments scattered throughout the preembryo surface rather than localized to one area. No ongoing pregnancy followed the transfer of these conceptuses

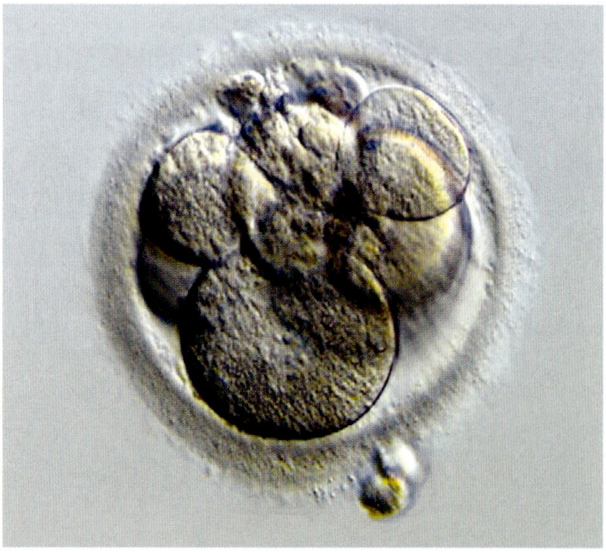

Figure 6.13 Grade 3 preembryo with blastomeres of distinctly unequal size and little or no fragmentation. One large, four intermediate, and two small blastomeres are present. The lower, larger blastomere is multinucleated

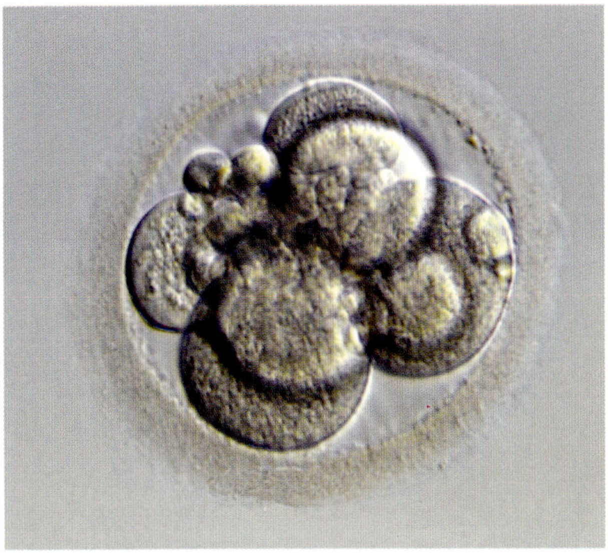

Figure 6.14 Grade 3 conceptus with two large, two intermediate, and three small blastomeres, and minor fragmentation

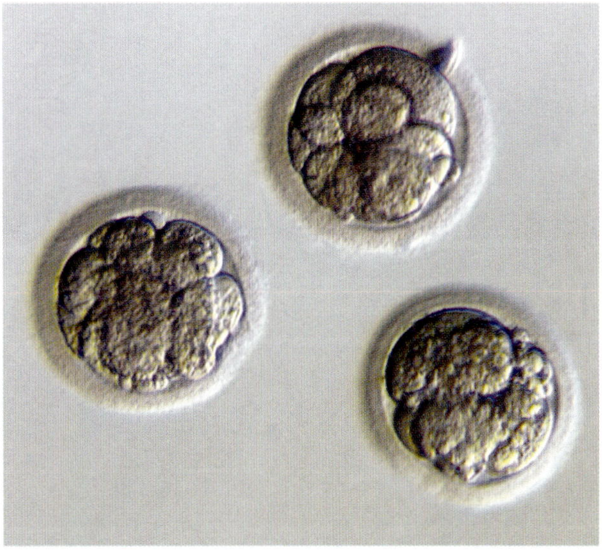

Figure 6.15 These three conceptuses were considered grade 3 on the basis of the irregularly sized blastomeres and overall morphology. Minor fragmentation can be seen in the lower two preembryos. None of these implanted after intrauterine transfer

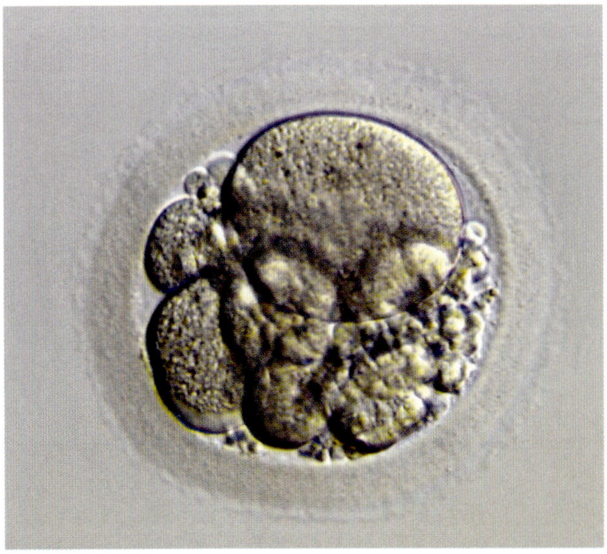

Figure 6.16 Very irregular blastomeres and significant cytoplasmic fragmentation (large and small fragments) contribute to a grading of 4 for this conceptus

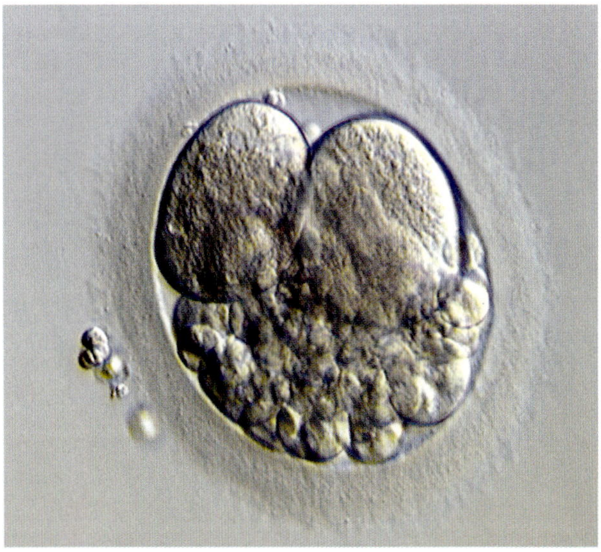

Figure 6.17 Nearly 50% of the surface of this grade 4 preembryo contains fragments. Only two blastomeres are present

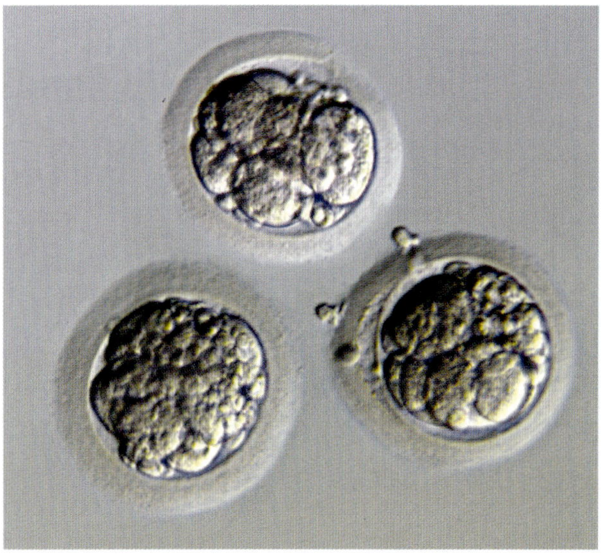

Figure 6.18 The two lowermost preembryos are grade 4 because of significant cytoplasmic fragmentation. The preembryo on the right has a bilayered zona

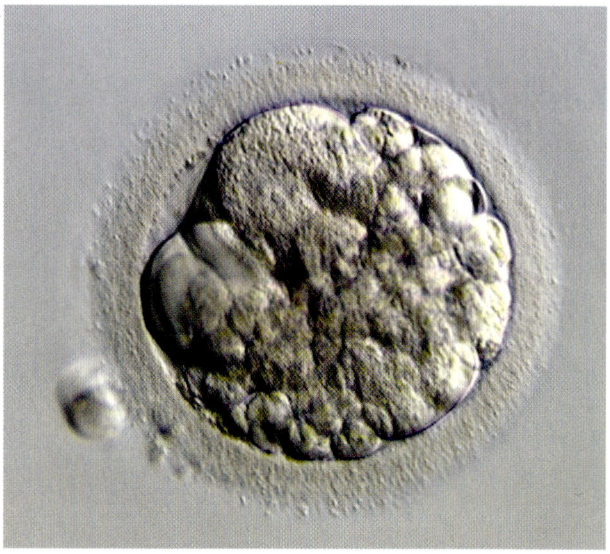

Figure 6.20 Grade 5 preembryo with approximately 80% cytoplasmic fragmentation. There is one blastomere, seen at eleven-o'clock, which has a large acytoplasmic fragment lying beneath it

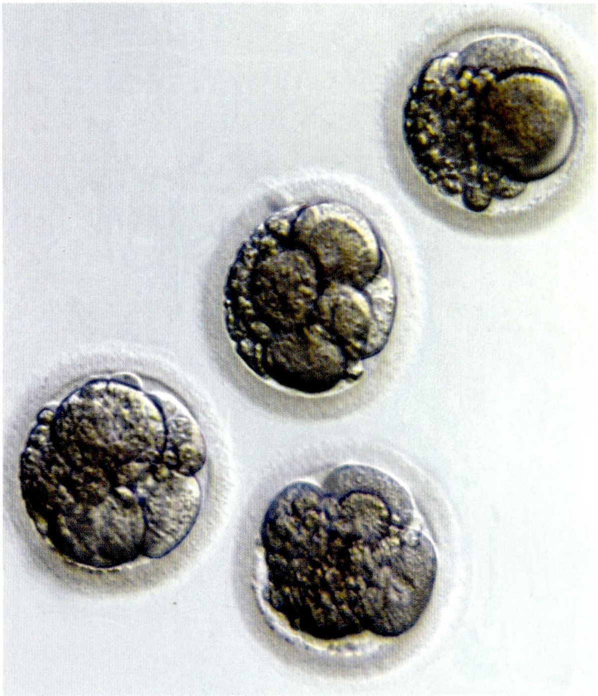

Figure 6.19 Grade 4 preembryos, three of which developed from germinal vesicle-bearing oocytes. Each shows significant cytoplasmic fragmentation, some in conjunction with irregular-sized blastomeres

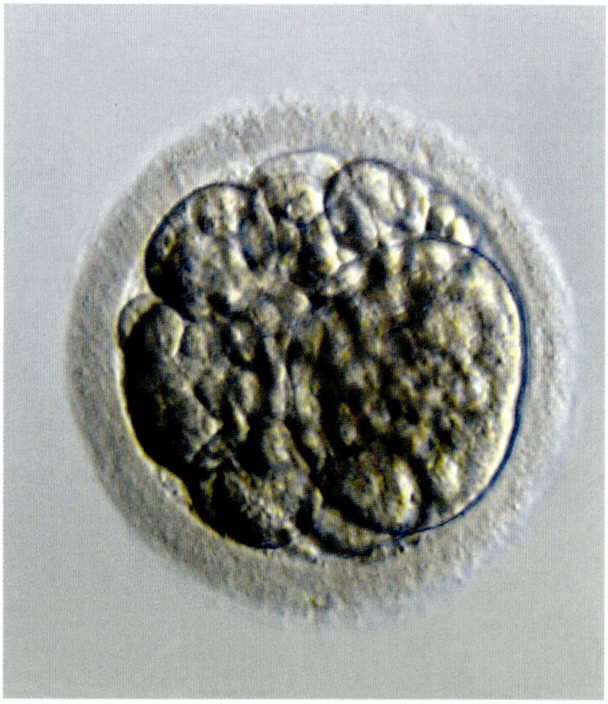

Figure 6.21 Grade 5 conceptus with a single large multinucleated blastomere associated with numerous large and small cytoplasmic fragments. Based on previous observation during growth, the structures to the left of the blastomere are probably fragments rather than small cells

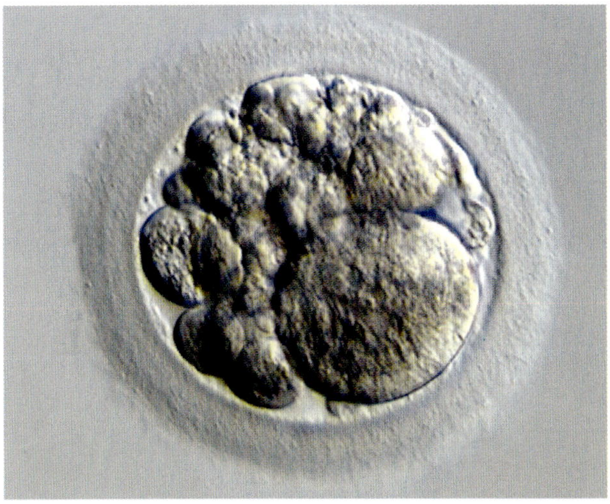

Figure 6.22 Grade 5 preembryo with a single multinucleated blastomere associated with numerous cytoplasmic fragments. Conceptuses bearing this morphology rarely contribute to pregnancy

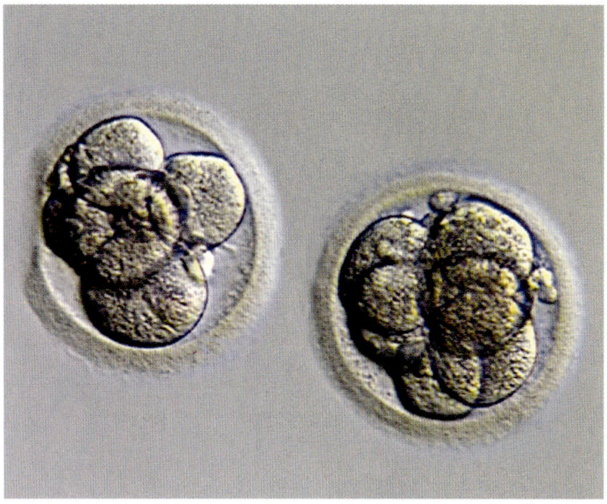

Figure 7.1 Two preembryos developed after ICSI with testicular spermatozoa. At testicular biopsy, a total of 13 spermatozoa were recovered. Because of localized fragmentation and slow growth, the upper preembryo underwent AHA and fragment removal. These two conceptuses were transferred to a 34-year-old woman on day 3 after harvest; both implanted in the uterus and led to fetal hearts on ultrasound. The twin pregnancy is now at >20 weeks of gestation without complications

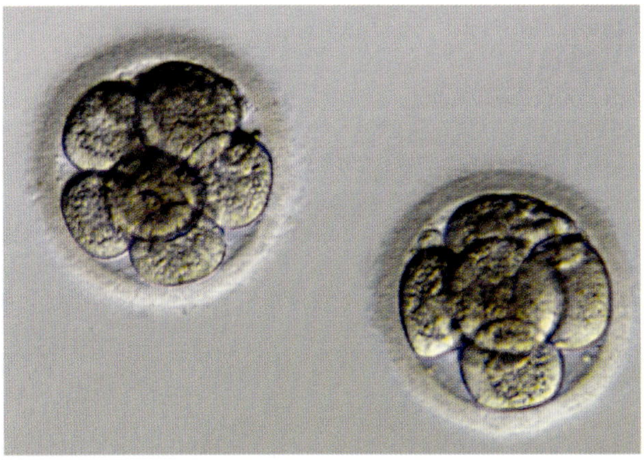

Figure 7.2 These two preembryos were transferred to a 37-year-old woman on day 3 after harvest. Both display some granularity and minor cytoplasmic fragmentation. The preembryo to the right has only six blastomeres and retains fragments at its upper pole. Both conceptuses implanted and led to fetal hearts by ultrasound, and resulted in the delivery of healthy females

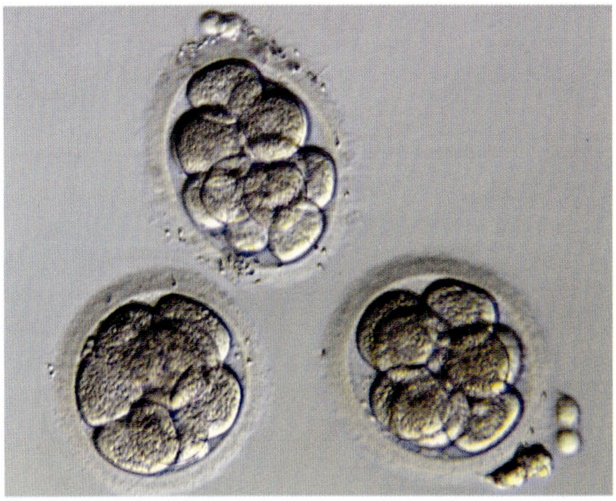

Figure 7.3 These three preembryos were transferred to a 31-year-old woman on day 3 after harvest. Each shows slightly granular blastomeres and none have fragments nor underwent AHA. After transfer, all implanted and led to fetal hearts by ultrasound. Another seven preembryos were frozen on day 3. The triplet pregnancy is now >20 weeks along without complications. Of interest is the correlation of the rapidly growing, *oval-shaped* preembryo with subsequent fetal development

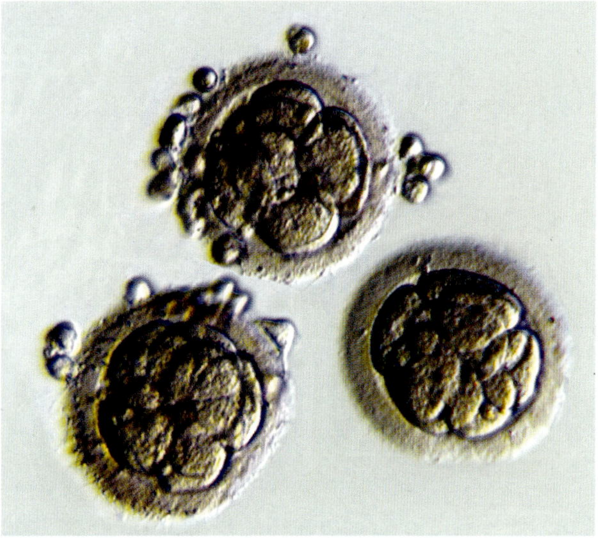

Figure 7.4 Three preembryos with slightly darkened zonae were transferred to a 29-year-old woman on day 3 after harvest. Nine other cleaved preembryos were frozen. Three fetal hearts were detected by ultrasound. The patient and her husband opted voluntarily to reduce the pregnancy to twins. Two healthy female infants were delivered by Cesarean section after an uneventful pregnancy

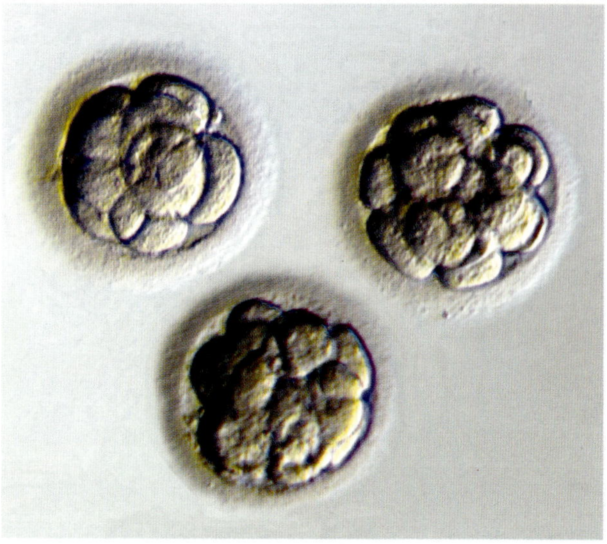

Figure 7.5 After ICSI with frozen epididymal spermatozoa, these three preembryos developed in culture. They were replaced in a 30-year-old woman following the freezing of another five prezygotes and four preembryos. None of these transferred conceptuses underwent AHA. A triplet pregnancy is now ongoing for >20 weeks without complications

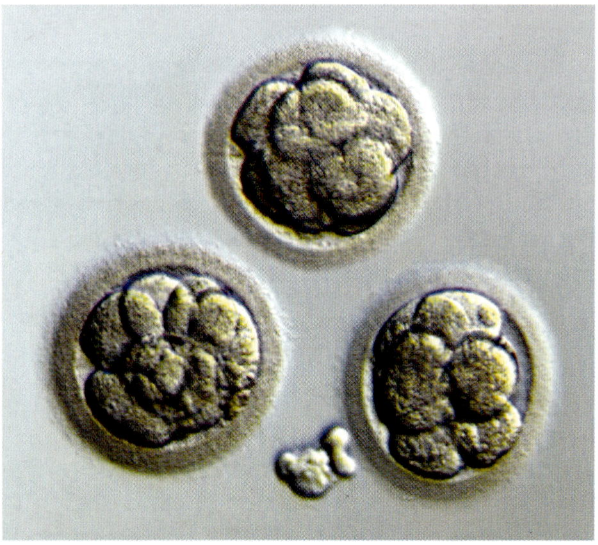

Figure 7.6 Each of these three preembryos led to the birth of a healthy child (two boys and one girl). All exhibit good morphology and acceptable growth rates; none were subjected to AHA. The 30-year-old mother also had five prezygotes and four preembryos frozen for future use

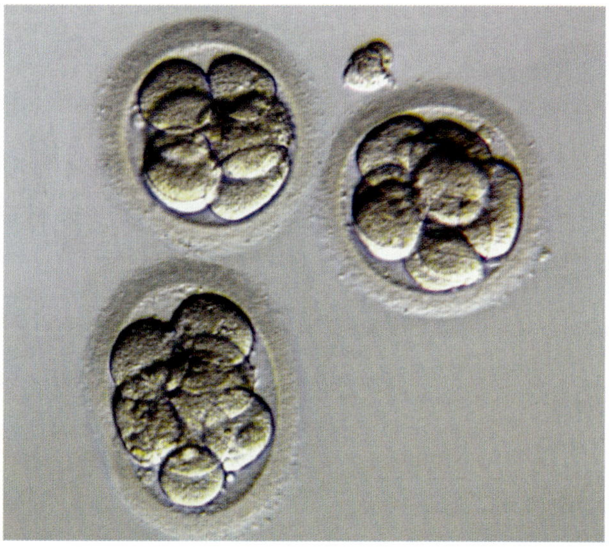

Figure 7.7 Three preembryos that led to the delivery of three healthy children, one boy and two girls. Only the lower preembryo, slightly irregular in shape, underwent AHA and was subjected to fragment removal. The 33-year-old mother had three other conceptuses frozen for potential future replacement

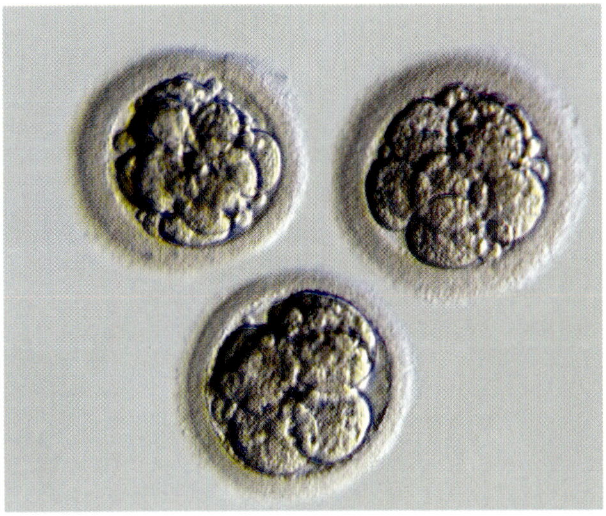

Figure 7.8 These three preembryos, all slightly fragmented, underwent AHA before transfer on day 3 to a 33-year-old woman. All three implanted. At 34 weeks, three underweight, but healthy, infant boys were delivered

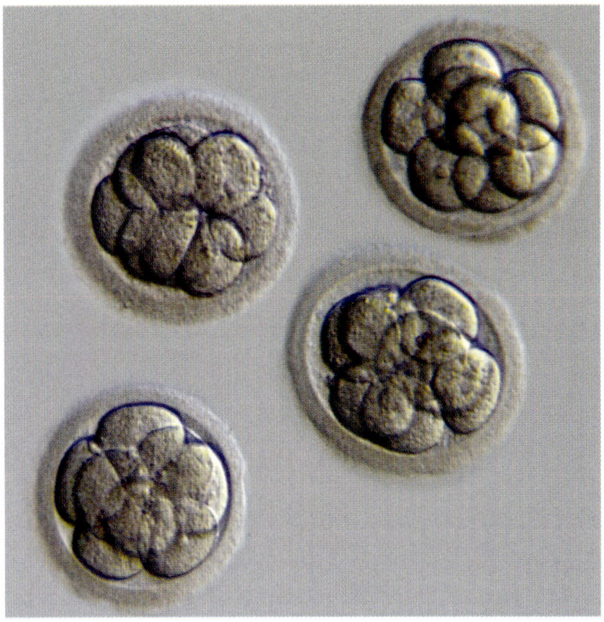

Figure 7.9 These four excellent preembryos were transferred to a 38-year-old woman on day 3 after harvest. Three of the four underwent AHA because of maternal age and previous failure of implantation in the mother. Upon discovering that all four conceptuses had implanted, the patient and her husband chose to undergo selective reduction to twins. Two boys were delivered without incident

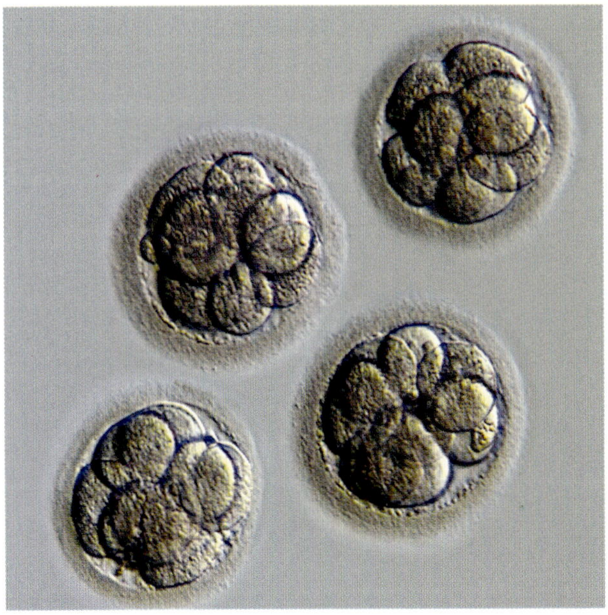

Figure 7.10 After fresh epididymal sperm collection, 13 preembryos developed in this cycle from a 36-year-old woman. Five prezygotes and four cleaved preembryos were cryopreserved before transfer. These four preembryos were replaced on day 3 after harvest. All underwent AHA and fragment removal, and all implanted in the patient's uterus. At this time, the quadruplet pregnancy is ongoing for >20 weeks

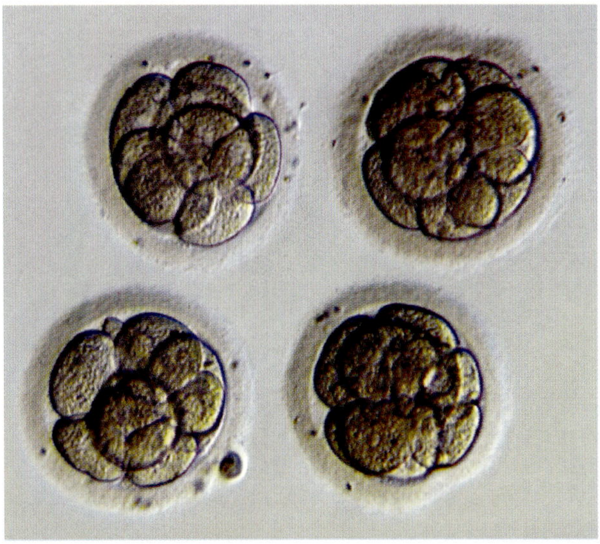

Figure 7.11 These four preembryos led to four fetal hearts in a 36-year-old woman. Two of the four conceptuses were subjected to AHA. After selective reduction to twins, the patient delivered two healthy children, a boy and a girl

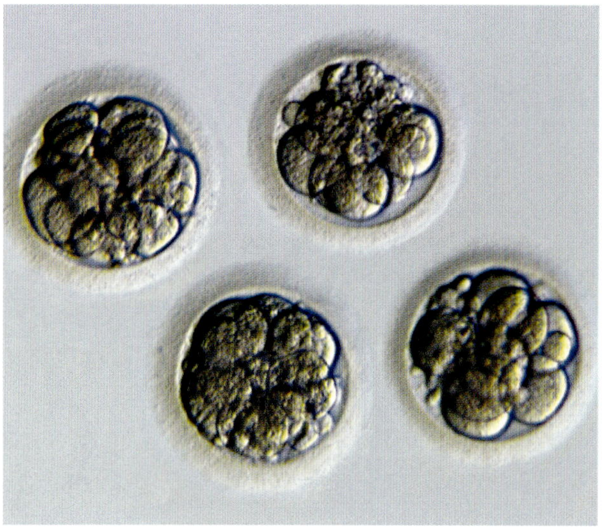

Figure 7.12 These four preembryos, three of which are slightly fragmented, led to four fetal hearts in a 35-year-old woman. Two of the four underwent selective AHA *in vitro*; seven other conceptuses were frozen. The quadruplet pregnancy was electively reduced to a single gestation; a healthy female child was delivered

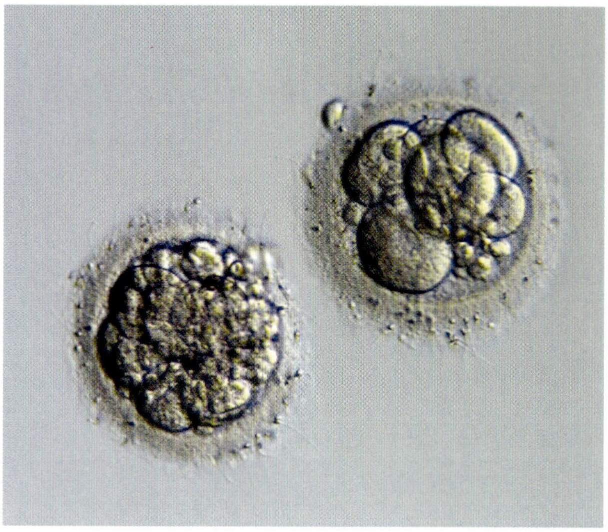

Figure 7.13 Two preembryos, neither of which underwent AHA due to lack of patient's consent, were transferred to a 39-year-old woman on day 3. One of these led to a fetal heartbeat and a normal pregnancy that is near term. The preembryo on the left is highly fragmented; the one on the right has irregularly sized blastomeres and localized fragments

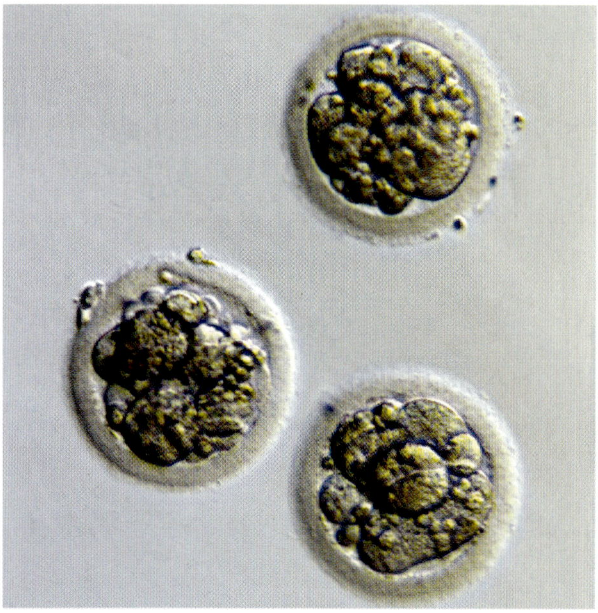

Figure 7.14 These fragmented preembryos were transferred to a 33-year-old woman on day 3. All three were subjected to AHA and fragment removal, but many fragments remain. One of these implanted and led to the birth of a healthy female child

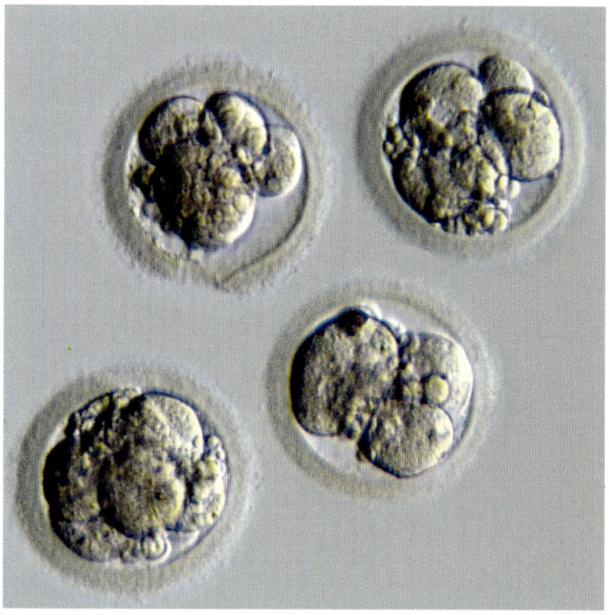

Figure 7.15 Four slow-growing and fragmented preembryos were transferred to a 43-year-old woman on day 3. Despite AHA, all four demonstrate poor morphology. One fetal heart was detected by ultrasound within a few weeks of replacement. The pregnancy is ongoing for >20 weeks

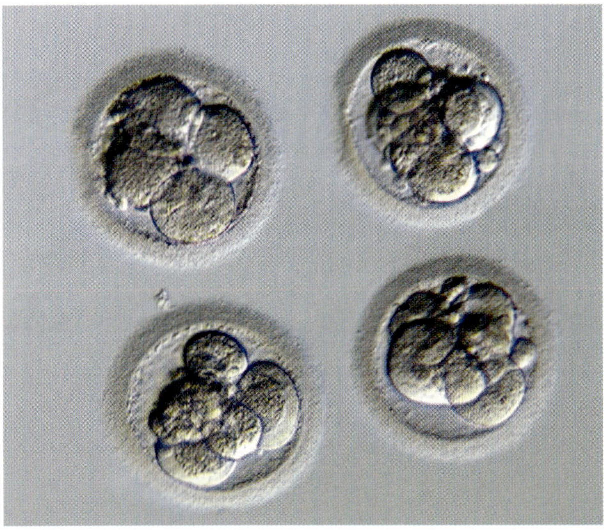

Figure 7.16 These slow-growing preembryos were transferred to a 36-year-old woman on day 3. All four were aggressively treated by fragment removal following AHA. The lower left conceptus displays intense cortical clearing of organelles and irregular-sized blastomeres. Surprisingly, one of these preembryos implanted and led to an ongoing pregnancy that is near term

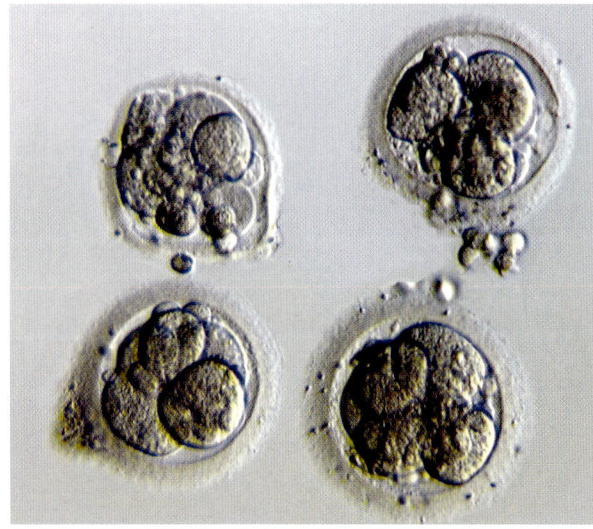

Figure 7.17 Slow growth, cytoplasmic fragments, and zonae defects mark this transfer of four preembryos on day 3. All underwent AHA. Nonetheless, the patient, aged 37 years, established an ongoing pregnancy that led to the birth of a normal boy. Note that the zona of the upper left preembryo is extraordinarily thin and fragile-looking. The zona of another preembryo is marred by a darkened bilayer zona defect

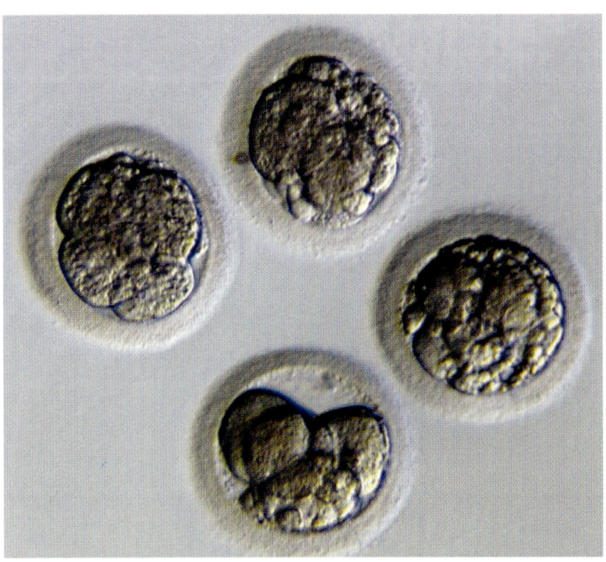

Figure 7.18 A 40-year-old woman received these preembryos on day 3 after harvest. Although all four underwent AHA and fragment removal, two (uppermost and on the right) retain an excessive number of fragments and have thick zonae. The conceptus on the left is intensely granular and has only four blastomeres; the lowermost preembryo displays the best morphology, but is slow-growing with a large perivitelline area from which fragments were removed. Two fetal hearts were detected by ultrasound after replacement. Chromosome analysis of both fetuses following amniocentesis was normal. Two healthy children, a boy and a girl, were delivered without incident

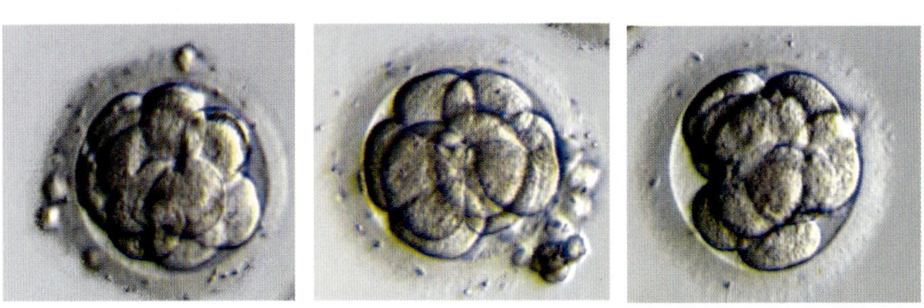

Figure 7.19 Three morphologically healthy preembryos, none of which underwent AHA, were replaced in a 31-year-old woman; all failed to implant

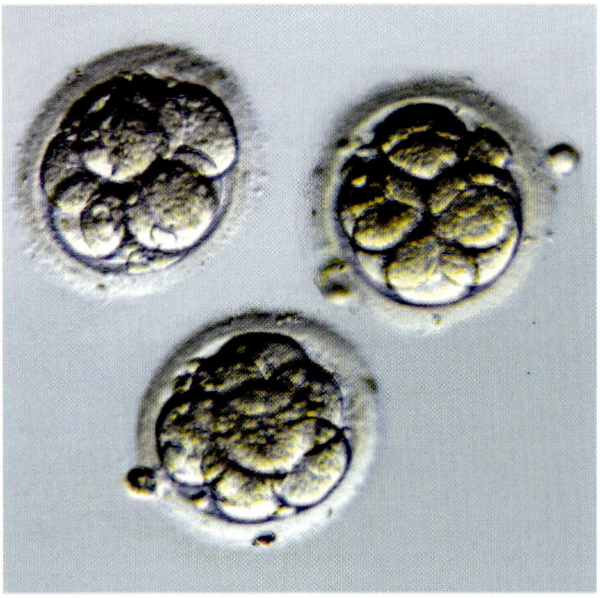

Figure 7.20 A 31-year-old woman received these three normally growing conceptuses, one of which underwent AHA. No pregnancy resulted from their replacement

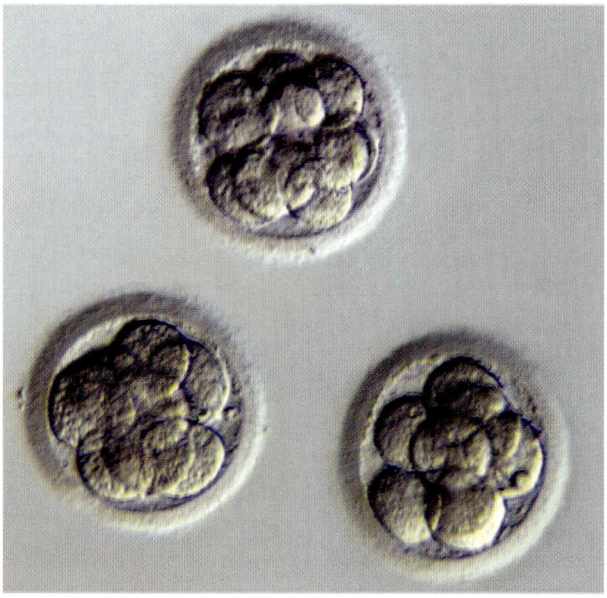

Figure 7.21 Good morphology and thin zonae characterize these three preembryos replaced in a 41-year-old woman. All three were subjected to AHA, but no pregnancy followed the transfer

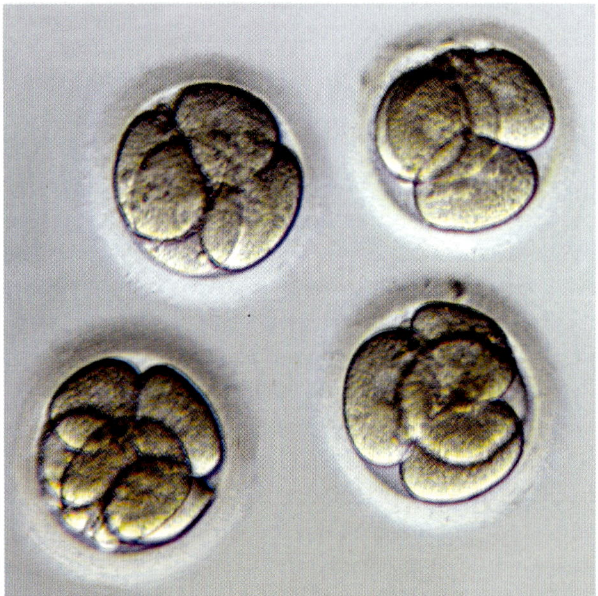

Figure 7.22 These healthy-looking day 2 preembryos were transferred to a 39-year-old woman after three of the four were subjected to AHA. No pregnancy was established

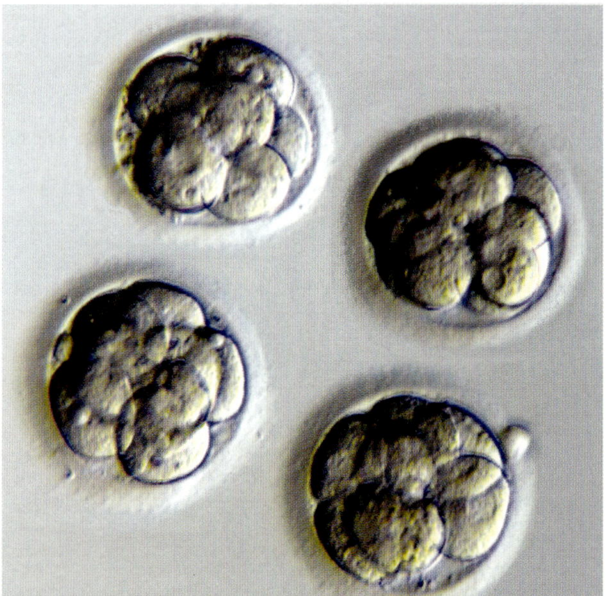

Figure 7.23 Four healthy-looking preembryos were transferred to a 38-year-old woman after three of the four underwent AHA. The upper right preembryo displays two small vacuoles in one of its blastomeres. No pregnancy followed this intrauterine transfer

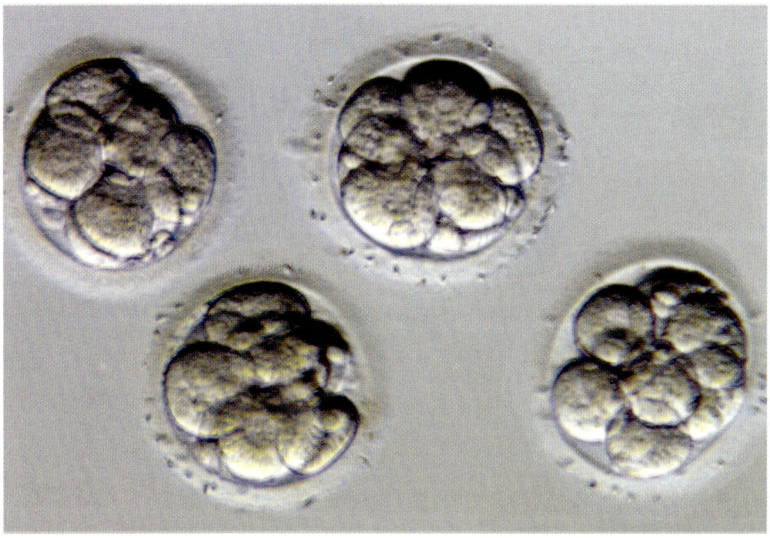

Figure 7.24 Good growth and minor fragmentation characterize these preembryos replaced in a 39-year-old woman on day 3. Three of the four conceptuses were subjected to AHA. No pregnancy was established

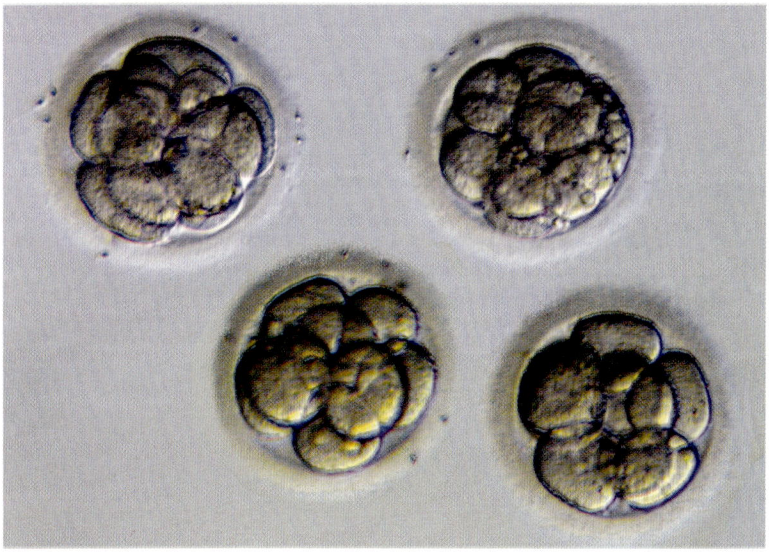

Figure 7.25 Three of four healthy-looking preembryos were subjected to AHA in this cycle from a 38-year-old patient. Because the preembryos displayed such excellent morphology and growth rate, it was surprising when implantation failed to occur. Seven other conceptuses were frozen during this attempt, one of which subsequently produced a healthy boy after thawing

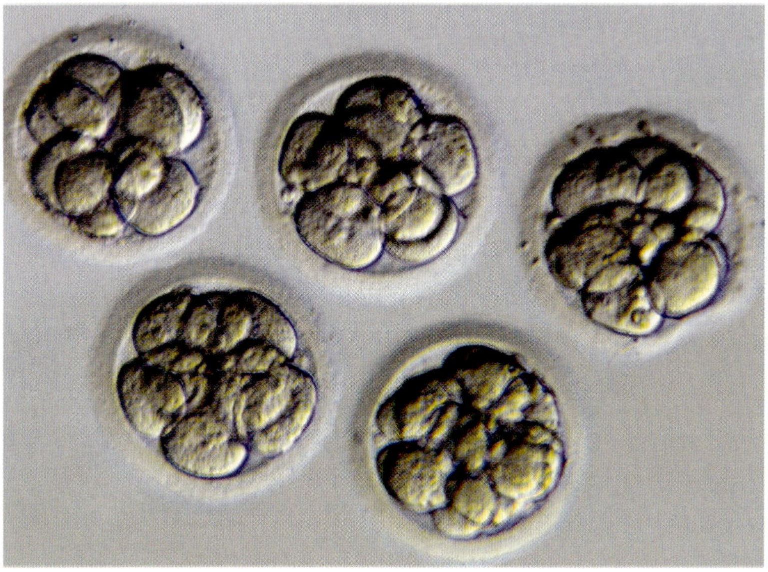

Figure 7.26 Five perfect conceptuses were replaced in a 41-year-old woman after a difficult intrauterine transfer. Despite good growth rate, excellent morphology, and thin zonae, none implanted. Four of the five had undergone AHA before transfer

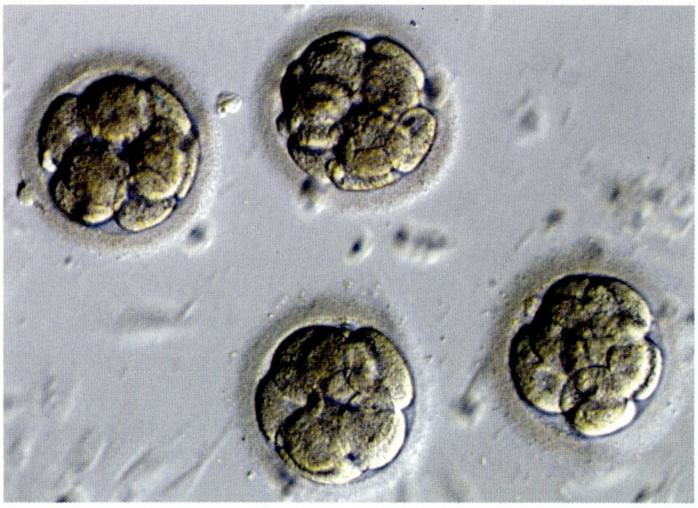

Figure 7.27 Preembryos growing on an endometrial cell coculture monolayer. One of these preembryos led to normal fetal development; the gestation is currently ongoing

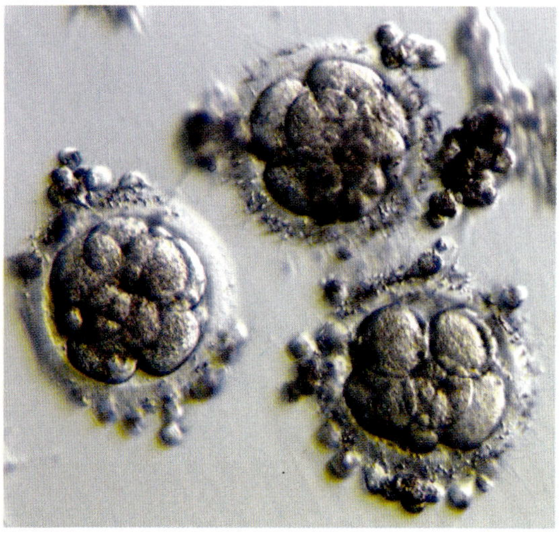

Figure 7.28 Preembryos growing on a granulosa cell coculture monolayer. After multiple previous failed attempts to become pregnant through IVF, the 41-year-old patient established a pregnancy, but underwent early pregnancy loss

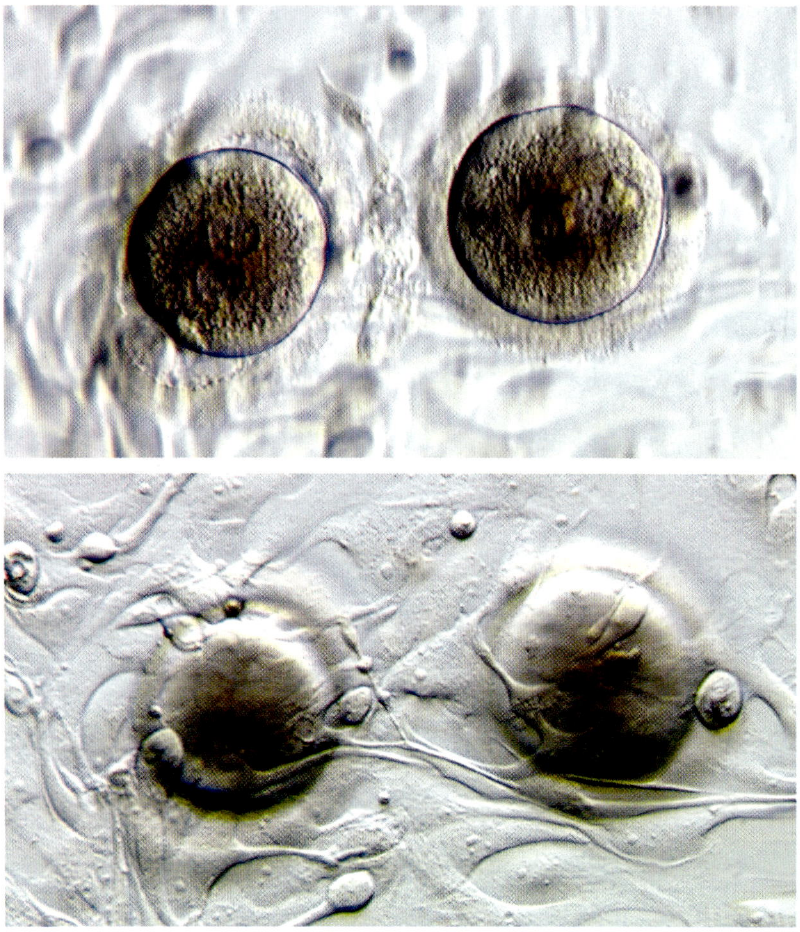

Figure 7.29 Different focal planes show prezygotes (upper) and endometrial coculture cells (lower). The prezygotes were cultured from a 40-year-old woman after multiple failed attempts at IVF. Her husband required testicular biopsy to retrieve spermatozoa for ICSI

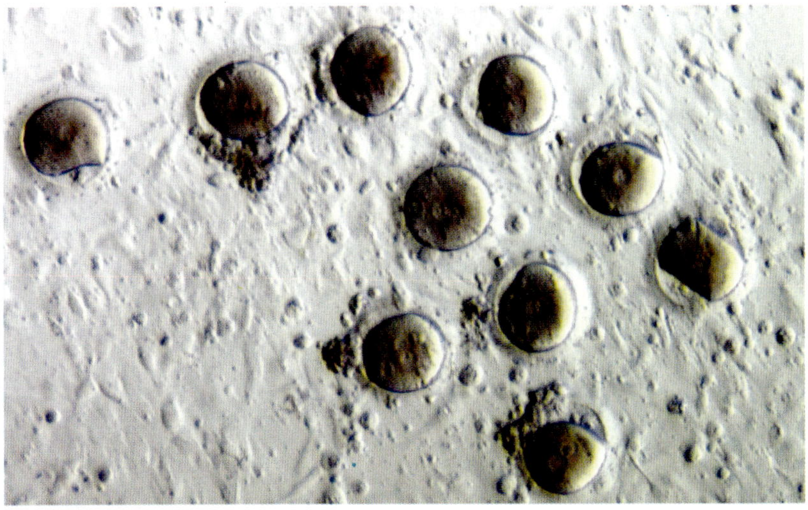

Figure 7.30 Ten prezygotes on a layer of endometrial coculture cells

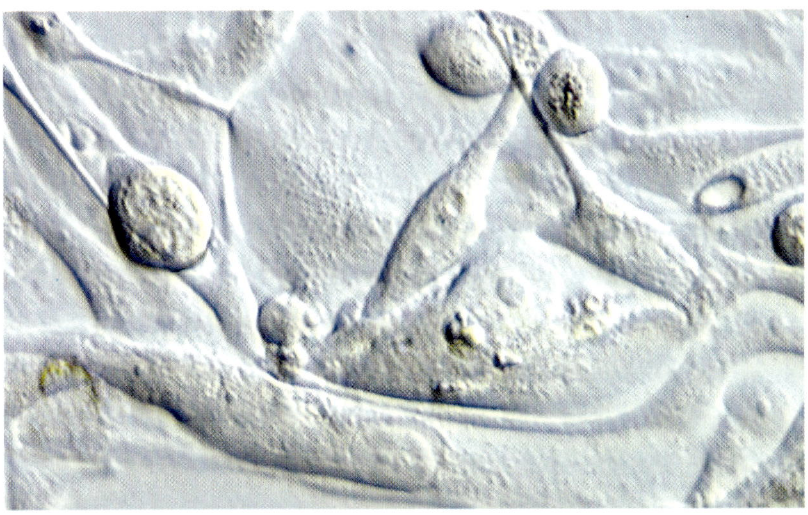

Figure 7.31 High-power view shows the typical morphology of endometrial cells growing in culture

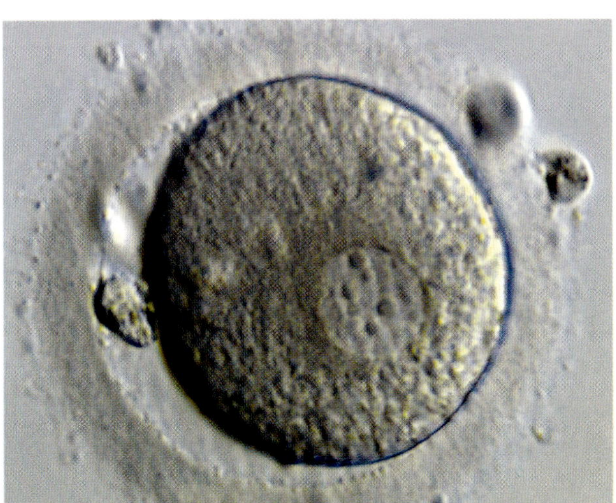

Figure 8.1 Single-pronucleate oocyte. The rather large single pronucleus displays several randomly located nucleoli

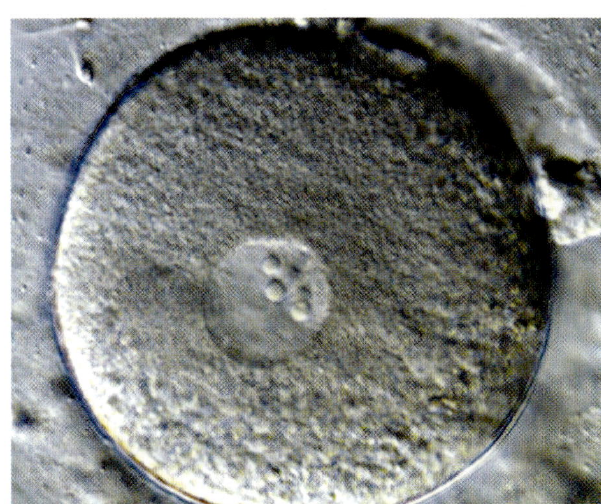

Figure 8.2 Oocyte with a single pronucleus and two polar bodies. The normal-sized pronucleus has five or six unilateral nucleoli

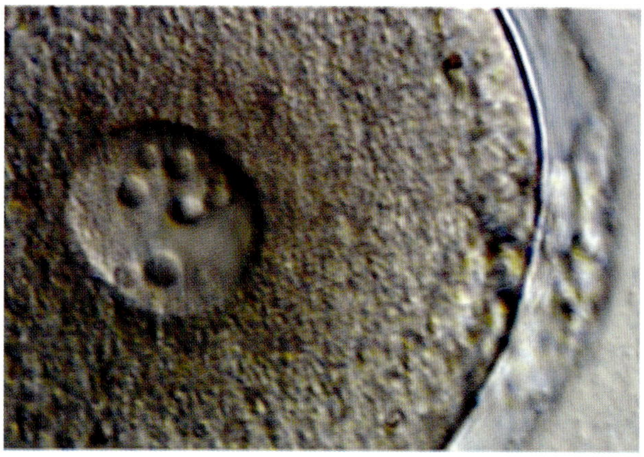

Figure 8.3 Oocyte with a single large distinct pronucleus with seven nucleoli. One or more fragmented polar bodies are seen to the right

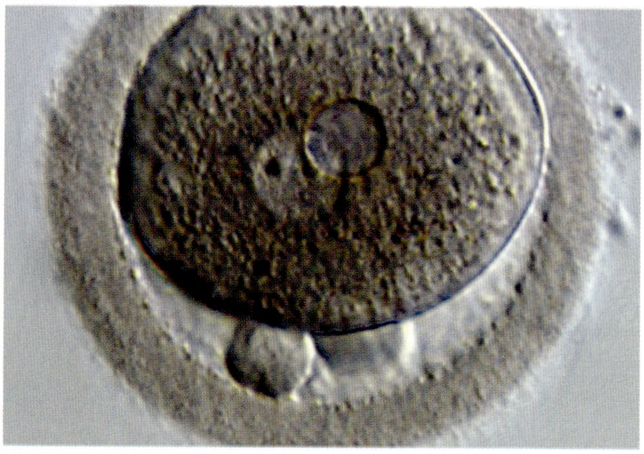

Figure 8.4 Oocyte with one pronucleus, one vacuole, and two large polar bodies. As the vacuole overlaps the single pronucleus, it appears to be a second pronucleus, but the vacuole contains no nucleoli and is different in both depth and content

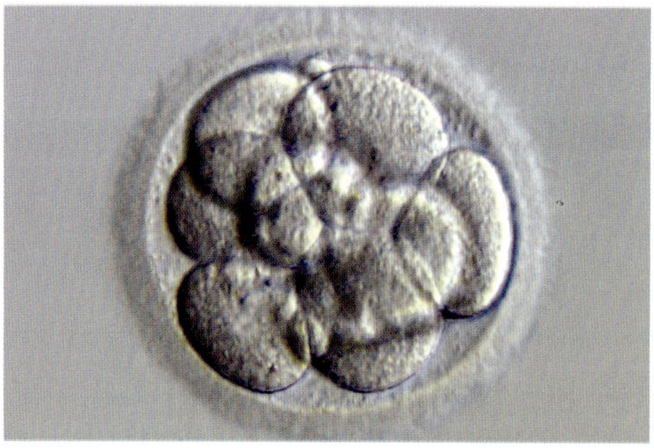

Figure 8.5 Eight-cell conceptus developed from a single-pronucleate oocyte. The morphology of these preembryos is often apparently normal. If generated after standard insemination, the oocyte exhibiting one pronucleus may, in fact, be diploid in DNA content[23]

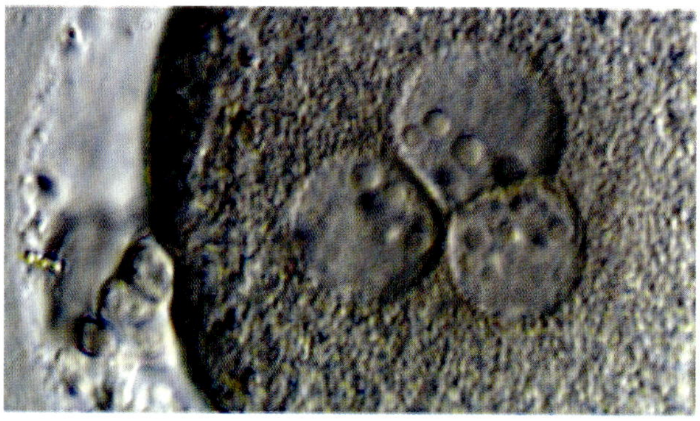

Figure 8.6 Triploid prezygote: Inseminated oocyte with one small and two large pronuclei. Although this suggests polyspermy, a larger pronucleus is located nearest the site of polar body extrusion

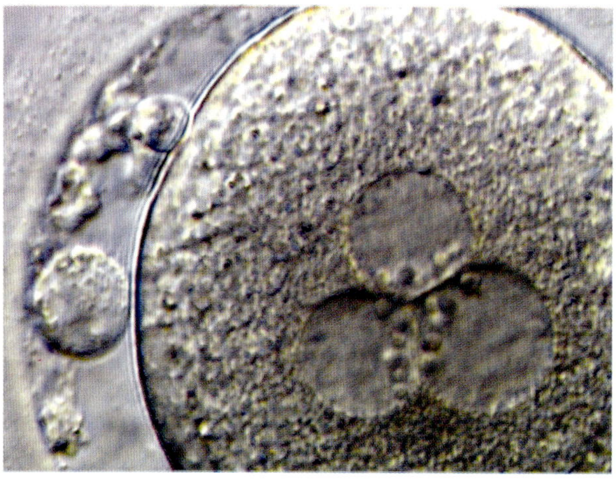

Figure 8.7 Triploid prezygote: Inseminated oocyte with one large and two smaller pronuclei. Polar body status is unclear because of the fragmented debris in the perivitelline space. Nucleoli within each pronuclear structure have aligned at adjacent pronuclear borders

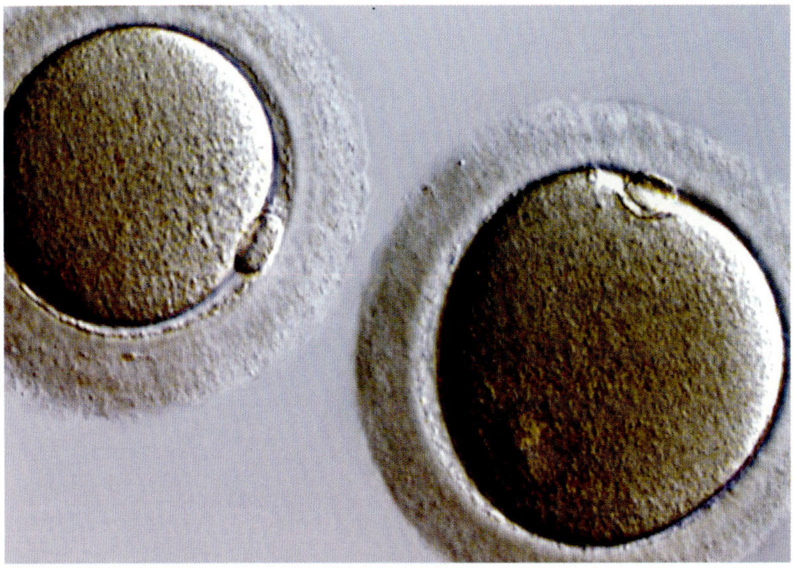

Figure 8.8 Uninseminated giant oocyte: Compared with its sibling, the cytoplasmic volume of the oocyte on the right is much greater. The size of the first polar body associated with the larger oocyte appears to be normal. Both oocytes possess rather thick zonae

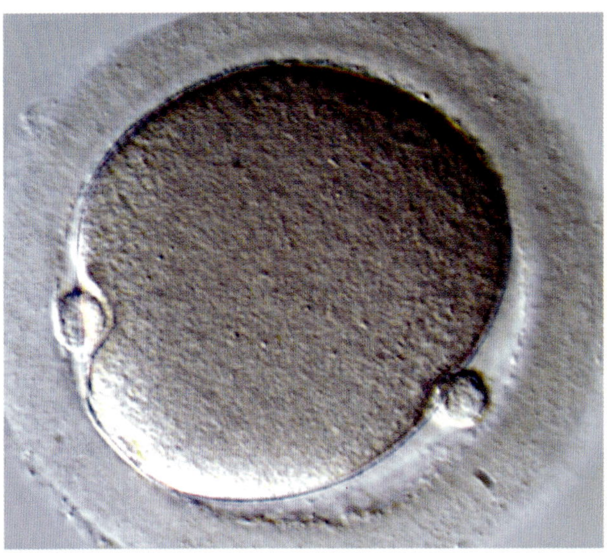

Figure 8.9 Uninseminated giant oocyte with two polar bodies located at opposite poles

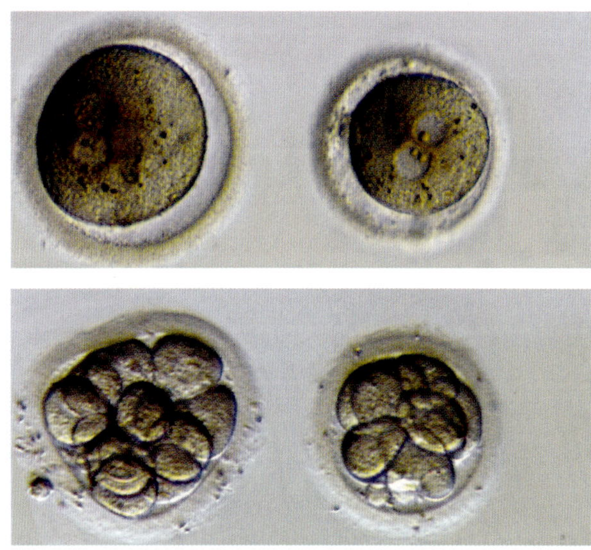

Figure 8.10 Overly large gametes and conceptuses: Pronuclear oocytes (upper), one of which is clearly larger than normal. Cleaved conceptuses (lower), one of which is clearly larger than the other (developed from an oocyte with four pronuclei before cleavage)

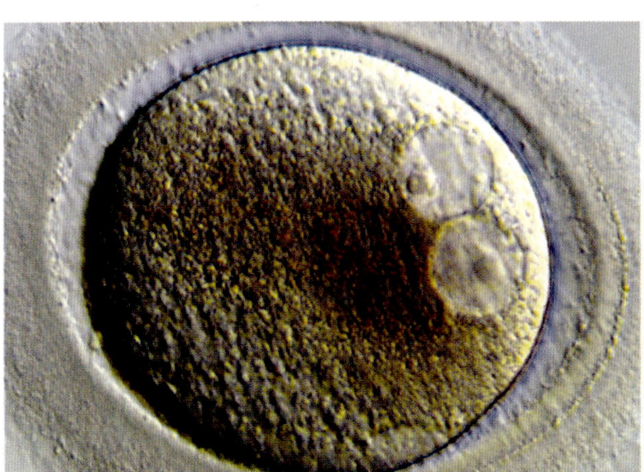

Figure 8.11 Binucleate germinal vesicle-bearing oocyte arrested at PI of maturation. Both undersized germinal vesicles show distinct nuceloli

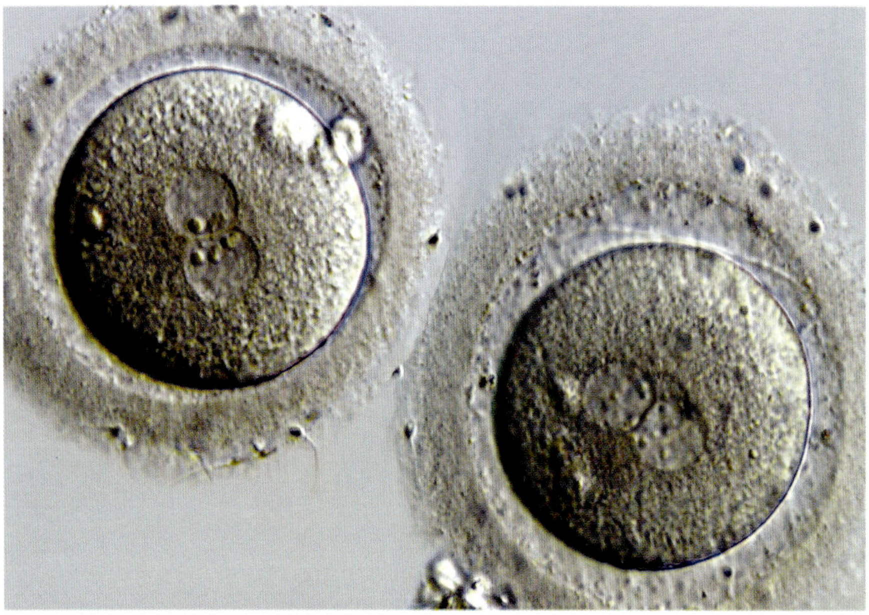

Figure 8.12 Comparison of pronuclear size in diploid and triploid prezygotes: The oocyte on the left has two pronuclei of normal size; that on the right has three pronuclei, all slightly smaller than those of the diploid conceptus

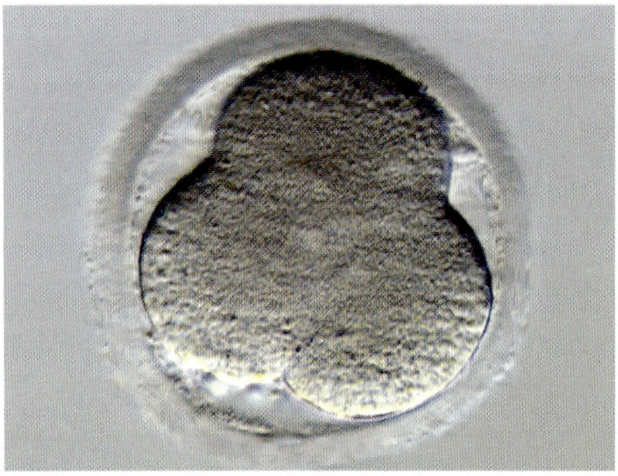

Figure 8.13 Early first cleavage of a zygote with a tripolar spindle. Three blastomeres are forming

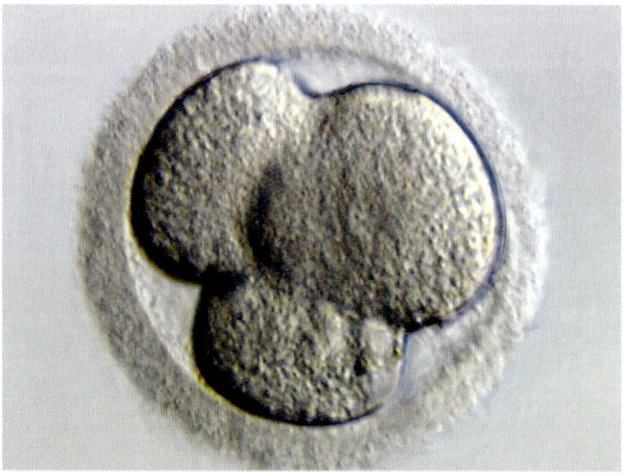

Figure 8.14 Telophase of the first mitotic cleavage of a zygote with a tripolar spindle. Direct cleavage into three blastomeres is not uncommon in triploid conceptuses

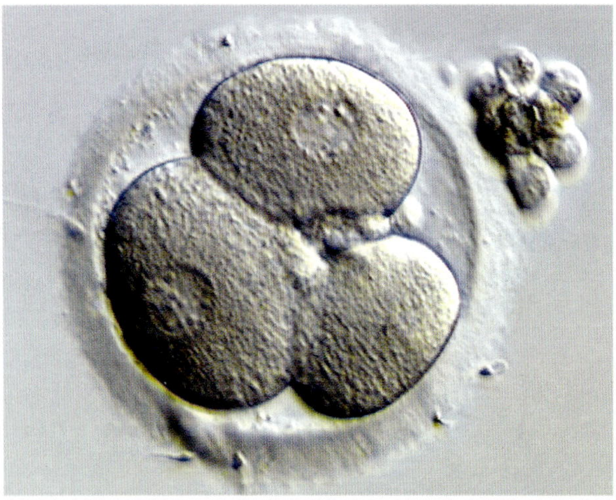

Figure 8.15 Result of first cleavage of a triploid prezygote. Three blastomeric structures are present, but only two possess nuclei. This is an example of the formation of two blastomeres and an extrusion mass (described by Kola *et al.*[29])

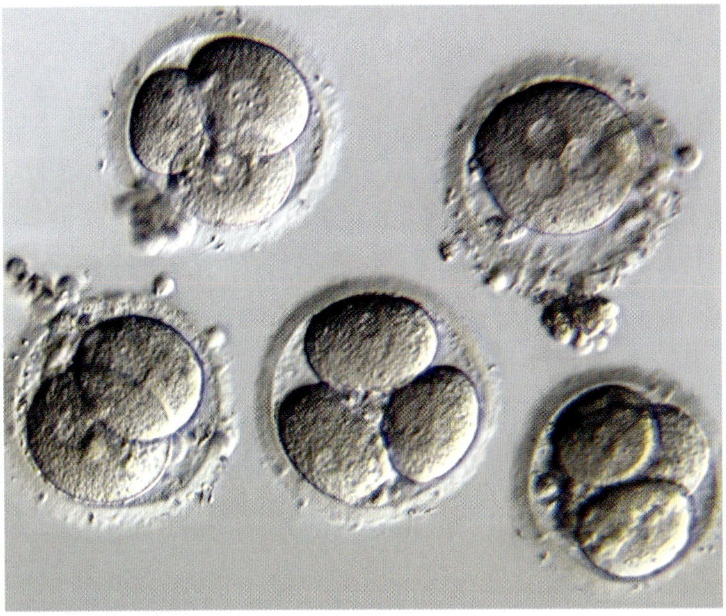

Figure 8.16 Various fates of tripronuclear prezygotes. One triploid specimen has failed to enter syngamy and proceed to the first cleavage; another has divided into two blastomeres; two have two blastomeres and an extrusion mass; and one has three multinucleated blastomeres

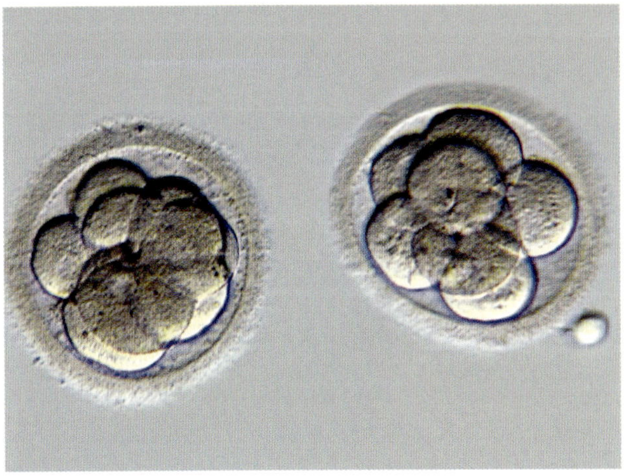

Figure 8.17 Two triploid conceptuses on day 3 after harvest. The generally normal morphological appearance of cleaved conceptuses developing from triploid prezygotes demands that ploidy be determined before cleavage occurs

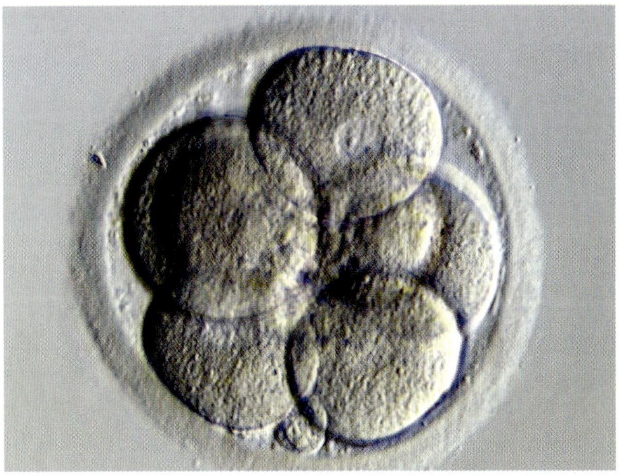

Figure 8.18 Preembryo generated from an oocyte possessing three pronuclei after insemination. Eight blastomeres are present in this apparently morphologically normal specimen

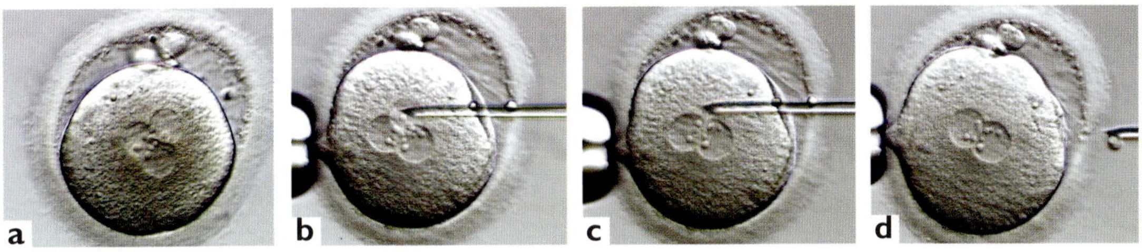

Figure 8.19 Pronucleus removal: (a) Prezygote with three proncuclei and two polar bodies following ICSI. (b) As digyny is strongly suspected, a micropipette is passed through the zona into the pronucleus nearest the polar bodies. (c) The pronucleus is gently aspirated into the micropipette. (d) The micropipette is withdrawn, restoring a diploid state. This procedure was followed by normal cleavage

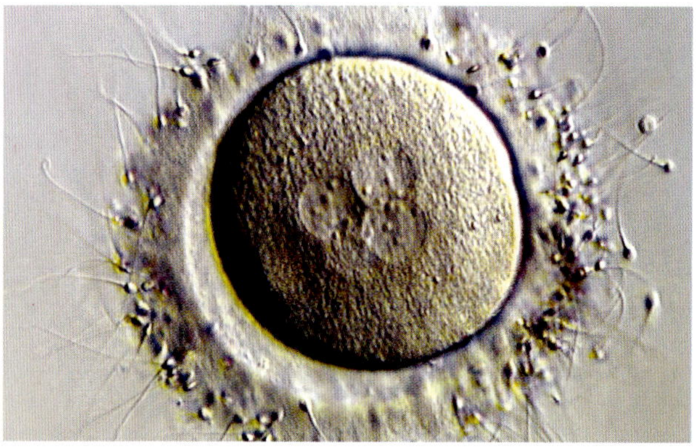

Figure 8.20 Tetraploid prezygote with four distinct pronuclei. The number of sperm bound to the zona is excessive despite the application of a standard inseminating sperm concentration

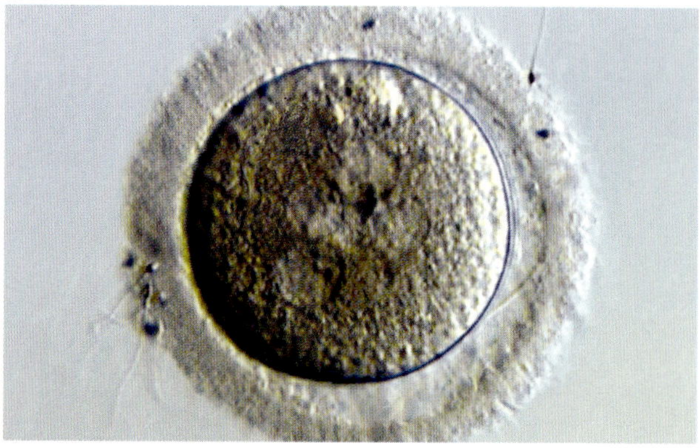

Figure 8.21 Oocyte displaying six pronuclei after standard insemination

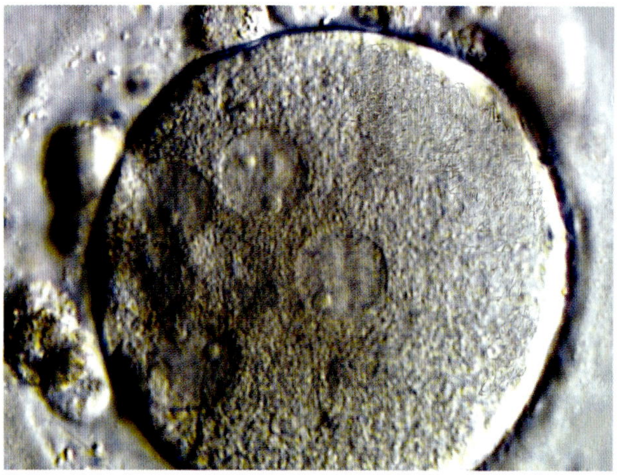

Figure 8.22 Oocyte with five to seven pronuclei after standard insemination. Large fragments, debris, and extraneous spermatozoa are present in the perivitelline space of this generally unhealthy-looking prezygote

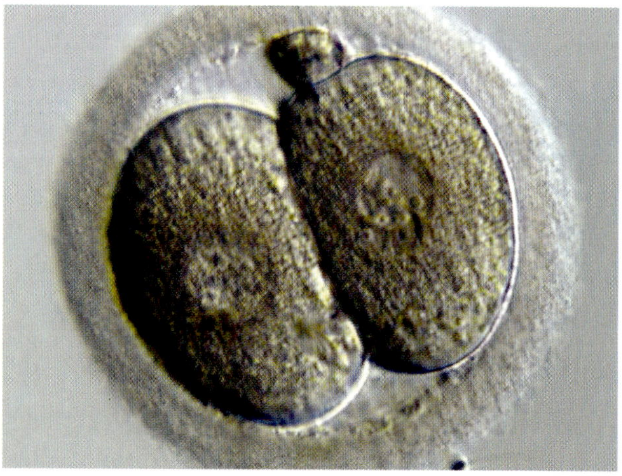

Figure 8.23 Two-cell conceptus with two multinucleated blastomeres. The blastomere on the right (in focus) shows one large and one small nucleus; that on the left is also multinucleated (but out of focus)

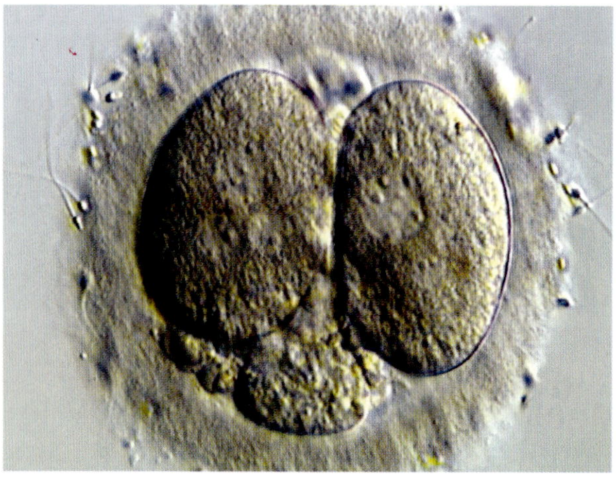

Figure 8.24 Triploid conceptus with two multinucleated blastomeres and an extrusion mass. The blastomere on the left contains at least three nuclei whereas the one on the right has two nuclei (one very faint small nucleus below the larger one)

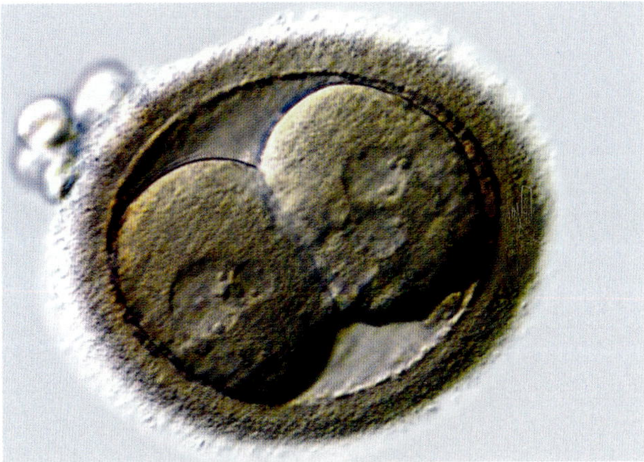

Figure 8.25 Extremely dark cytoplasm and zona accompany this unhealthy-looking multinucleated preembryo. Each blastomere possesses at least three nuclei or nuclear fragments

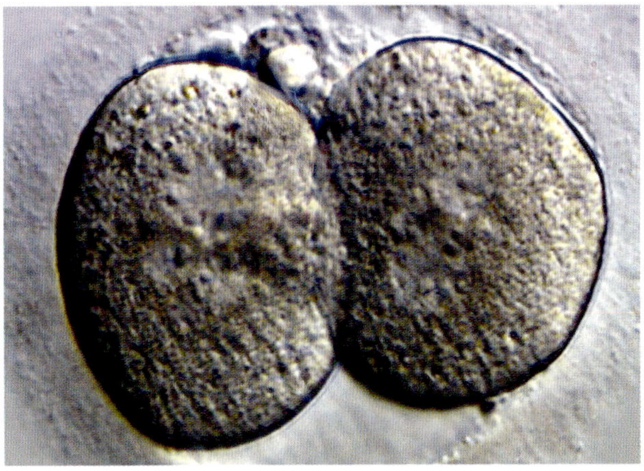

Figure 8.26 Two-cell conceptus with two multinucleated blastomeres

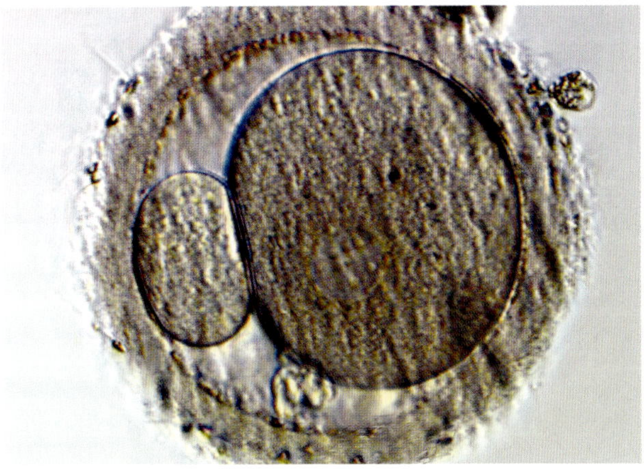

Figure 8.27 Abnormally large polar-body-like structure seen 18h after insemination. A second polar body is at the six-o'clock position. The large structure was first noted at the time of oocyte harvest; no other smaller structure was identifiable as a first polar body. A single, albeit faint, pronucleus is present near the center of the oocyte

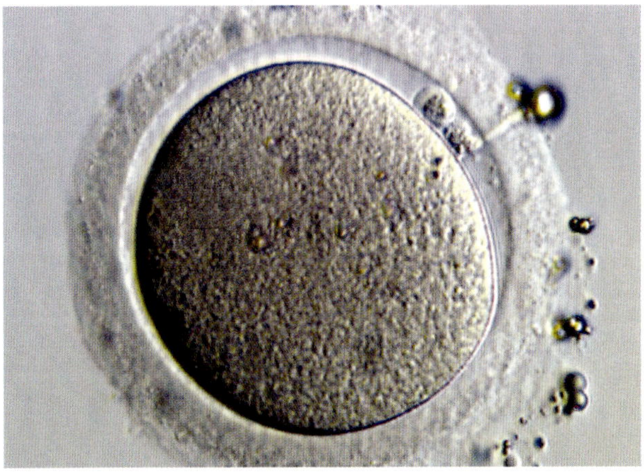

Figure 8.28 Small, fragmented first polar body

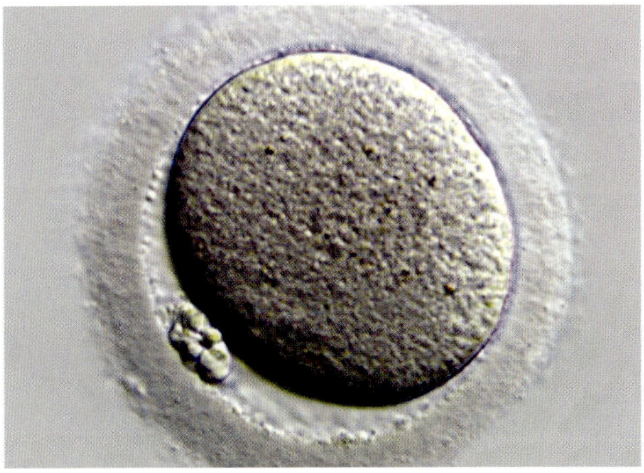

Figure 8.29 Fragmented first polar body associated with a slightly granular oocyte

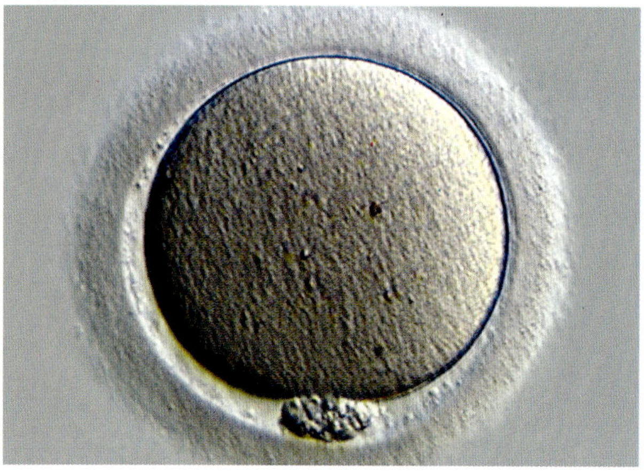

Figure 8.30 Fragmenting first polar body

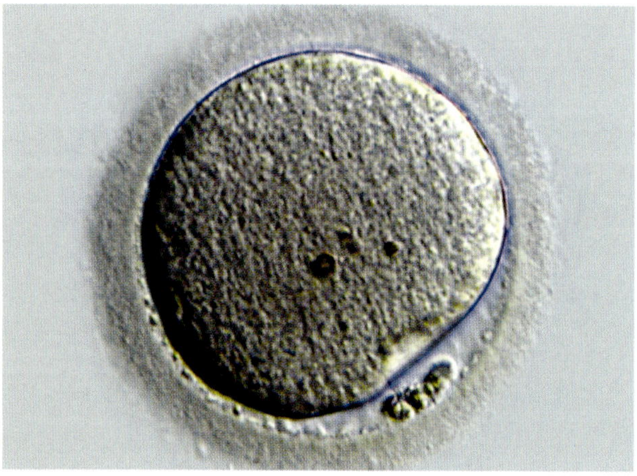

Figure 8.31 Completely detached and fragmented first polar body

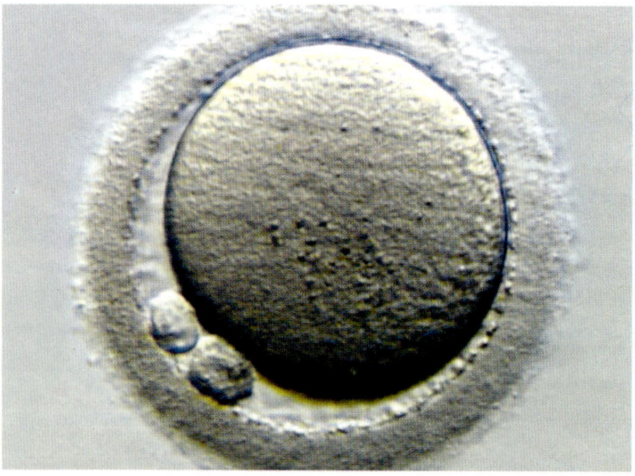

Figure 8.32 Uninseminated oocyte with two polar bodies

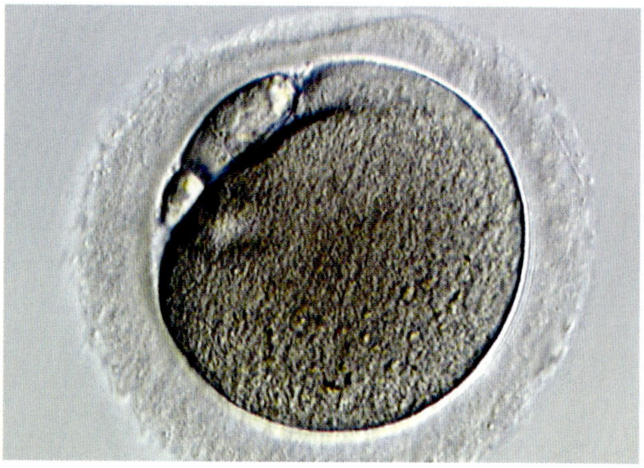

Figure 8.33 'Immature' first polar body as described by Xia[53]. Note the flattened configuration. This oocyte matured *in vitro* from PI of maturation

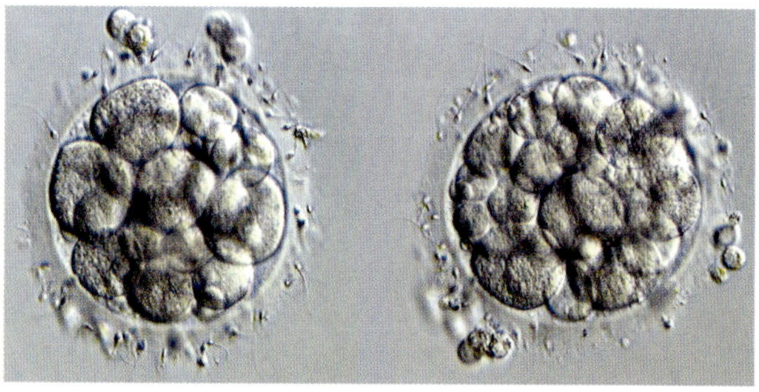

Figure 8.34 Complete cytoplasmic fragmentation of two sibling oocytes at 15 h postinsemination

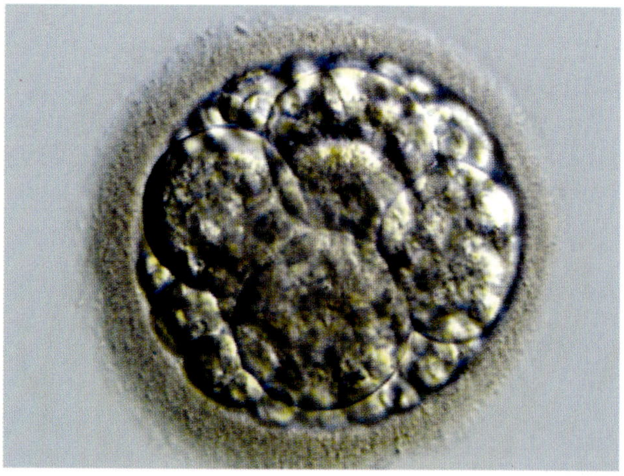

Figure 8.35 Severe fragmentation of a five-cell conceptus at 68 h post-ICSI. Fragments scattered throughout the preembryo surface surround and intermingle with the blastomeres

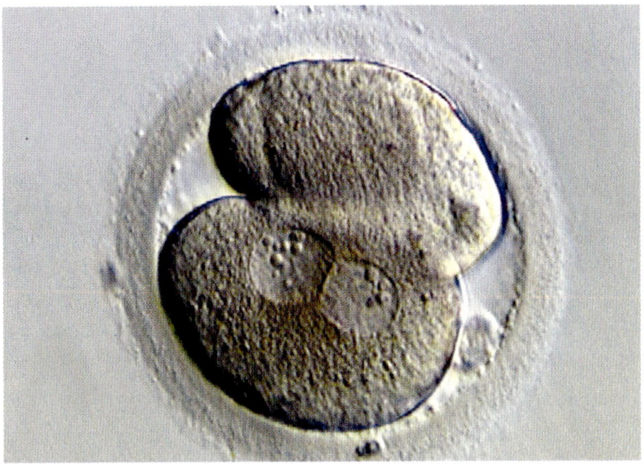

Figure 8.36 Early fragmentation of a diploid pronuclear oocyte. This type of early and equal fragmentation resembles cleavage. Such prezygotes generally display significant cytoplasmic fragmentation after true nuclear division

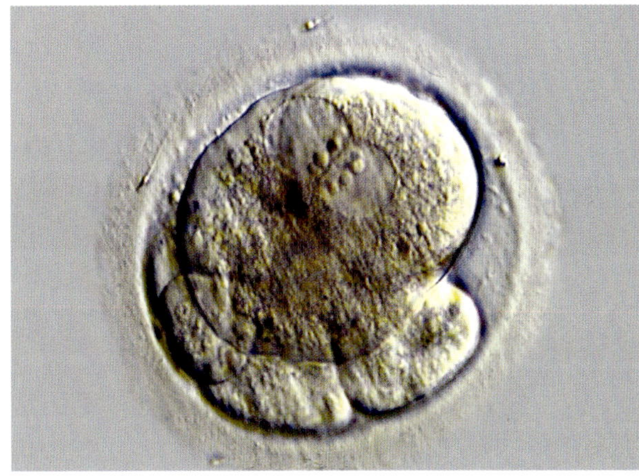

Figure 8.37 Early fragmentation: The ooplasm of this prezygote, with its two pronuclei, has fragmented into several large segments before syngamy

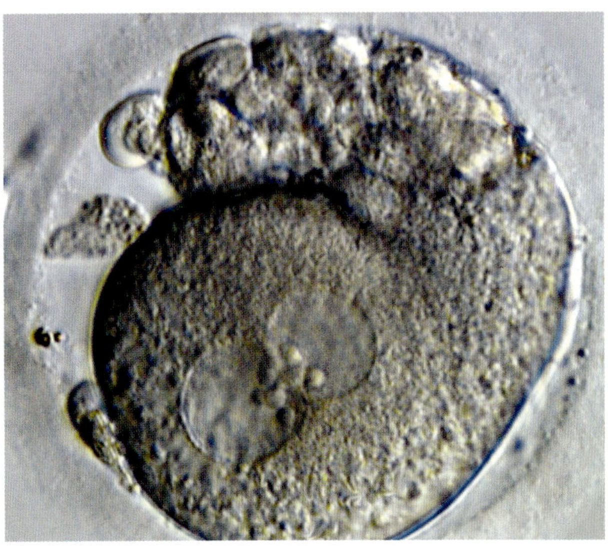

Figure 8.38 Early fragmentation: While still showing two pronuclei, this conceptus has begun to fragment excessively along one pole

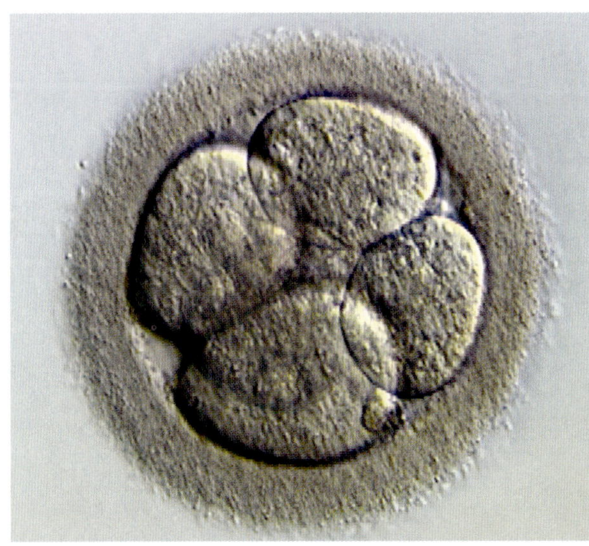

Figure 8.39 The zona pellucida of this five-cell conceptus is extremely dark in color and appears to be ragged and porous

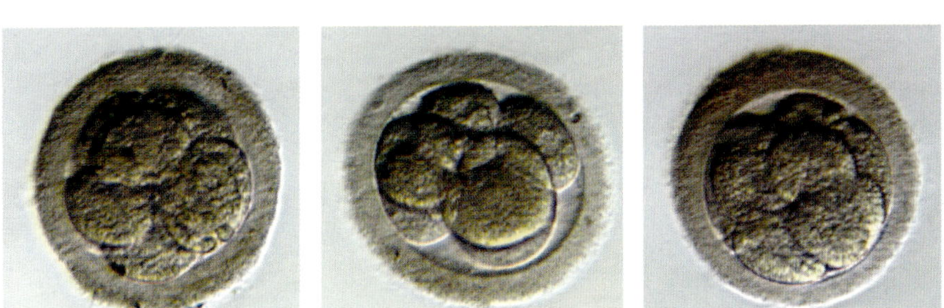

Figure 8.40 These three preembryos with dark and thick zonae underwent AHA and were subsequently transferred. Twin boys were delivered after the intrauterine transfer of these conceptuses

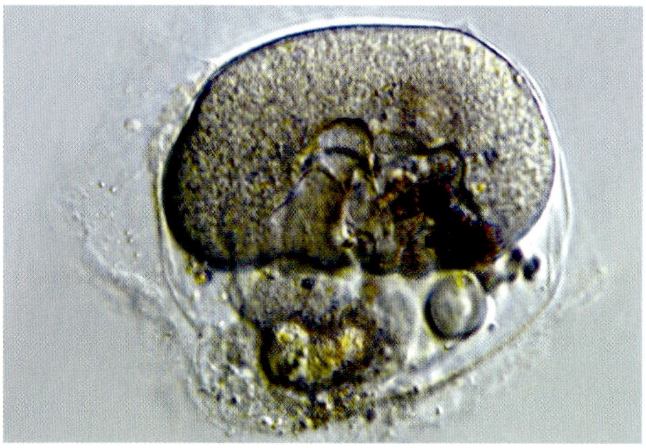

Figure 8.41 An abnormally thin and fragile zona surrounds an irregular, fragmented, and vacuolated oocyte

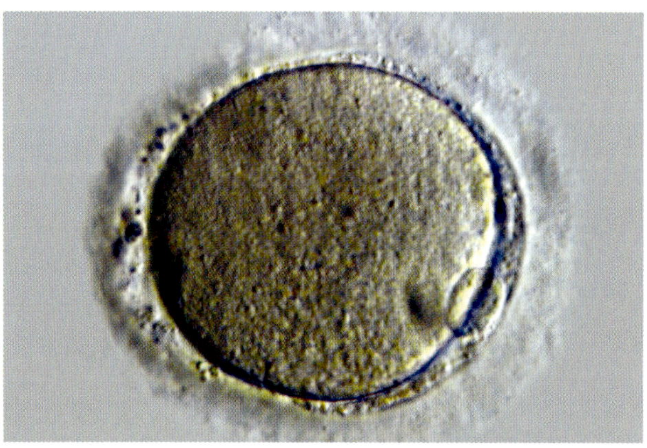

Figure 8.42 Perivitelline debris lines the internal zona surface of this oocyte. The zona is varied in thickness and appears to be disintegrating

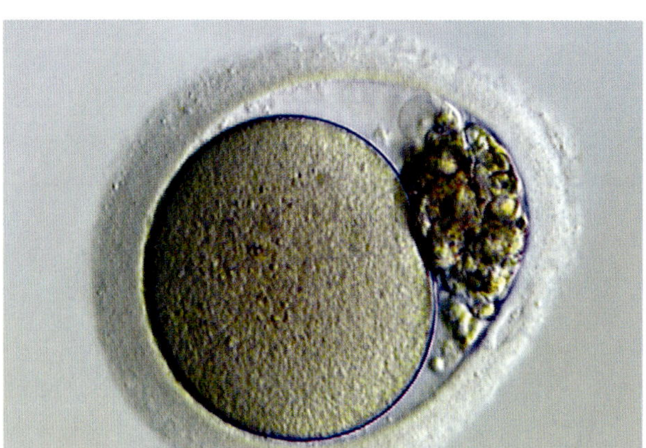

Figure 8.43 Cumulus cells are present within the perivitelline space of this healthy-looking oocyte. These can easily be removed by micromanipulative techniques

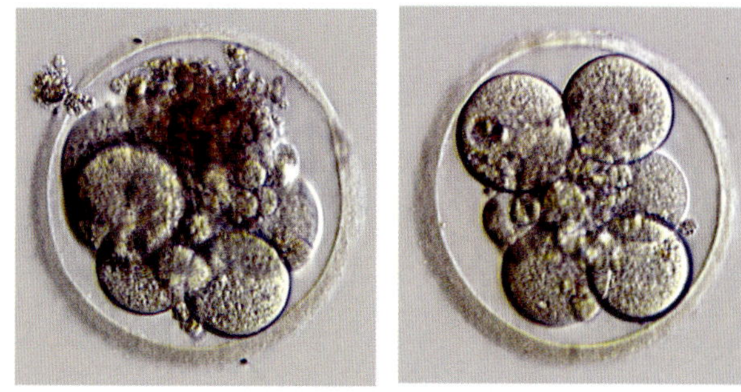

Figure 8.44 Before (left) and after (right) views of a conceptus with degenerating cumulus cells trapped within its zona. Before removal of these cells by aspiration through an opening in the thin zona, the preembryo showed significant degenerative material at the 12-o'clock position

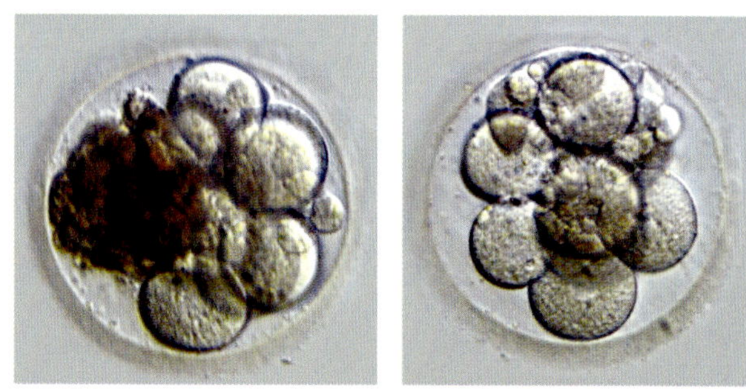

Figure 8.45 Before (left) and after (right) views of a conceptus with degenerating trapped cells, which were microsurgically removed to enhance development of the cleaving eight-cell conceptus. Its appearance has been greatly improved after cleaning

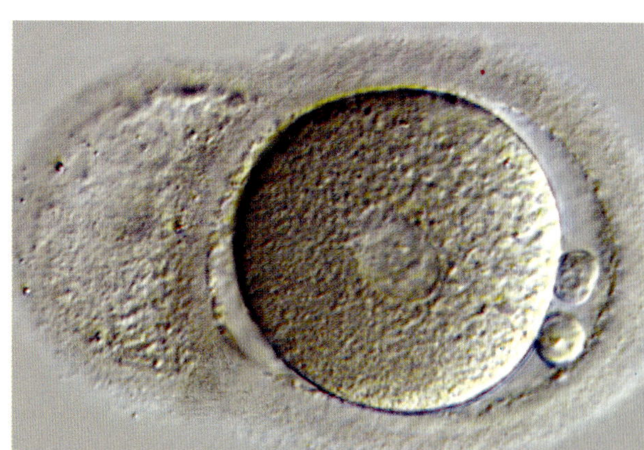

Figure 8.46 Two different zona layers are attached to the left of an otherwise typical zona associated with a fertilizing prezygote (one pronucleus overlaps the other)

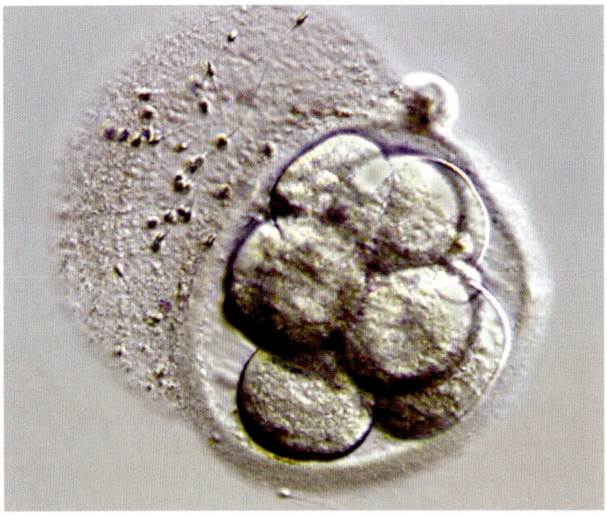

Figure 8.47 Significant thickening and distortion of one area of the zona in an eight-cell preembryo

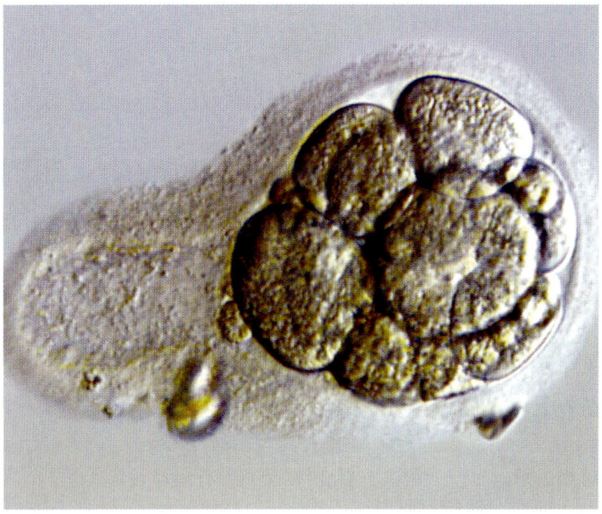

Figure 8.48 Irregular thickening and extreme distortion of the zona of a cleaved conceptus

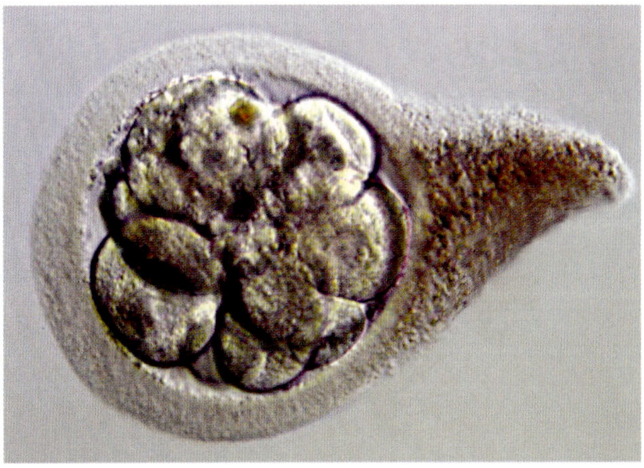

Figure 8.49 Dark thickening of the zona is localized to only one part of its circumference

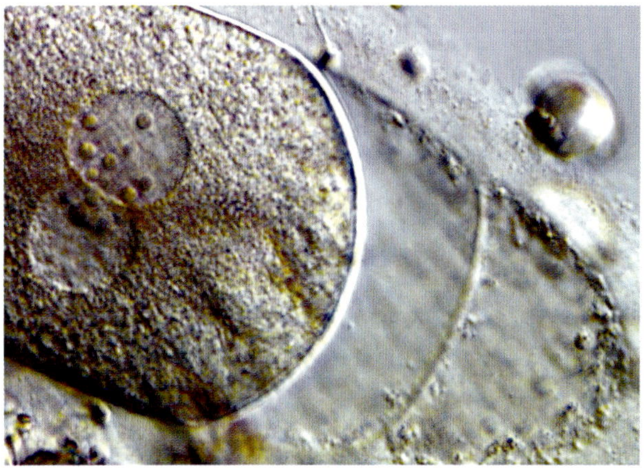

Figure 8.50 Area of bilayering associated with an abnormal zona. The shape of this pronuclear oocyte is clearly distorted by the defect

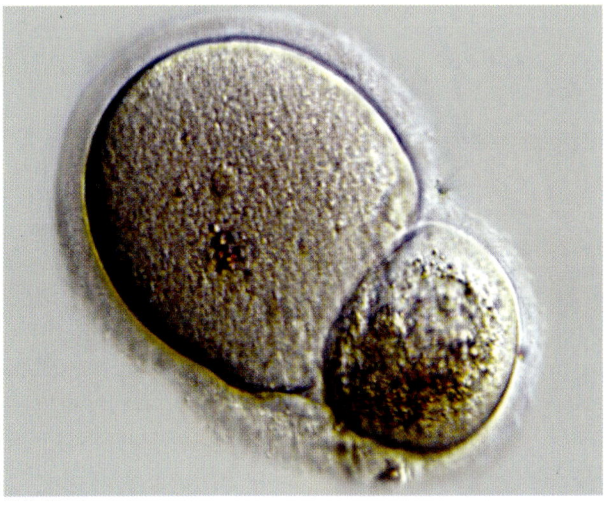

Figure 8.51 Example of the not-so-uncommon finding of two oocytes sharing a common or conjoined zona. In most such cases, a primary oocyte (small in size with chromosomes at PI of maturation) is attached to a maturing one. Here, an MI oocyte is bound to a smaller germinal vesicle-bearing oocyte. Often, the larger oocyte is fertilized whereas the primary oocyte generally demonstrates developmental arrest. The two gametes may be easily separated using microsurgical procedures, but the separation leaves a large breach in the zona

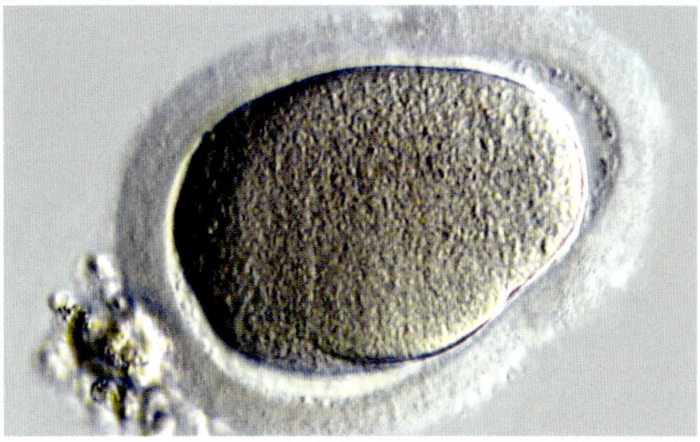

Figure 8.52 Oval-shaped oocyte at MI of maturation. Some distortion of the zona is present on the right; the ooplasm appears to be fragmenting

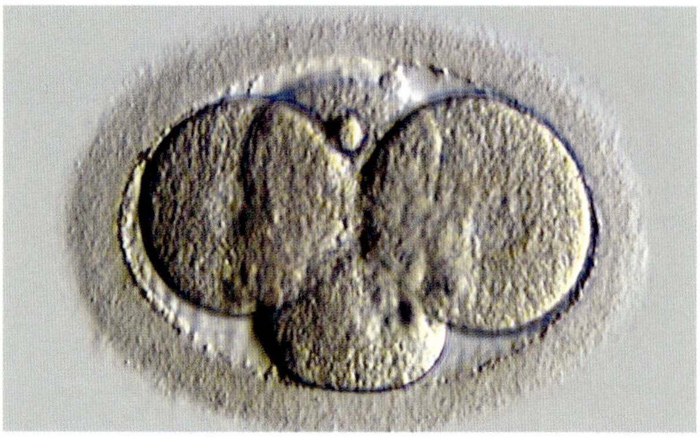

Figure 8.53 Oval-shaped four-cell conceptus with larger, or less constricted, blastomeres along one plane. The zona is darkened and uniformly porous

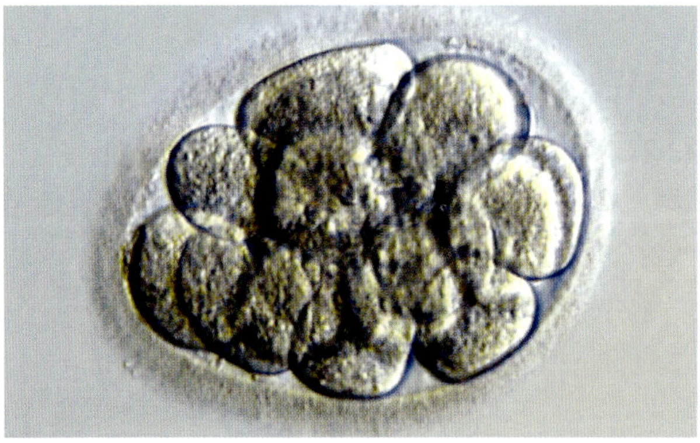

Figure 8.54 Sixteen-cell conceptus with a slight oval or teardrop configuration

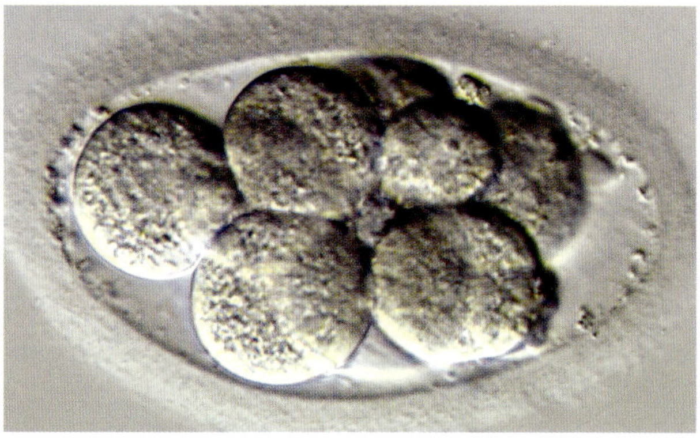

Figure 8.55 Preembryo with an extremely elliptical shape displays nine granular blastomeres

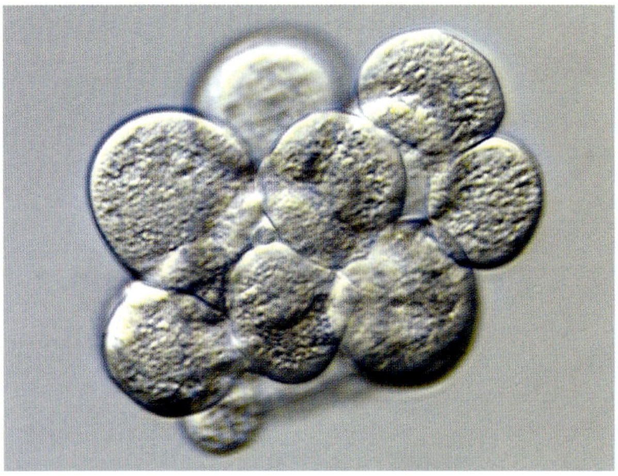

Figure 8.56 Zona-free conceptus at approximately the ten-cell stage developed normally in culture despite the loss of its zona at the pronuclear stage. Its blastomeres remain conjoined

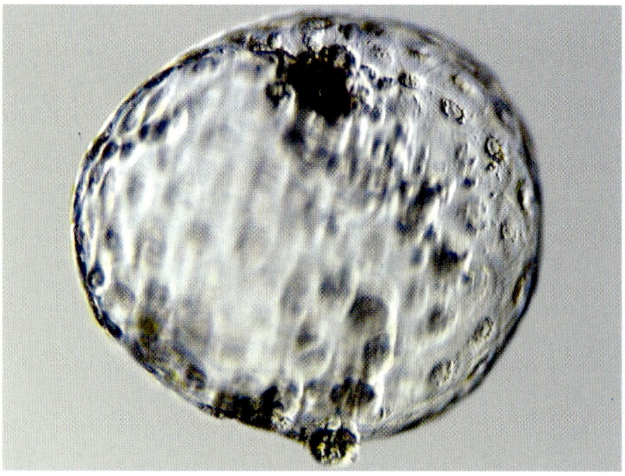

Figure 8.57 Same conceptus as in Figure 8.56 after an additional three days of culture. A relatively normal-looking blastocyst developed and persisted for >24 h in culture, albeit with a small inner cell mass. The structure expanded as expected for a typical naturally hatched blastocyst

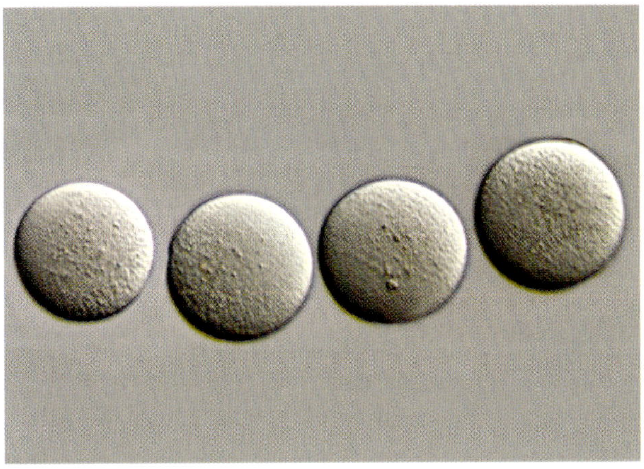

Figure 8.58 Four oocytes from a patient whose gametes all lacked zonae. First polar bodies were lost during enzymatic and mechanical clearing of obscuring cumulus cells

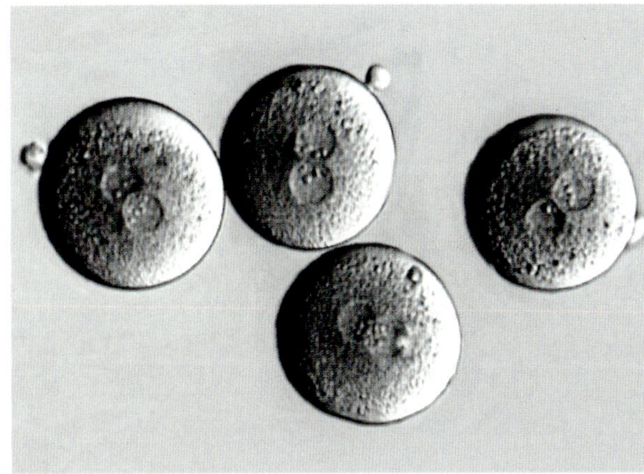

Figure 8.59 After ICSI, four normal-looking pre-zygotes developed in culture. Note that the second polar bodies remain attached to the oocytes

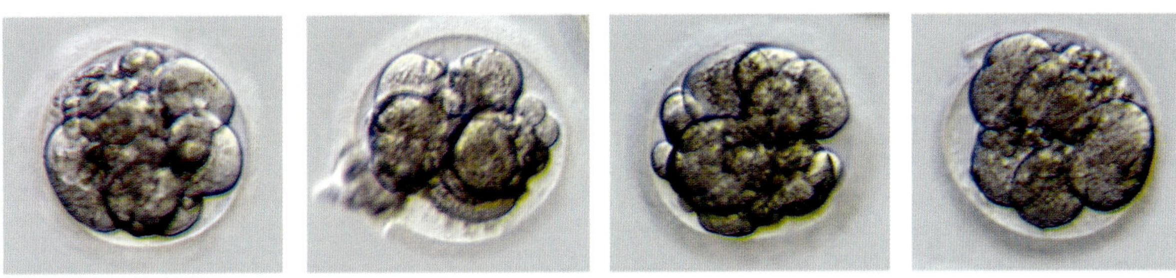

Figure 8.60 After placing the cleaving conceptuses in donor zonae, four slightly fragmented pre-embryos were prepared for intrauterine transfer

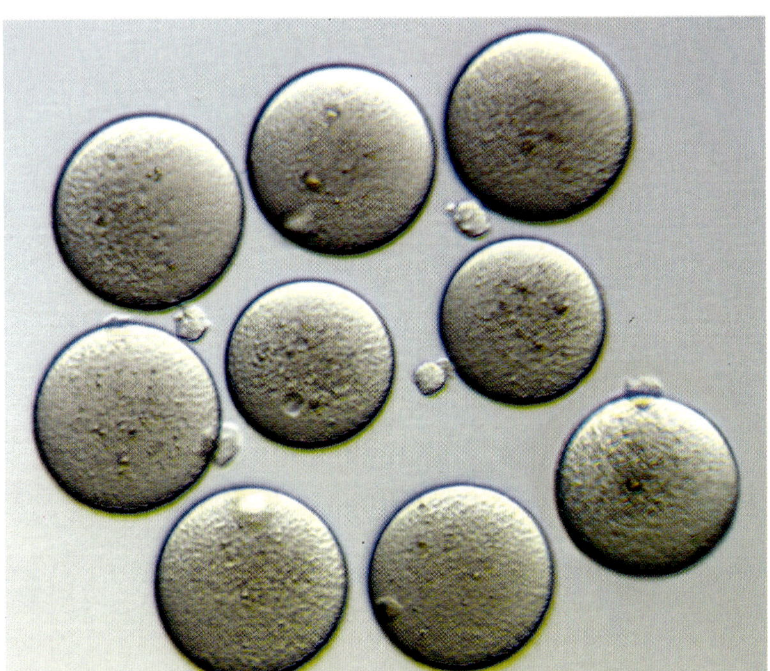

Figure 8.61 Nine zona-free oocytes recovered from the patient in Figure 8.58 on a subsequent attempt. As the cleaning of obscuring cells was carried out with extreme care, first polar bodies remain attached to the oocytes. The difference in oocyte diameter observed in the two central oocytes is the result of a minor loss of cytoplasm during cleaning

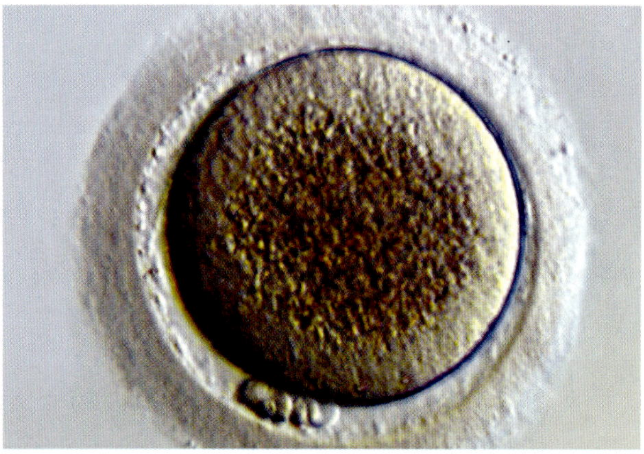

Figure 8.62 Oocyte displaying significant central cytoplasmic granularity

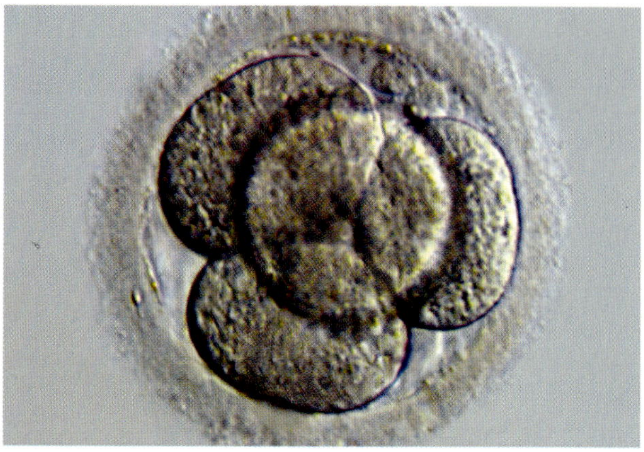

Figure 8.63 Intensely granular / mottled four-cell stage conceptus

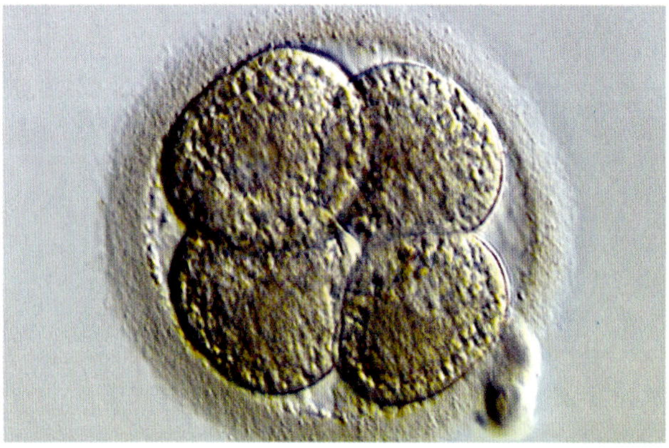

Figure 8.64 Typical appearance of a four-cell preembryo after development in commercially available culture media. Surprisingly, pregnancy potential is not adversely affected by this morphological condition

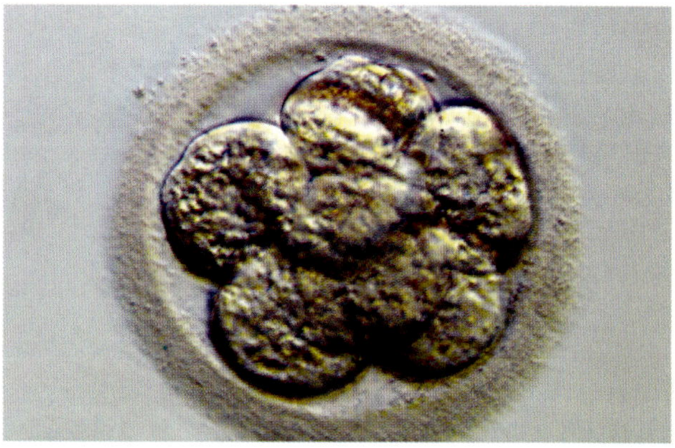

Figure 8.65 Another conceptus developed in commercially available media. Note the mottled appearance of the cytoplasm and the dark zona

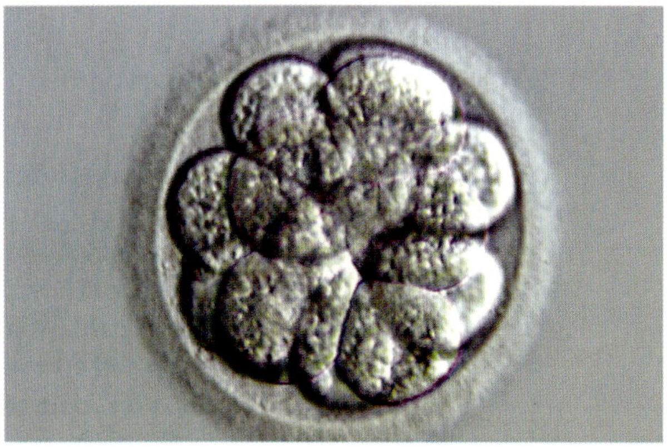

Figure 8.66 Mottled cytoplasm in a regularly cleaving thirteen-cell conceptus

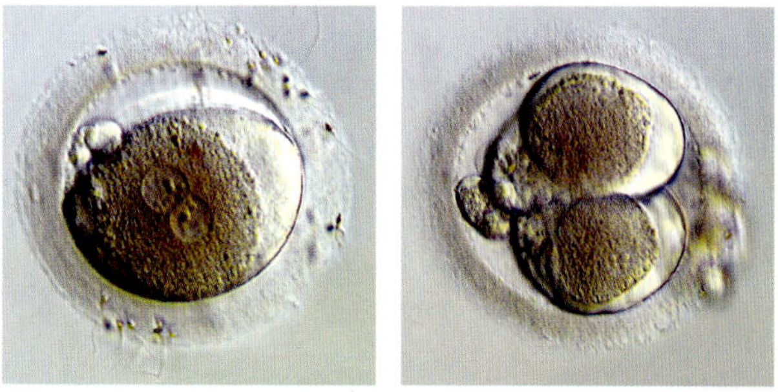

Figure 8.67 Centralized granularity associated with an acytoplasmic peripheral cortex: Pronuclear oocyte with a granular center and clear periphery (left); two-cell conceptus with granular blastomeres and clear cortical areas (right)

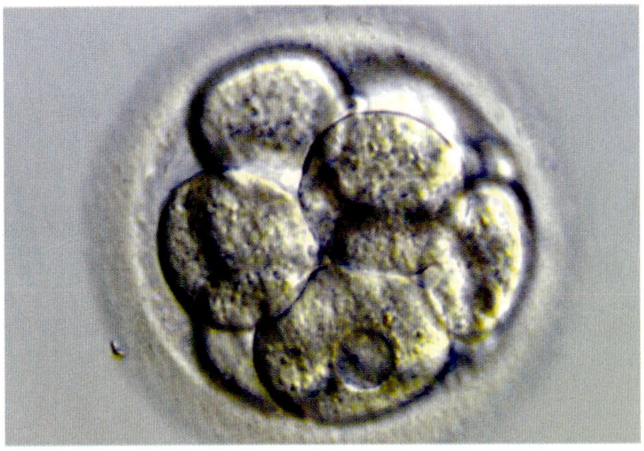

Figure 8.68 One blastomere of this nine-cell conceptus has a medium-sized cytoplasmic vacuole (six-o'clock position)

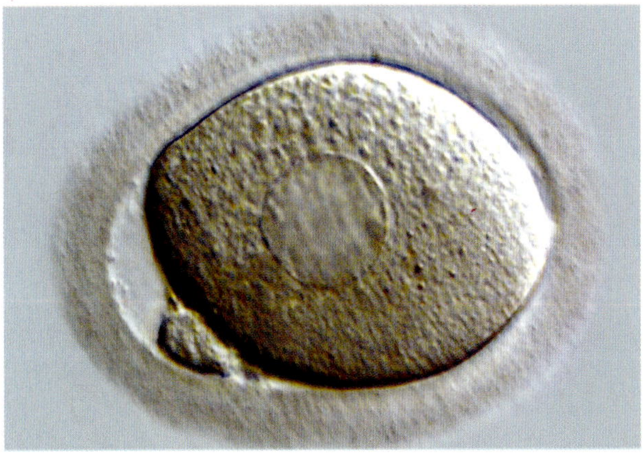

Figure 8.69 A large vacuole centrally located in an oval-shaped M II oocyte

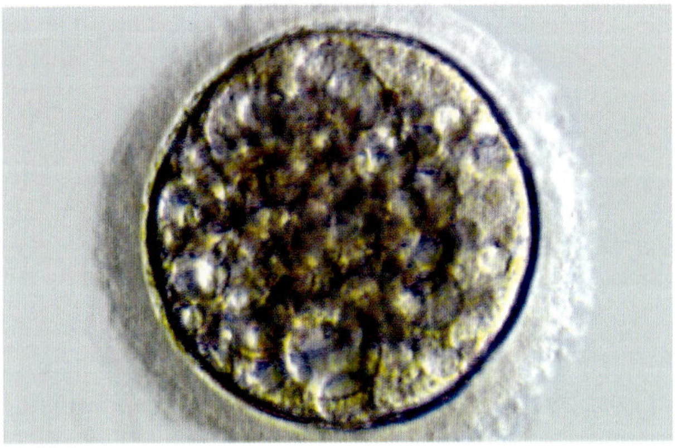

Figure 8.70 Degenerative oocyte with multiple small- and medium-sized vacuoles throughout its necrotic cytoplasm

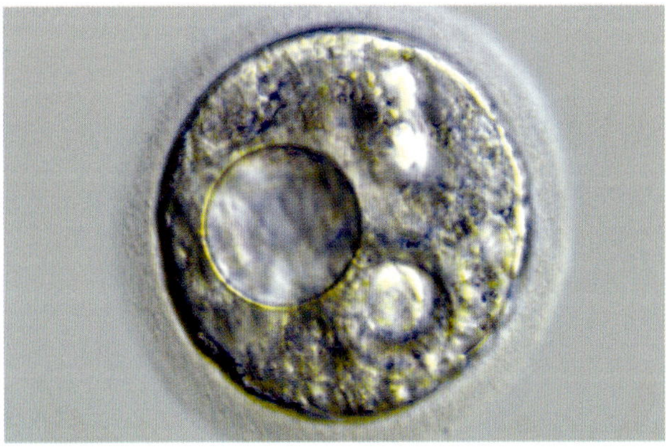

Figure 8.71 Degenerating oocyte with several medium-sized and large vacuoles in degenerating necrotic cytoplasm

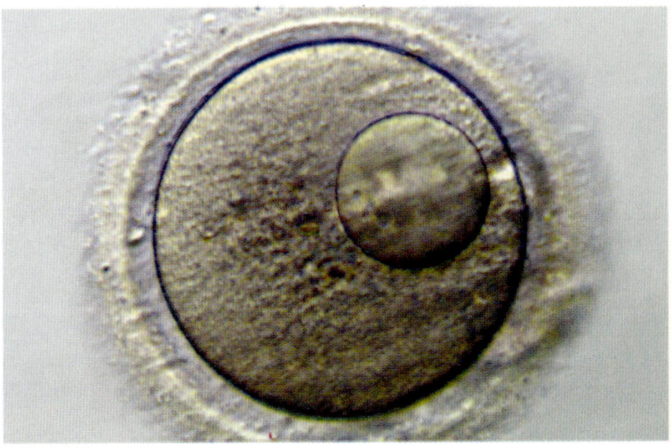

Figure 8.72 M II oocyte with a vacuolar structure which is large and rounded, rather than the typical flattened or concave shape; it may represent a fluid-filled inclusion. This morphology is rarely observed

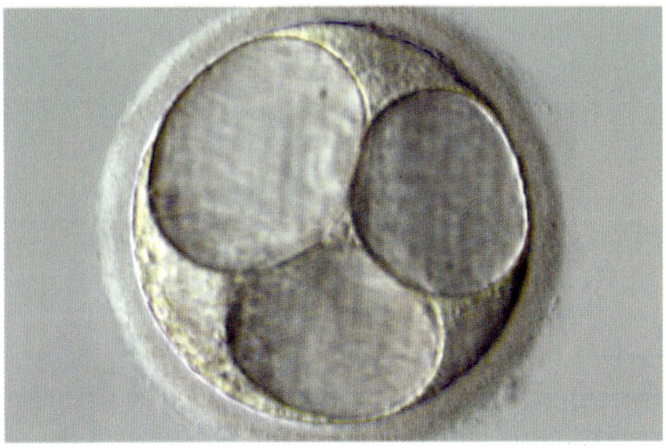

Figure 8.73 Three extremely large cytoplasmic vacuoles within a degenerating oocyte

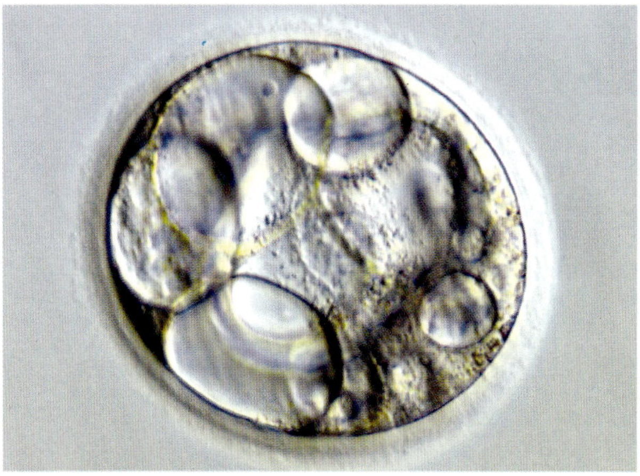

Figure 8.74 Multiple large cytoplasmic vacuoles developing within a degenerating oocyte

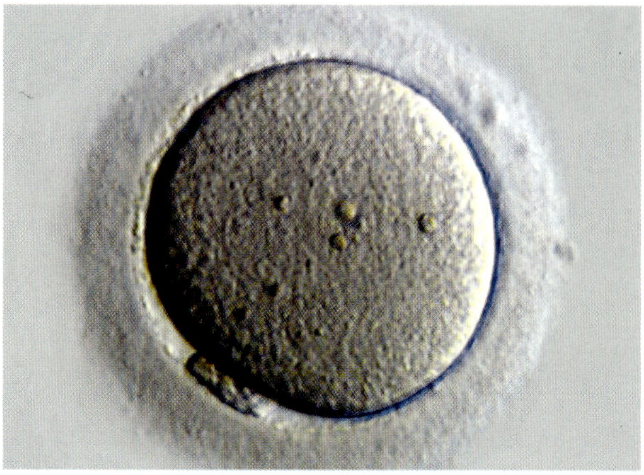

Figure 8.75 Small normal inclusions typically associated with mature oocytes. The patient who produced this oocyte and others with similar inclusions delivered a child after ICSI

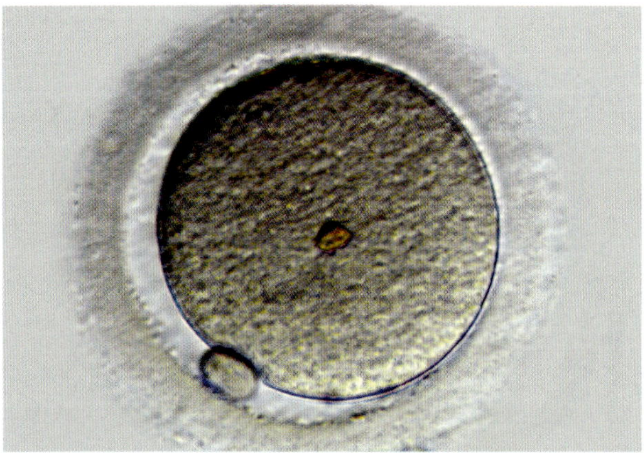

Figure 8.76 A large brown central inclusion within an M II oocyte. Similar inclusions were found in all 17 oocytes collected from this patient. As the husband of this patient produced no spermatozoa at testicular biopsy, the fertilization and pregnancy potentials for these oocytes are unknown

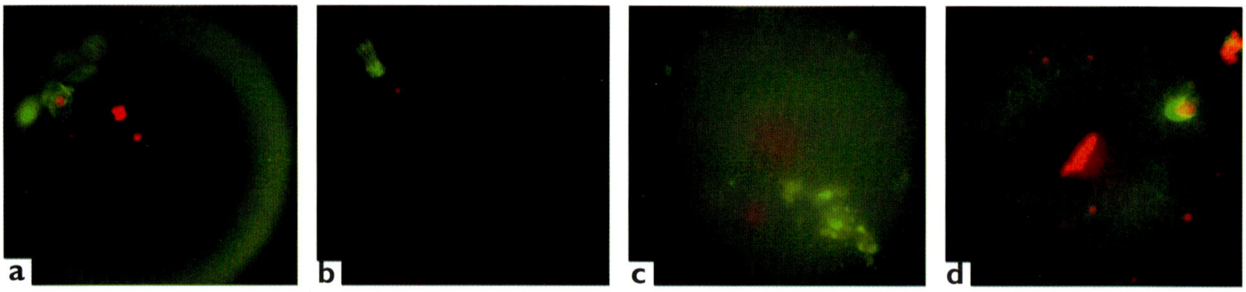

Figure 8.77 Immunofluorescent cytochemical staining of non-fertilized and single-pronucleate oocytes: (a) Typical unfertilized oocyte following IVF insemination shows a few peripheral cytoskeletal fibers (green) and a contracted fragmented nucleus(i) (red). (b) Oocyte which failed fertilization due to developmental arrest at M I of maturation. Scant chromatin accompanies the otherwise apparently normal meiotic spindle (green). (c) Post-ICSI oocyte showed a single pronucleus on LM. Immunofluorescent cytochemical staining reveals two faint nuclei (red) of discordant sizes with a complete cytoskeletal assembly. The disorganized or possibly damaged spindle/aster fibers (green) are close to, but not associated with, either nucleus. (d) Post-ICSI single-pronucleate oocyte with dyssynchrony between the aster (green) of the condensed sperm head (red oval) and the aligned condensed maternal chromosomes (red linear array). Courtesy of Maureen Moomjy, MD

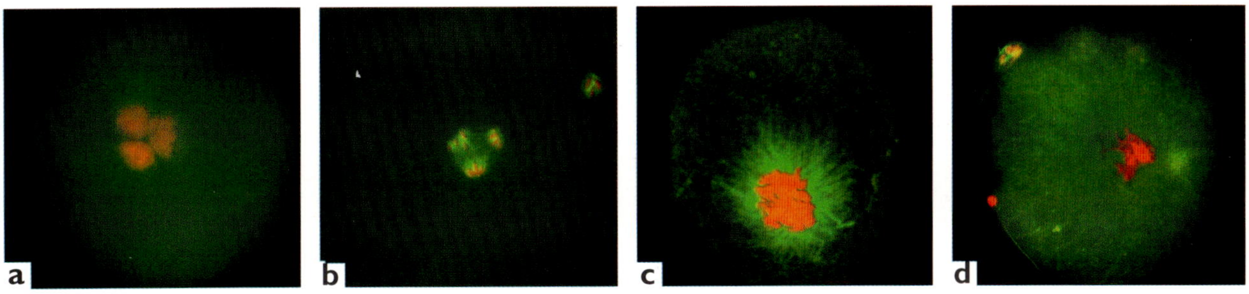

Figure 8.78 Immunofluorescent cytochemical staining of tripronucleate prezygotes after standard insemination: (a) Three decondensed and apposed nuclei (red) with a complete cytoskeletal assembly, but without apparent spindle formation. (b) Tripolar spindle with condensed chromosomes and negligible cytoskeletal assembly. (c) Concentrated astral array of spindle fibers emanating from a large collection of condensed chromosomes. (d) Two apposed vacuolated nuclei (red) and one faint contracted nucleus on a different focal plane (four-o'clock position). A complete cytoskeletal assembly is seen, but with no apparent spindle or aster fibers. A spermatozoon is adherent to the oolemma. Courtesy of Maureen Moomjy, MD

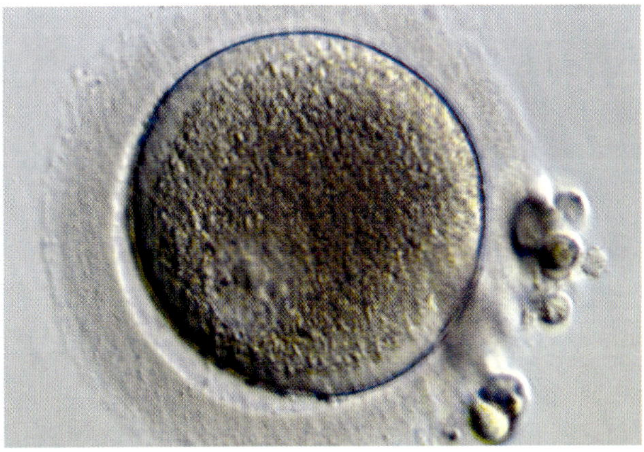

Figure 9.1 Germinal vesicle-bearing oocyte frozen and thawed under a research protocol using 1,2-propanediol. Although darkened in appearance, the oolemma and zona are intact. This oocyte underwent germinal vesicle breakdown in culture over the next 24 h

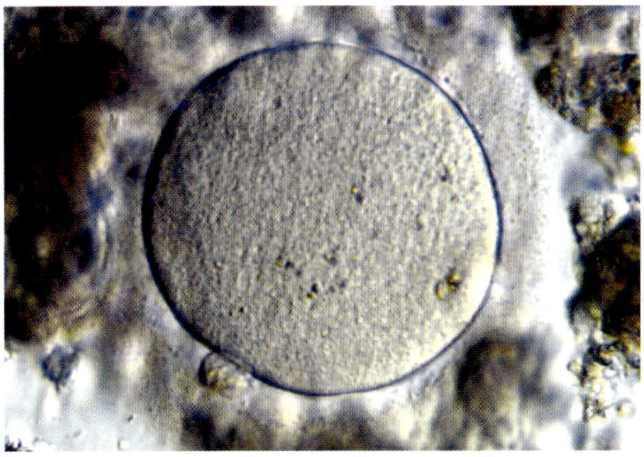

Figure 9.2 Human MII oocyte, cryopreserved with 1,2-propanediol and thawed under research conditions. The general morphology is good. Cumulus cells remain associated with the oocyte despite the manipulations

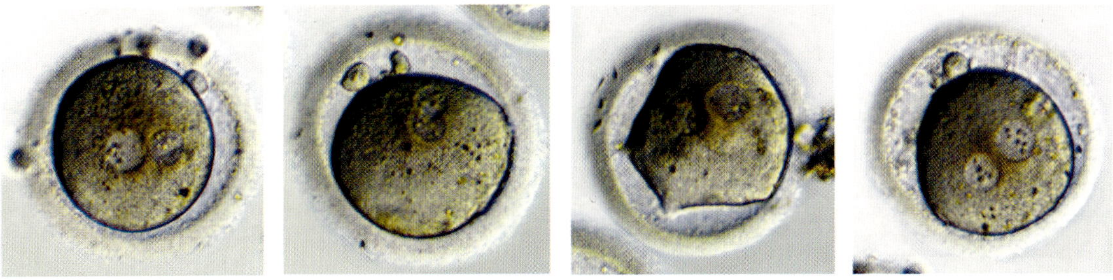

Figure 9.3 Four prezygotes immediately after thawing. These were frozen using 1,2-propanediol without sucrose as the cryoprotectant. Although one prezygote is grossly misshapen, it regained its normal round shape within a short time. All four display intact zonae and oolemmae

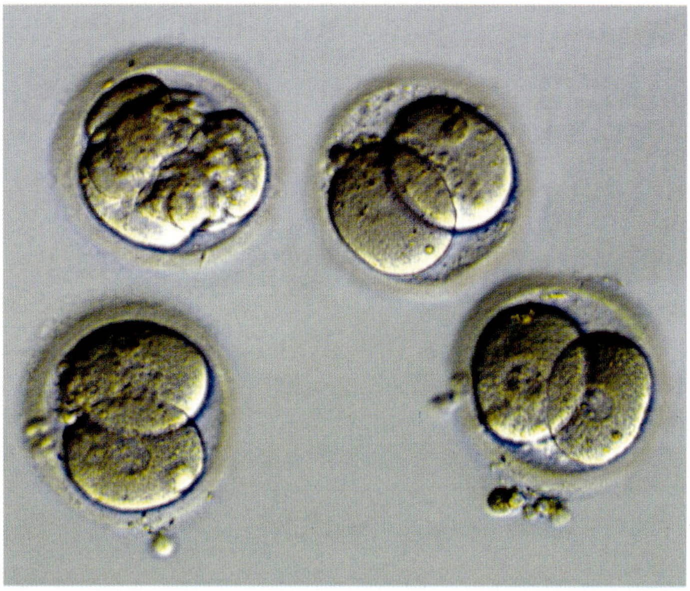

Figure 9.4 Same prezygotes as in Figure 9.3 after 24 h of culture. Three have developed to the two-cell stage, and one is cleaving to four cells. After intrauterine replacement, two gestational sacs were identified by ultrasound. A pregnancy is currently ongoing

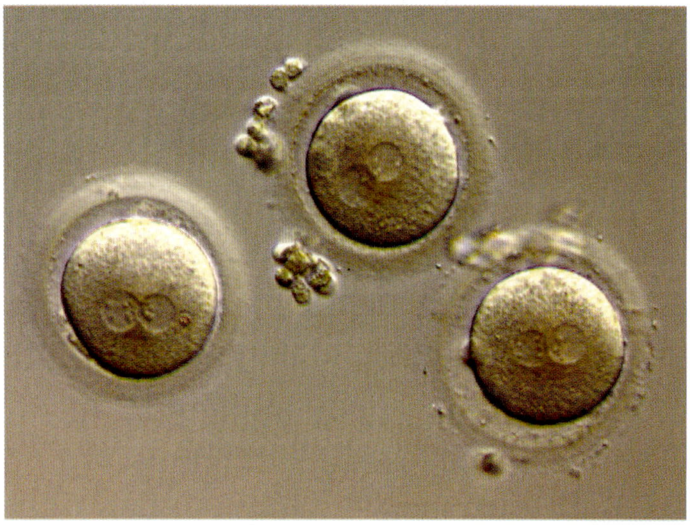

Figure 9.5 Three prezygotes shown immediately after thawing. These were frozen using 1,2-propanediol without sucrose as the cryoprotectant and stored for 553 days. All three show normal morphology

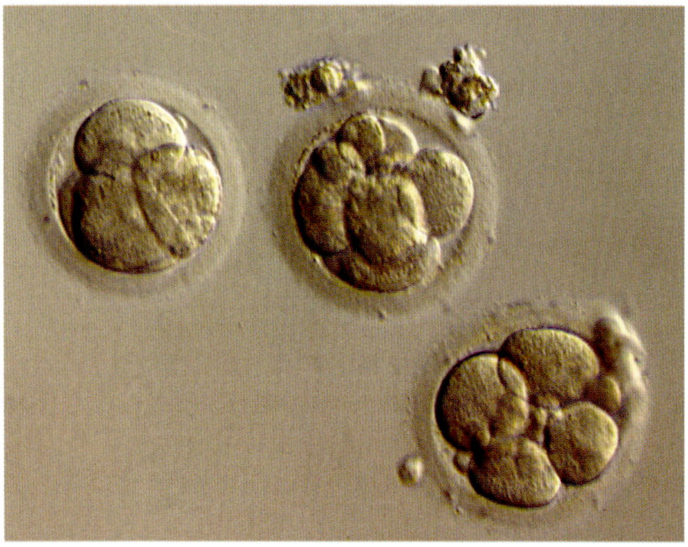

Figure 9.6 Same conceptuses as in Figure 9.5 after 24 h of culture. Because of the attached cells, it may be assumed that these prezygotes are oriented in the same succession. Each exhibits minor cytoplasmic fragmentation, but has an acceptable overall morphology. A twin pregnancy was established after transferring these three conceptuses to a 26-year-old woman, leading to the birth of two healthy infants, one boy and one girl

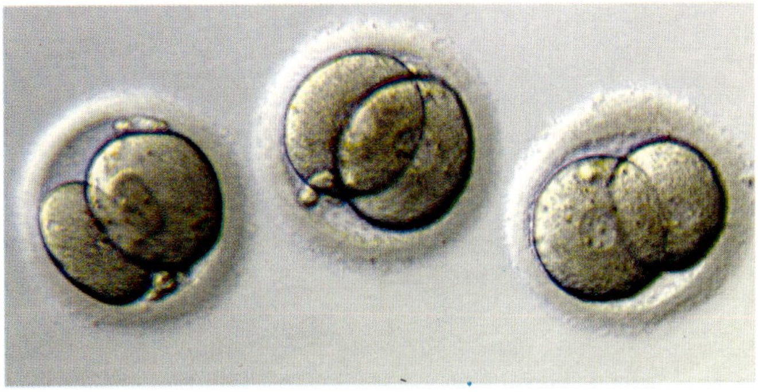

Figure 9.7 Three conceptuses developing from frozen/thawed prezygotes stored for 482 days. One of these implanted in the uterus of the 38-year-old mother and led to the birth of a normal girl

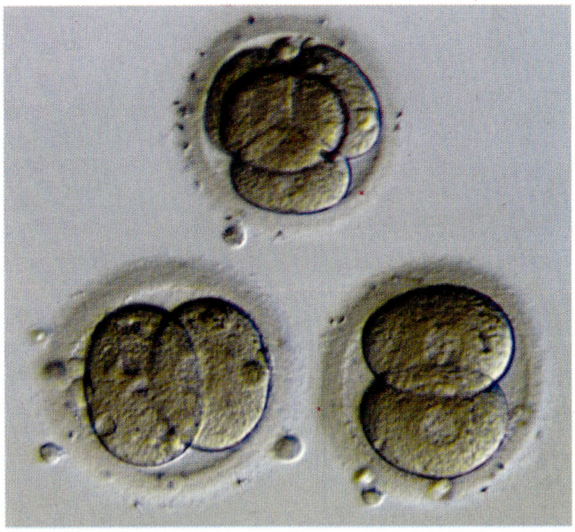

Figure 9.8 Three conceptuses developing from frozen/thawed prezygotes stored for 961 days. Despite their pleasing morphology, the transfer of these preembryos to a 35-year-old woman failed to result in pregnancy

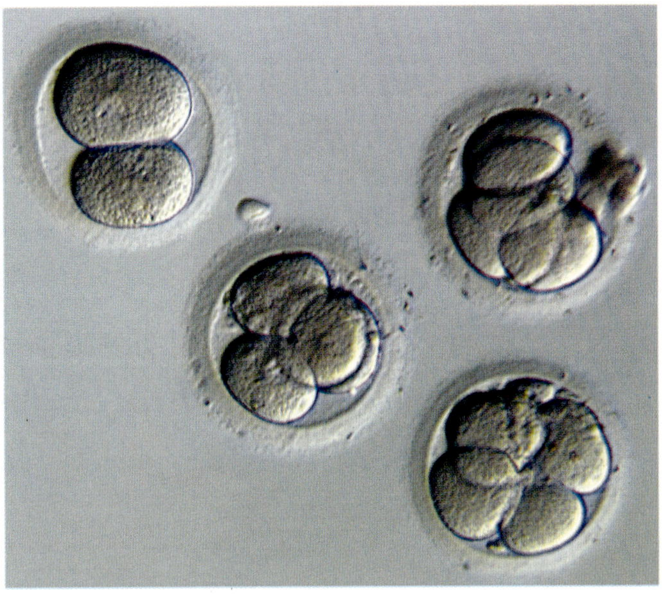

Figure 9.9 Four conceptuses developed from frozen/thawed prezygotes stored for 834 days. Although the patient delivered a child from her fresh cycle and produced these high-quality pre-embryos, their transfer failed to result in an ongoing pregnancy

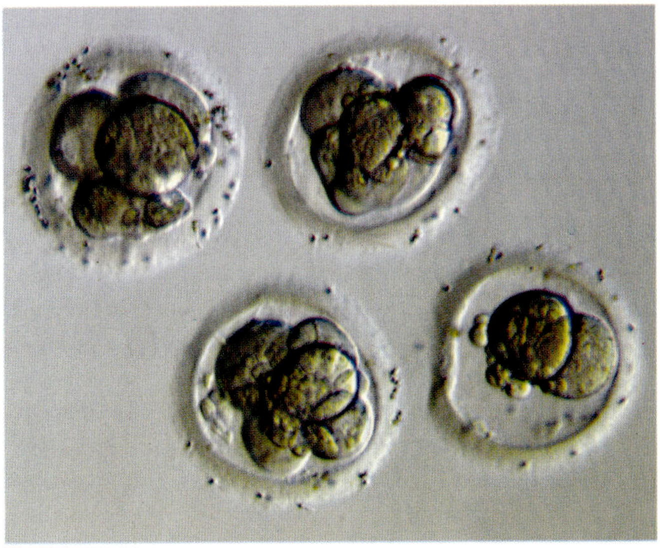

Figure 9.10 Four conceptuses developed from frozen/thawed prezygotes stored for 203 days. All four underwent AHA to remove extensive cytoplasmic fragments (note the empty space in the lower right conceptus from where fragments were removed). The 41-year-old donor-oocyte recipient became pregnant, but miscarried

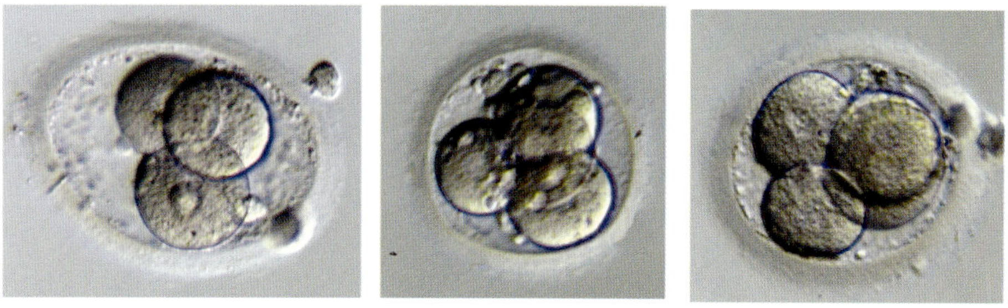

Figure 9.11 These three preembryos were frozen for >5 years. Upon thawing, two of the three were completely intact (middle and right). The one on the left had three surviving blastomeres out of four. The degenerated blastomere was removed by micromanipulation. Following the difficult transfer of the three conceptuses to a 42-year-old woman who had conceived in her fresh cycle, implantation failed to occur

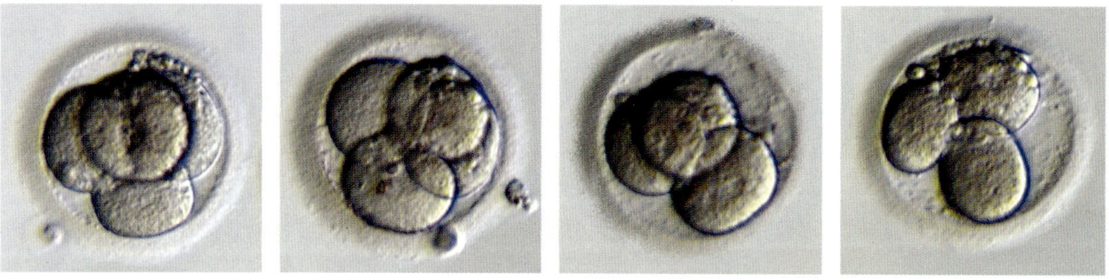

Figure 9.12 In this example, two of four preembryos (left), stored for 861 days, survived thawing with all blastomeres intact. The remaining two conceptuses lost a single blastomere during the process (right). Degenerative cells were removed before intrauterine transfer to a 35-year-old woman. A healthy female child was delivered

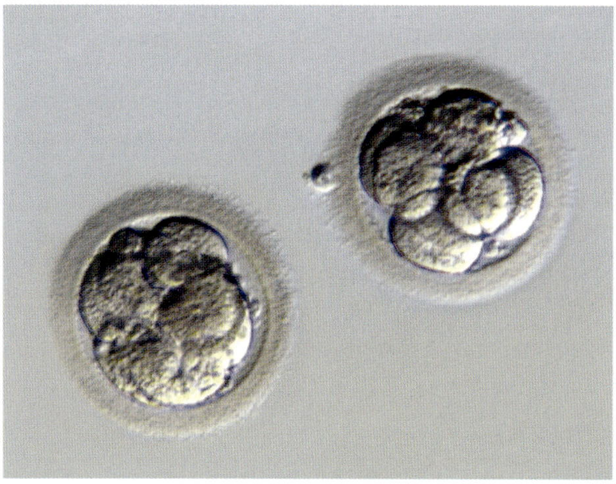

Figure 9.13 Two day-3 preembryos shown just before freezing

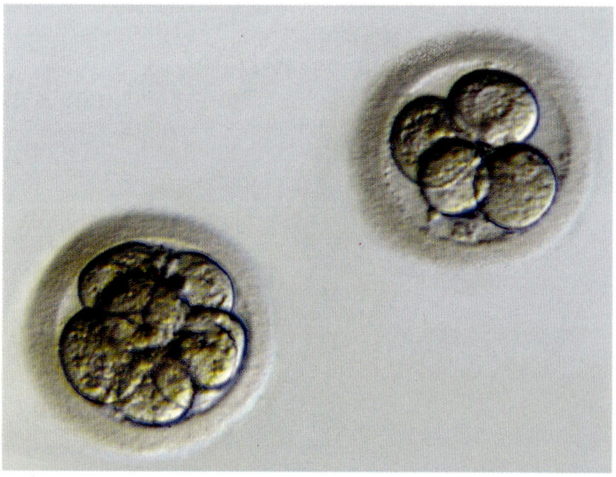

Figure 9.14 The same preembryos as in Figure 9.13 after cryostorage for 144 days. Both survived although, in the conceptus on the right, two blastomeres were damaged and had to be microsurgically removed. The 38-year-old recipient failed to achieve pregnancy with these preembryos, but returned for a second attempt with thawed prezygotes and subsequently conceived

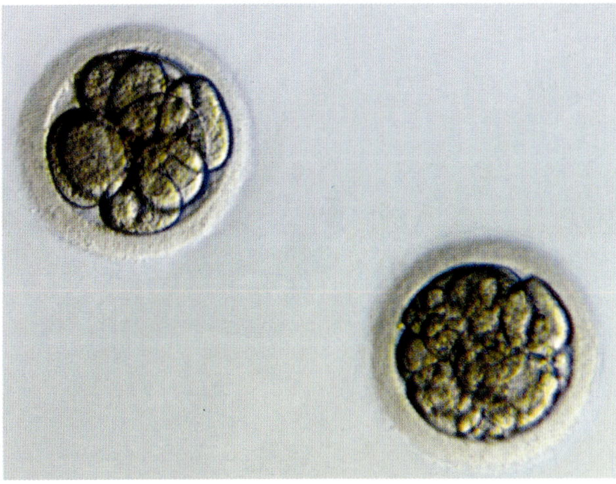

Figure 9.15 Two preembryos cryopreserved on day 3 after harvest, shown just before freezing. One possesses no fragments; the other is moderately fragmented

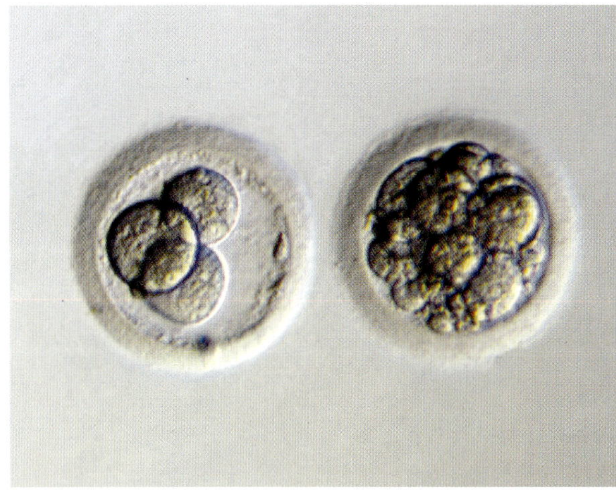

Figure 9.16 The same preembryos as in Figure 9.15 after thawing 122 days later. Only three of eight blastomeres survived in the less fragmented preembryo. Surprisingly, the second preembryo, which was more fragmented, survived with all blastomeres intact. Pregnancy and miscarriage followed the transfer of these conceptuses to a 39-year-old woman

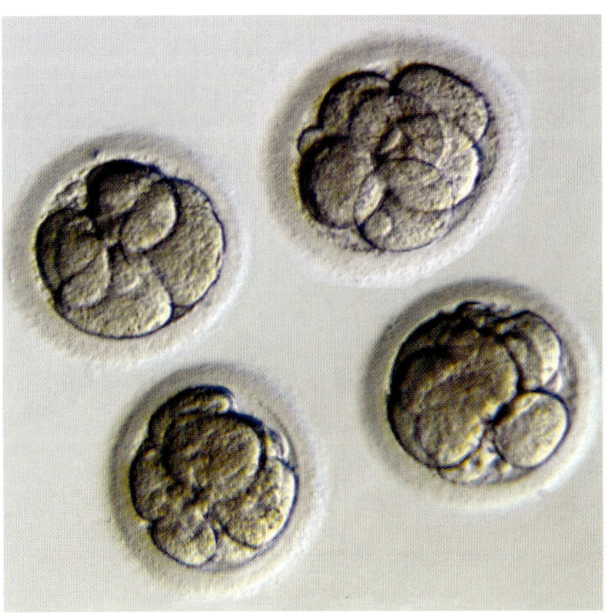

Figure 9.17 Four preembryos shown just before freezing on day 3 after harvest

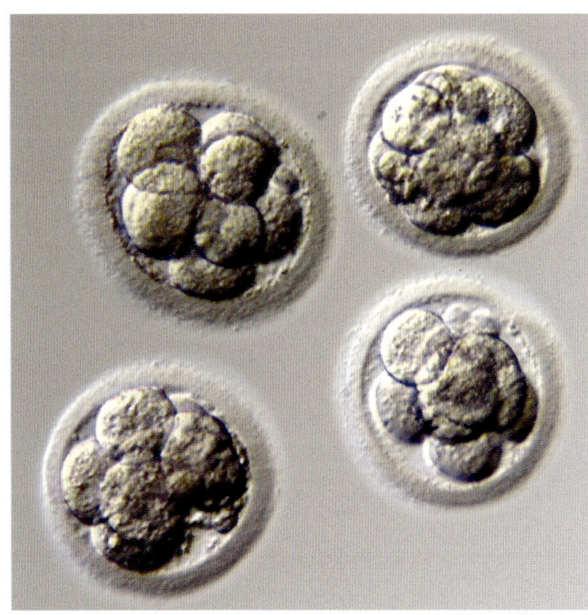

Figure 9.18 The same preembryos as in Figure 9.17 shown a few hours after thawing 94 days later. All tolerated the freezing and thawing procedures well. After intrauterine transfer, the 35-year-old mother became pregnant from this cohort and subsequently delivered a healthy boy

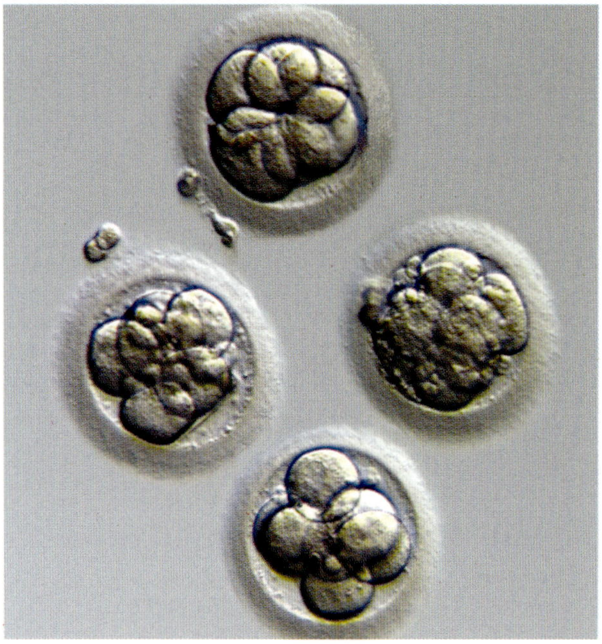

Figure 9.19 Four preembryos shown just before freezing on day 3 after harvest

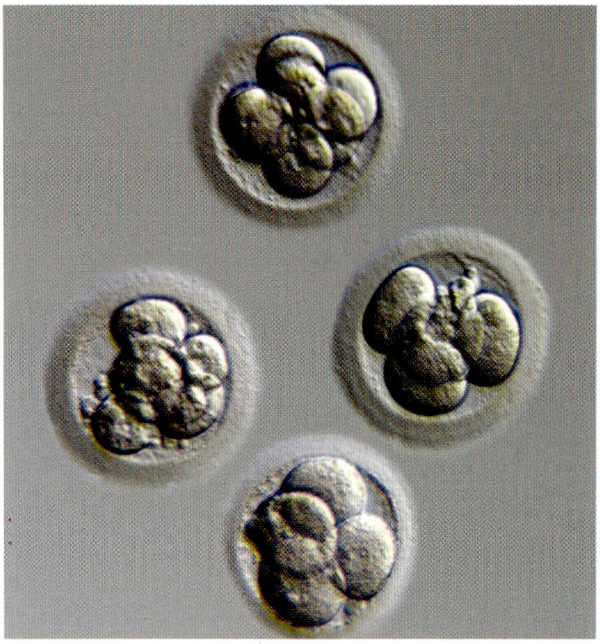

Figure 9.20 The same preembryos as in Figure 9.19 shown a few hours after thawing 68 days later. Two of these conceptuses have had degenerative blastomeres and fragments removed. The 37-year-old recipient became pregnant after transfer, showing two sacs and one fetal heart by ultrasound. A singleton pregnancy has been ongoing for >20 weeks

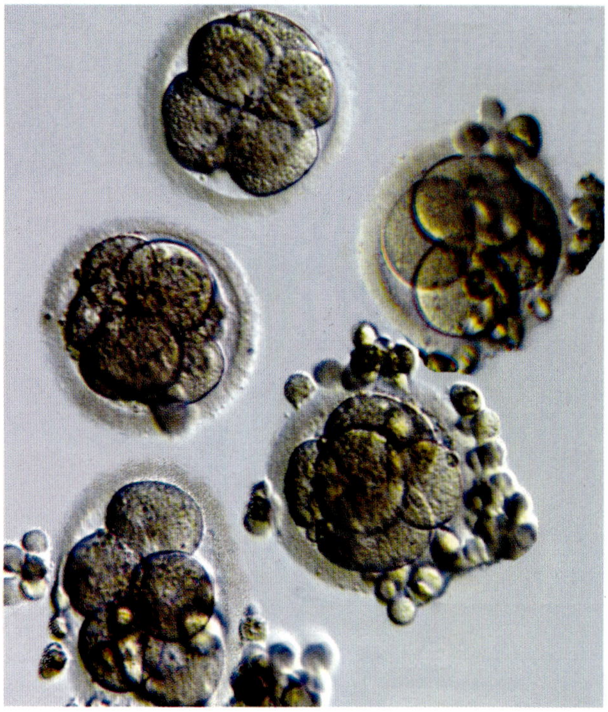

Figure 9.21 Five conceptuses shown just before freezing on day 3 after harvest

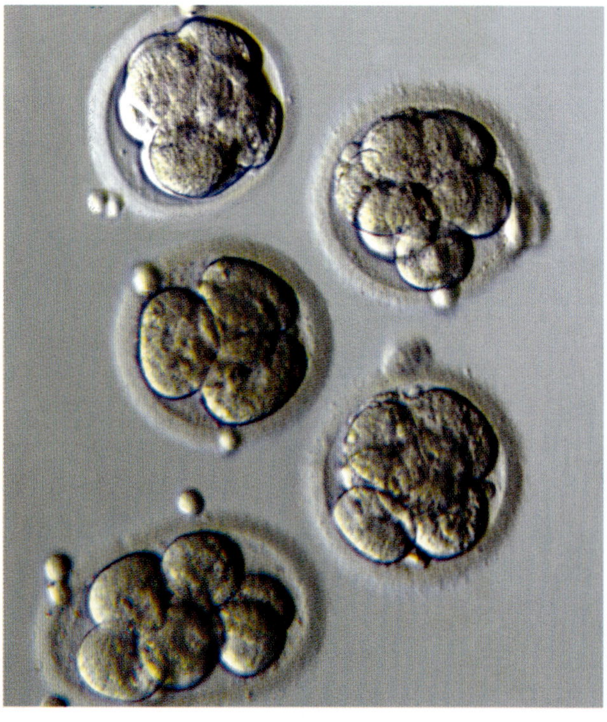

Figure 9.22 Same preembryos as in Figure 9.21 after thawing 68 days later; all survived. A preclinical pregnancy and loss were experienced by the 38-year-old recipient after transfer

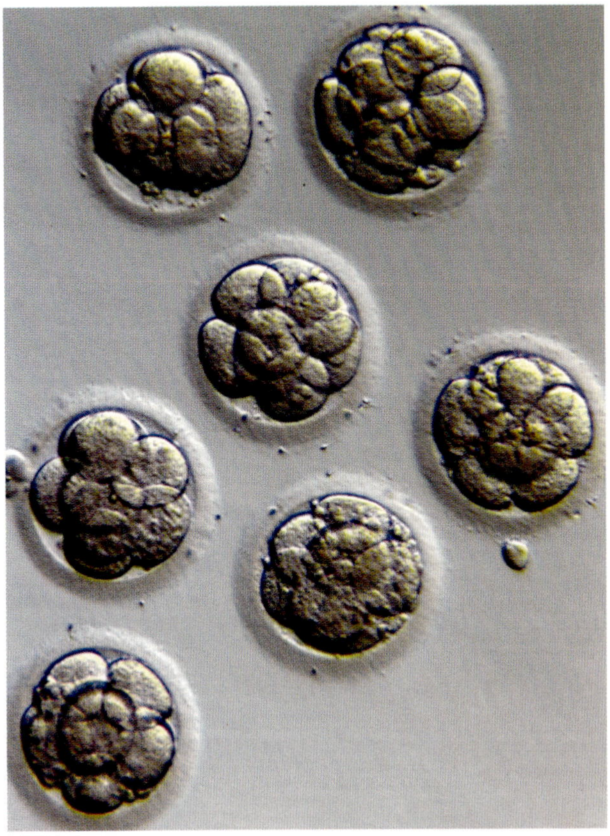

Figure 9.23 Seven apparently healthy conceptuses shown before freezing on day 3 after harvest

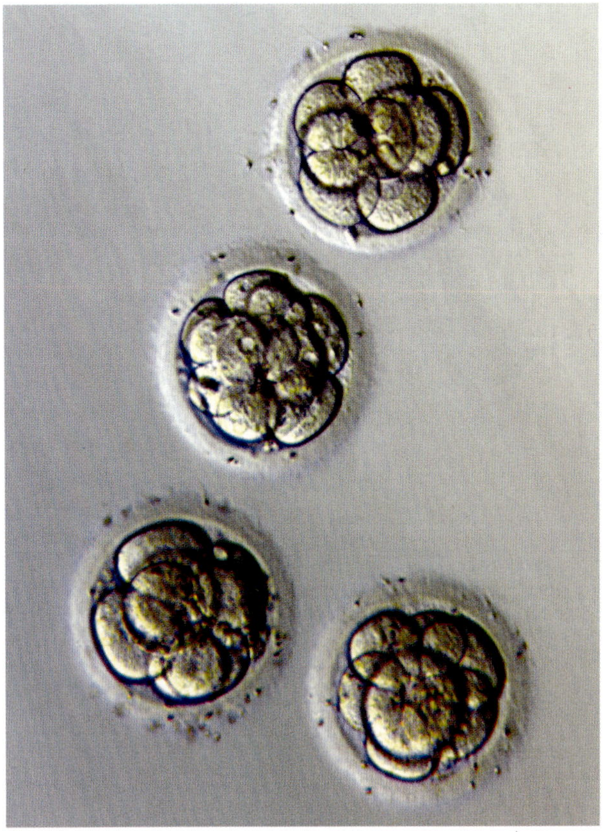

Figure 9.24 Four of the preembryos seen in Figure 9.23 were thawed 122 days later; all survived. Unfortunately, no pregnancy was established in the 38-year-old woman who produced these conceptuses

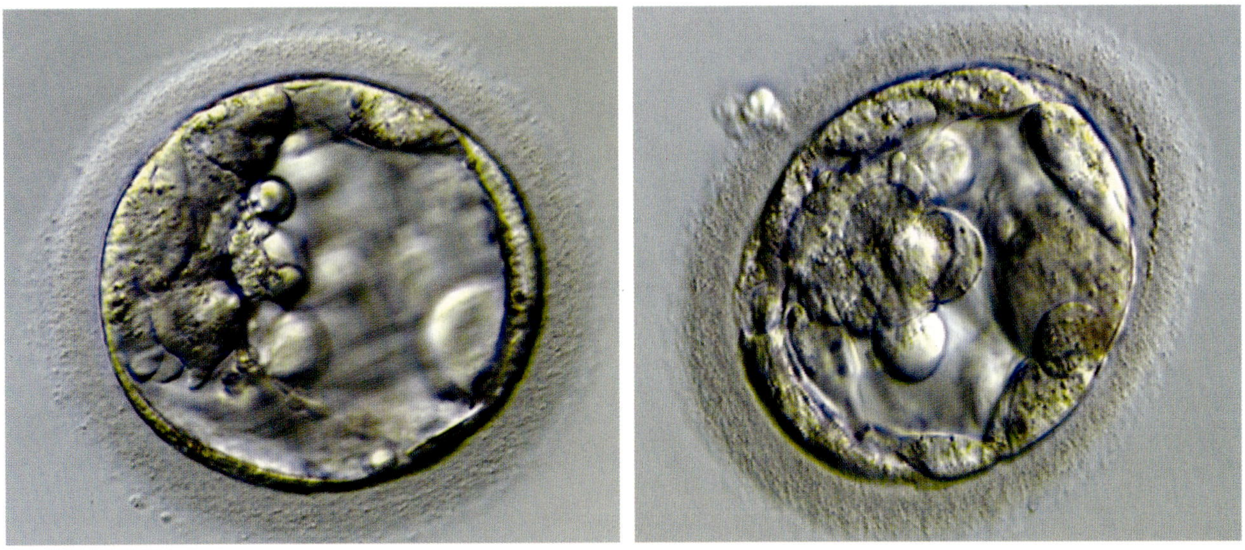

Figure 9.25 Early blastocysts, frozen for 3 years in 10% glycerol, shown just after thawing. Despite a relatively normal appearance, their transfer to a 42-year-old woman failed to result in pregnancy

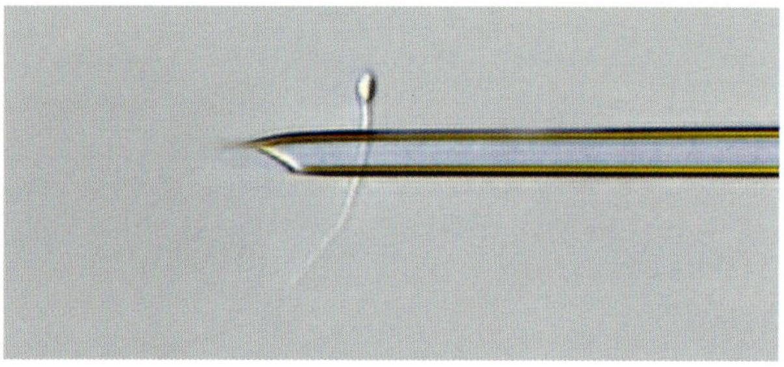

Figure 10.1 The spermatozoon is immobilized by gently lowering the tip of the injection pipette to compress the midregion of the sperm flagellum against the bottom of the dish

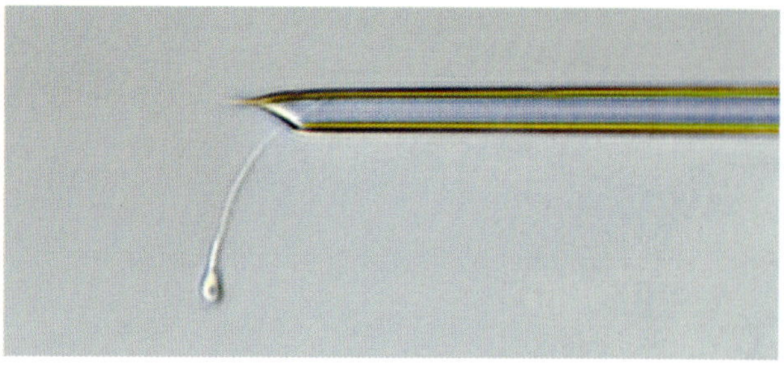

Figure 10.2 The spermatozoon is aspirated tail first into the injection pipette

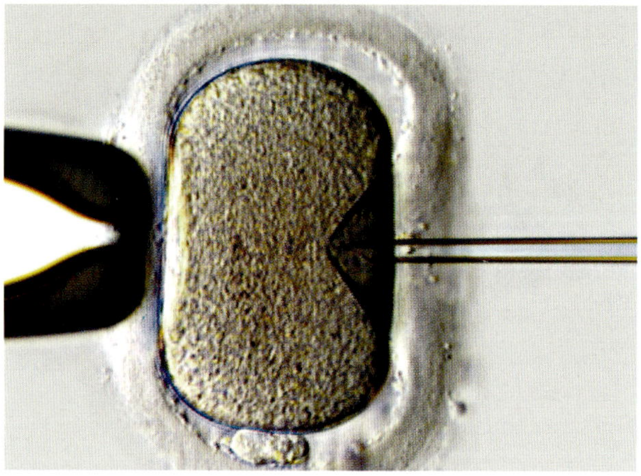

Figure 10.3 The zona pellucida is transversed

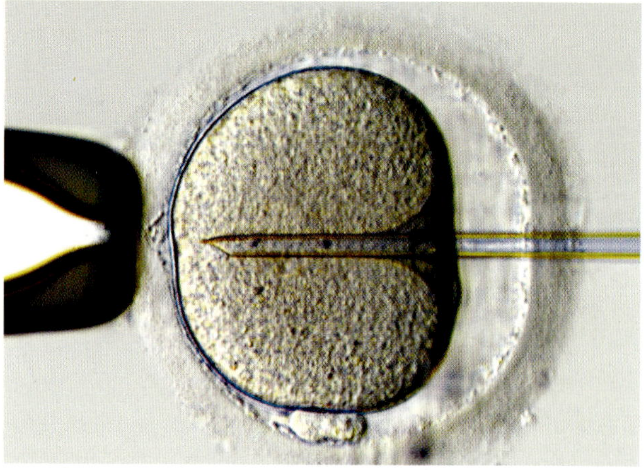

Figure 10.4 The injection pipette is plunged deeply into the ooplasm in an effort to pierce the oolemma

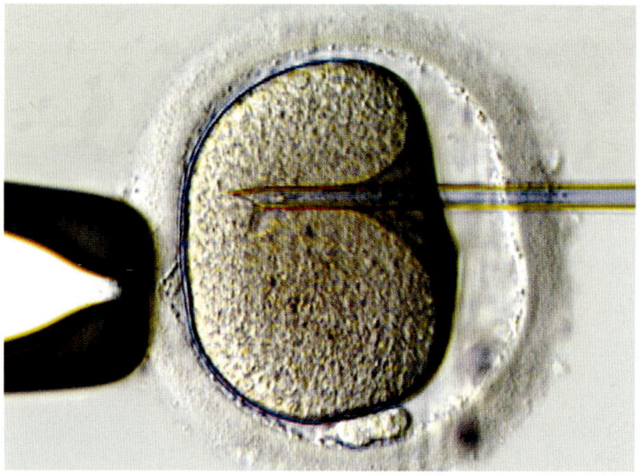

Figure 10.5 If the oolemma proves to be elastic and resists breakage, the injection pipette may be repositioned, hooking the upper or lower border of the invagination with the spike to penetrate the oocyte in a line parallel to its equatorial plane

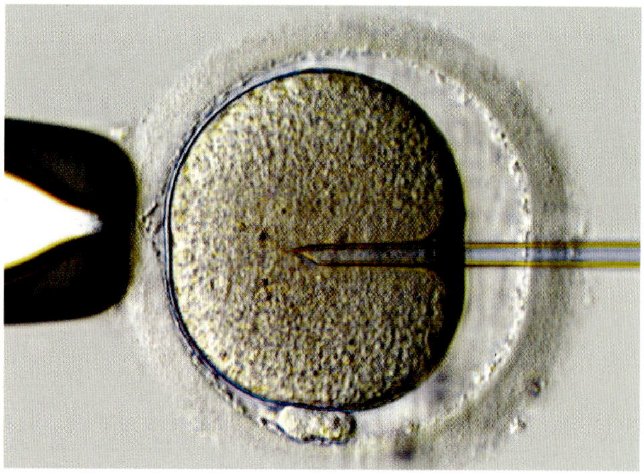

Figure 10.6 Once the spermatozoon is deposited and a bit of ooplasm has been aspirated and expelled, the injection pipette is gently withdrawn. Withdrawal is accomplished by exerting a slight negative pressure, leaving a nearly closed funnel-shaped formation in the ooplasm

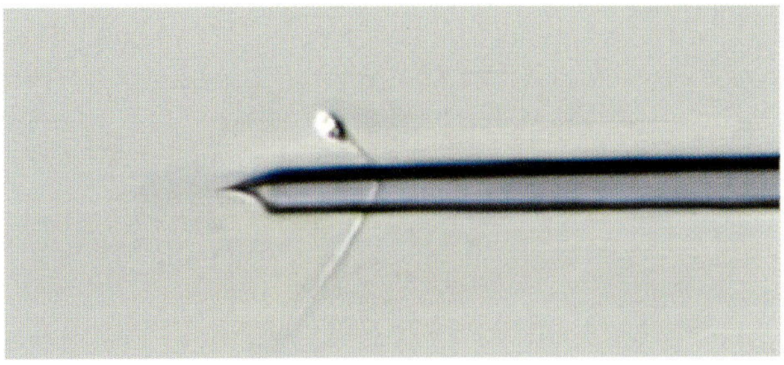

Figure 10.7 The immobilization procedure may briefly distort the spermatozoon flagellum. This is easily remedied by aspiration of the sperm one or more times in and out of the injection pipette

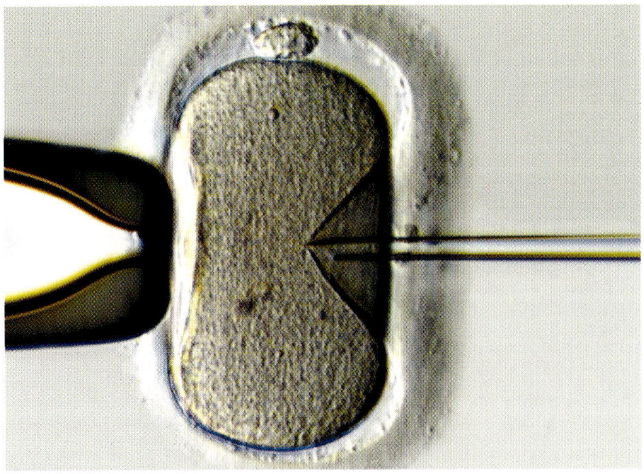

Figure 10.8 The zona pellucida is pierced

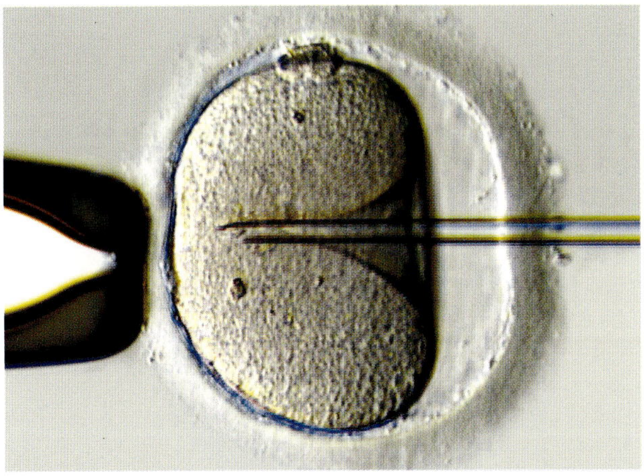

Figure 10.9 An elastic membrane is evident by the distinct funnel-shaped formation produced with pressure of the injection pipette

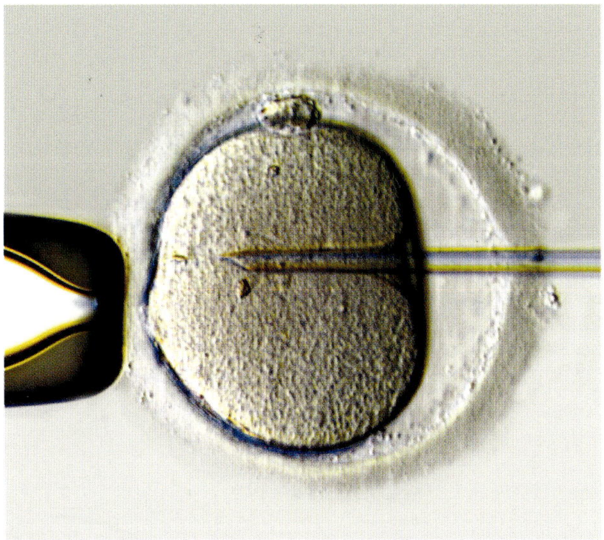

Figure 10.10 When the membrane is broken, the spermatozoon is deposited deep within the ooplasm after aspiration and expulsion of a small amount of cytoplasm

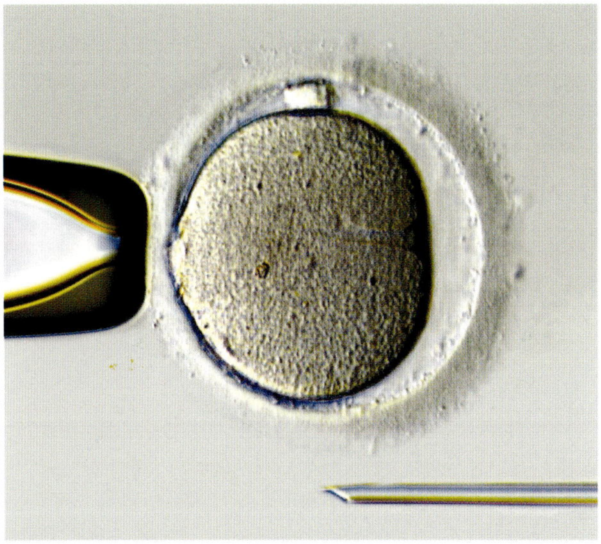

Figure 10.11 When the injection pipette is withdrawn properly (with application of a slight negative pressure), the funnel-shaped formation becomes less evident

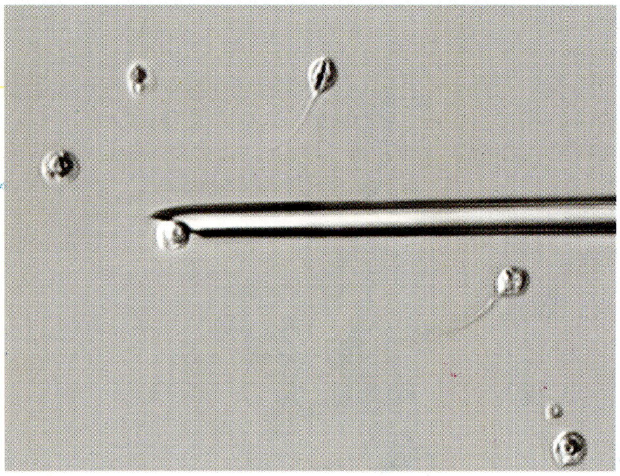

Figure 10.12 A round spermatid is aspirated into the injection pipette. Elongated spermatids have also been selected for potential injection

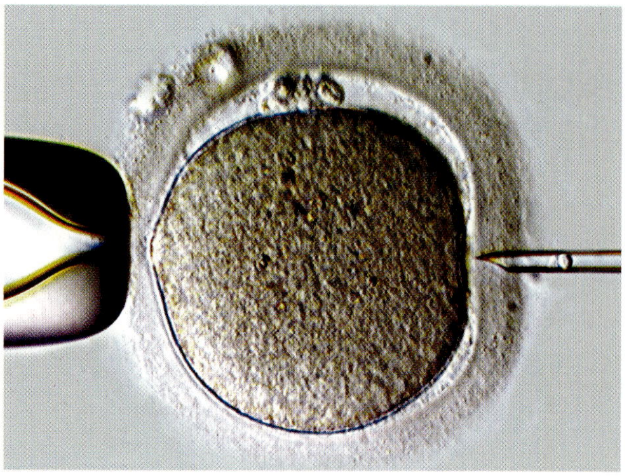

Figure 10.13 The spermatid is brought to the tip of the injection pipette

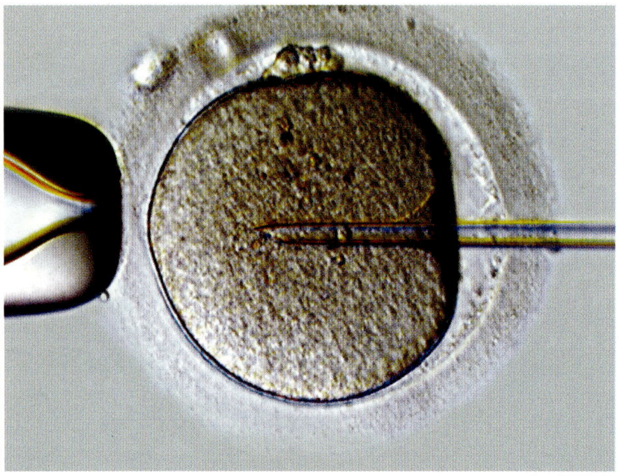

Figure 10.14 The injection pipette is inserted deeply into the ooplasm

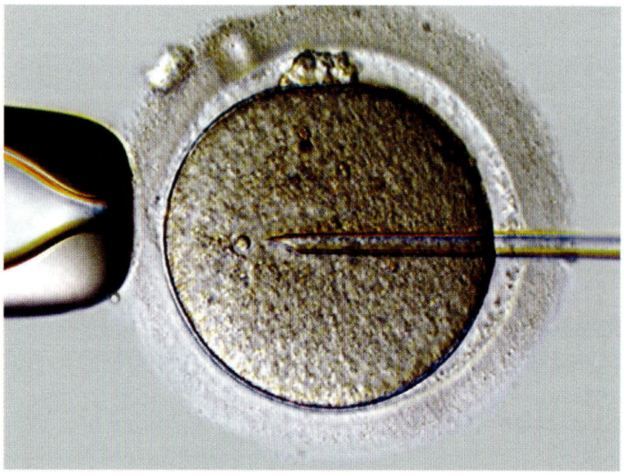

Figure 10.15 The spermatid is expelled into the ooplasm after aggressive aspiration and expulsion of a small amount of cytoplasm

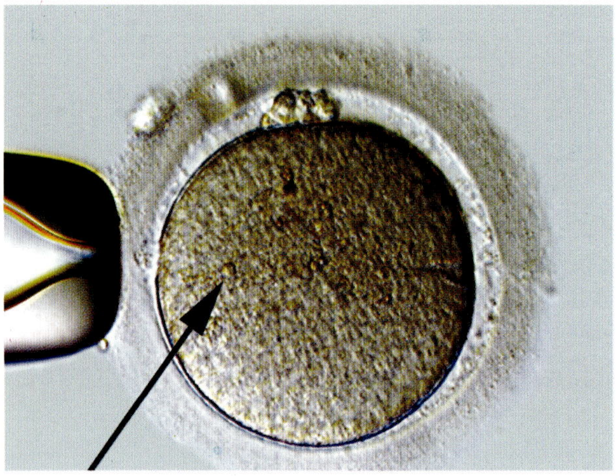

Figure 10.16 The spermatid can be visualized (arrowed) within the ooplasm after the injection pipette is removed

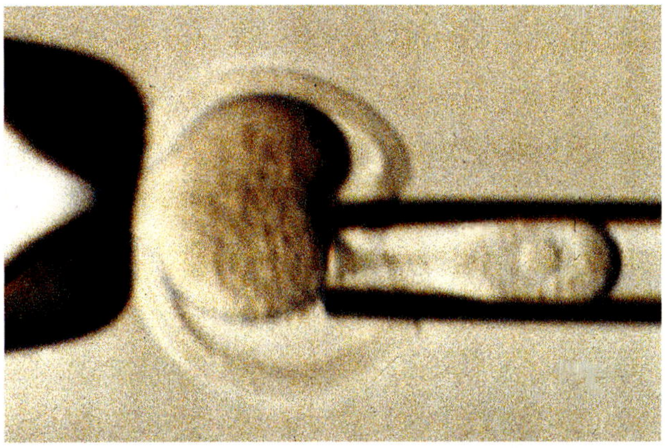

Figure 10.17 Enucleation of mouse oocyte number I for nuclear transplantation

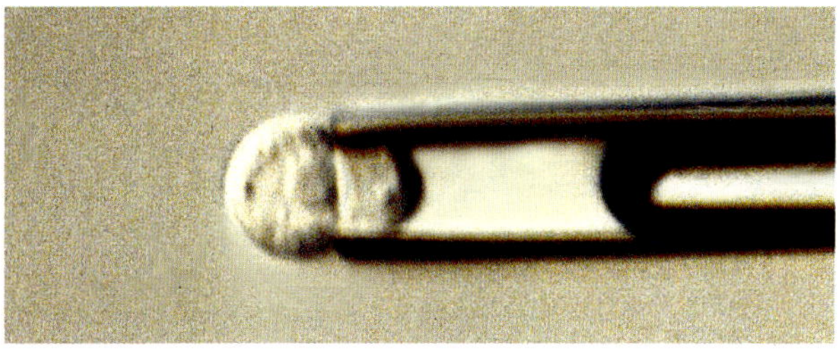

Figure 10.18 Enucleated nucleus from second oocyte in micropipette

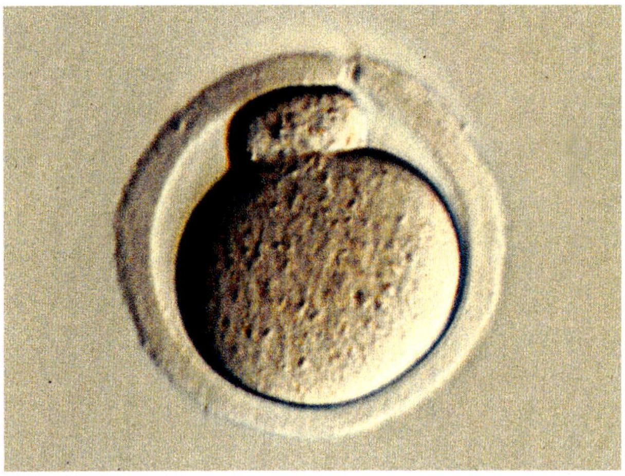

Figure 10.19 Electrofused oocyte number I and nucleus number 2

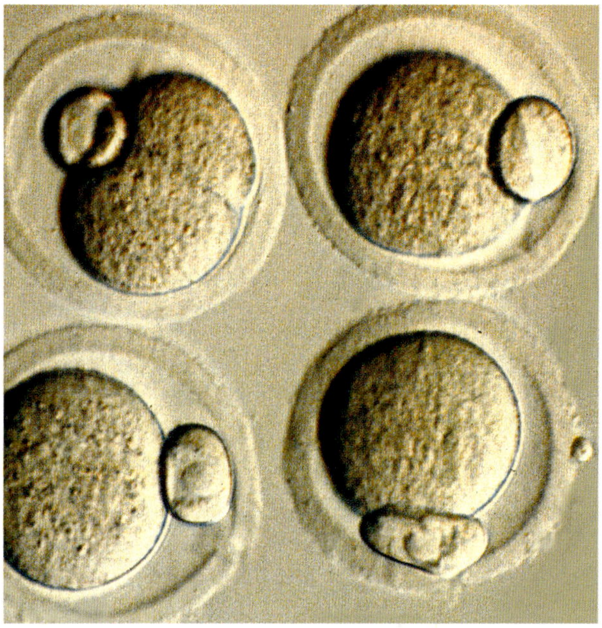

Figure 10.20 The reconstituted oocytes

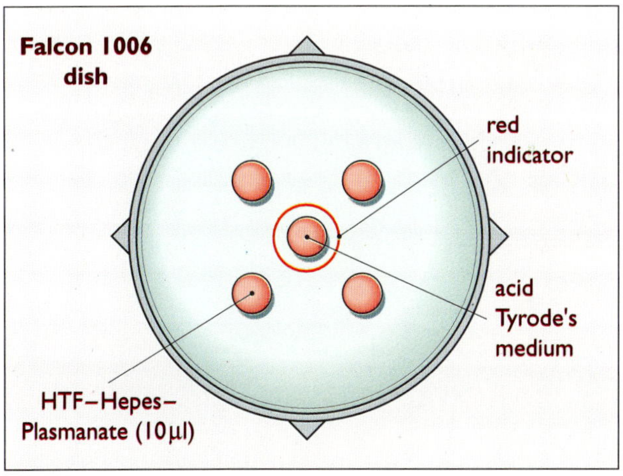

Figure 11.1 Diagrammatic representation of an AHA dish containing one drop of acid Tyrode's (AT) medium and four working droplets

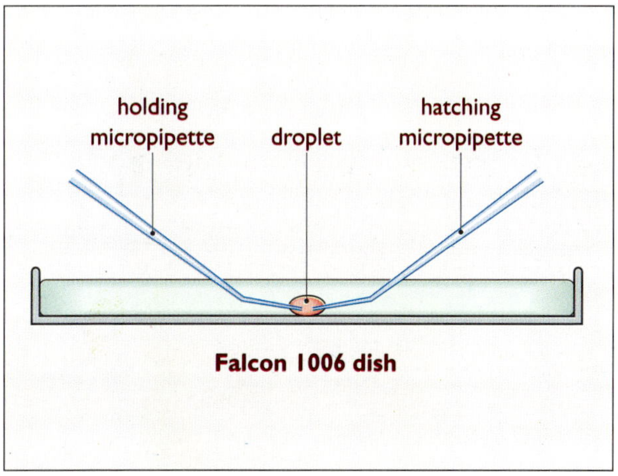

Figure 11.2 Diagrammatic representation of micropipette alignment in the AHA dish

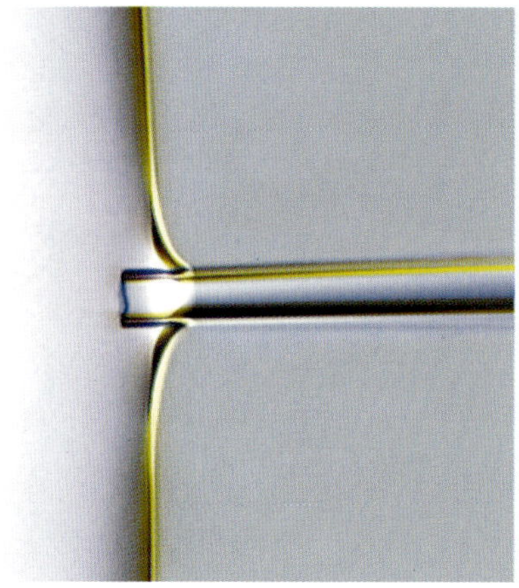

Figure 11.3 The AHA micropipette is loaded with AT solution

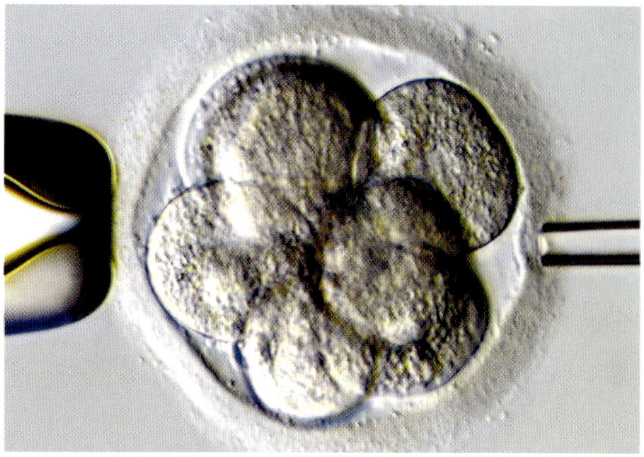

Figure 11.4 The preembryo is positioned so that the AHA micropipette aims at a space between the blastomeres

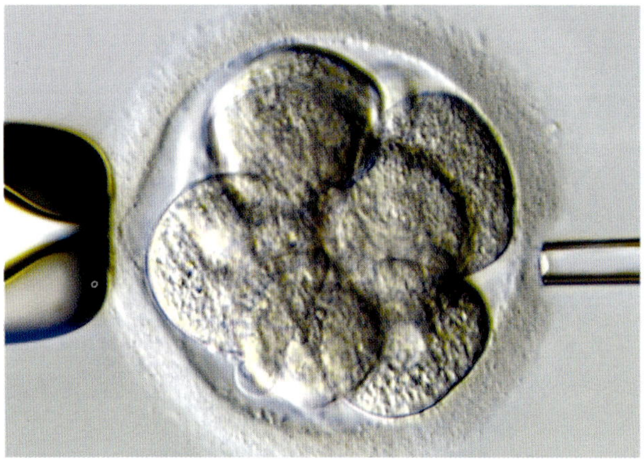

Figure 11.5 AT solution is gently expelled over a small area (20–30μm) of the zona pellucida

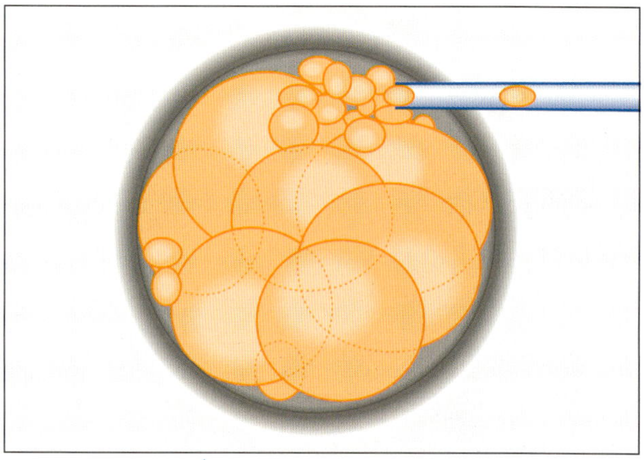

Figure 11.6 Diagrammatic representation of fragment removal

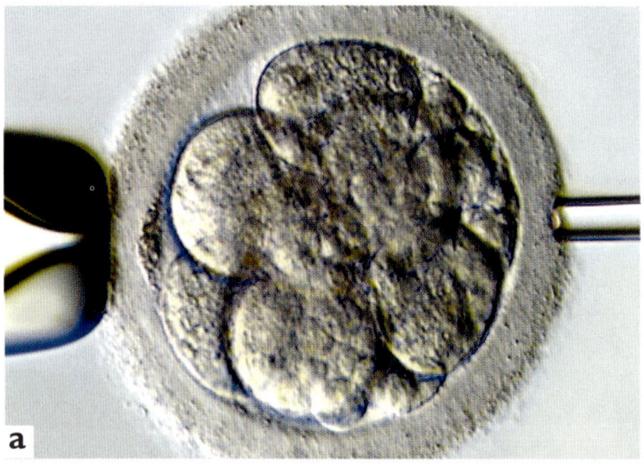

a

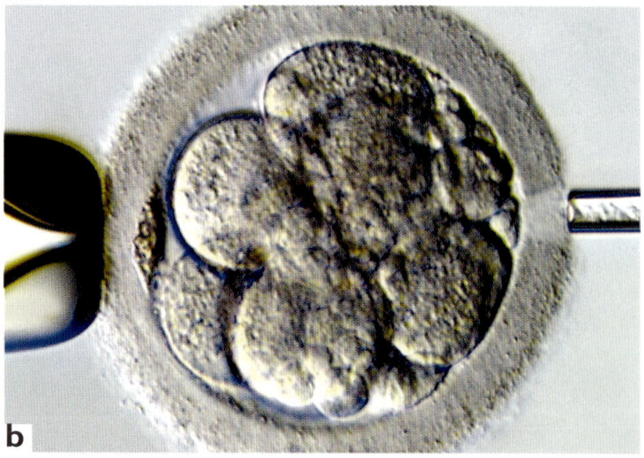

b

Figure 11.7 The preembryo is positioned so that the AHA micropipette aims at an area of fragmentation between blastomeres (a). Once the zona is open, expulsion of AT solution is immediately stopped. Gentle suction removes traces of AT from the immediate area (b)

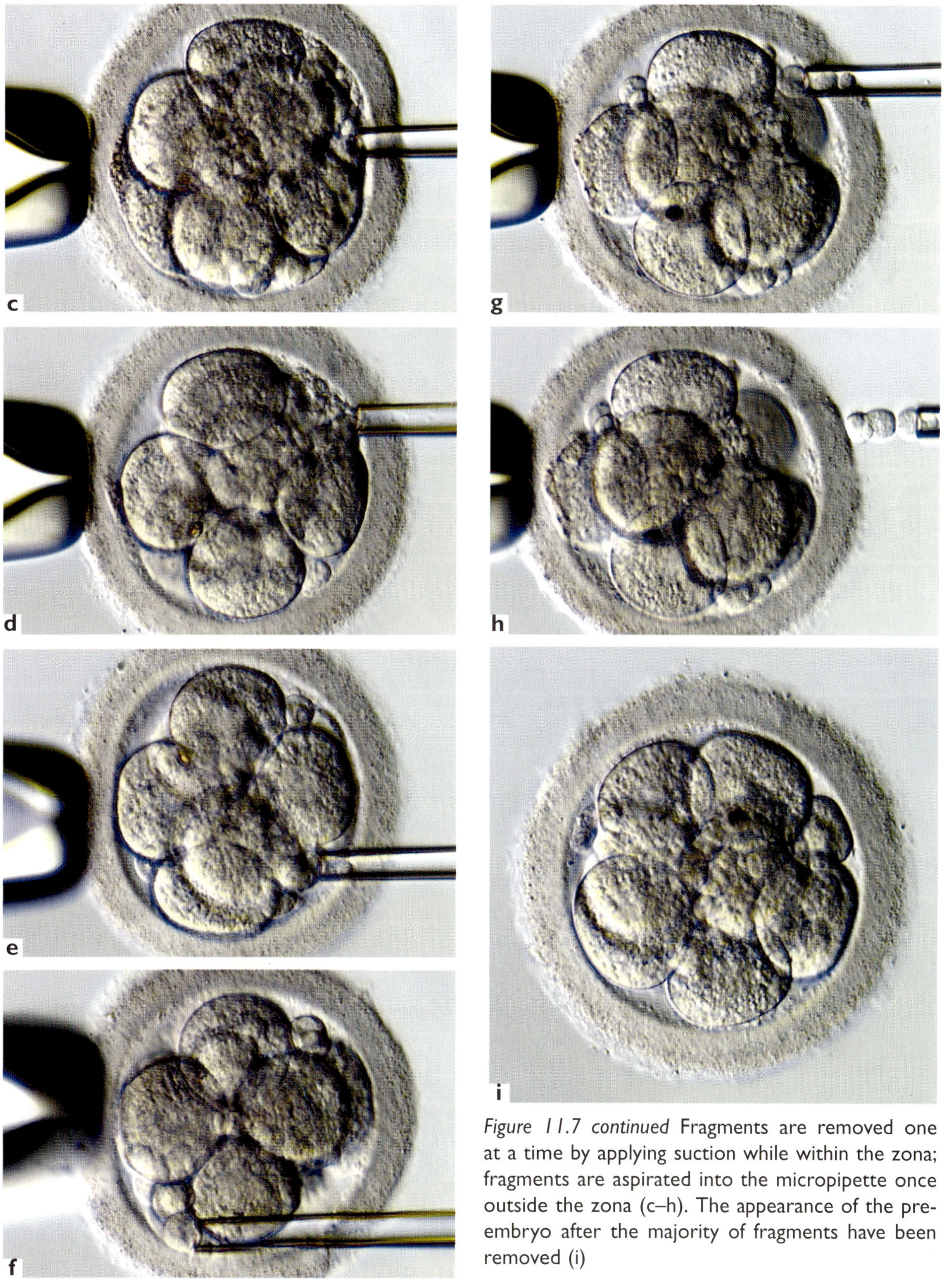

Figure 11.7 continued Fragments are removed one at a time by applying suction while within the zona; fragments are aspirated into the micropipette once outside the zona (c–h). The appearance of the pre-embryo after the majority of fragments have been removed (i)

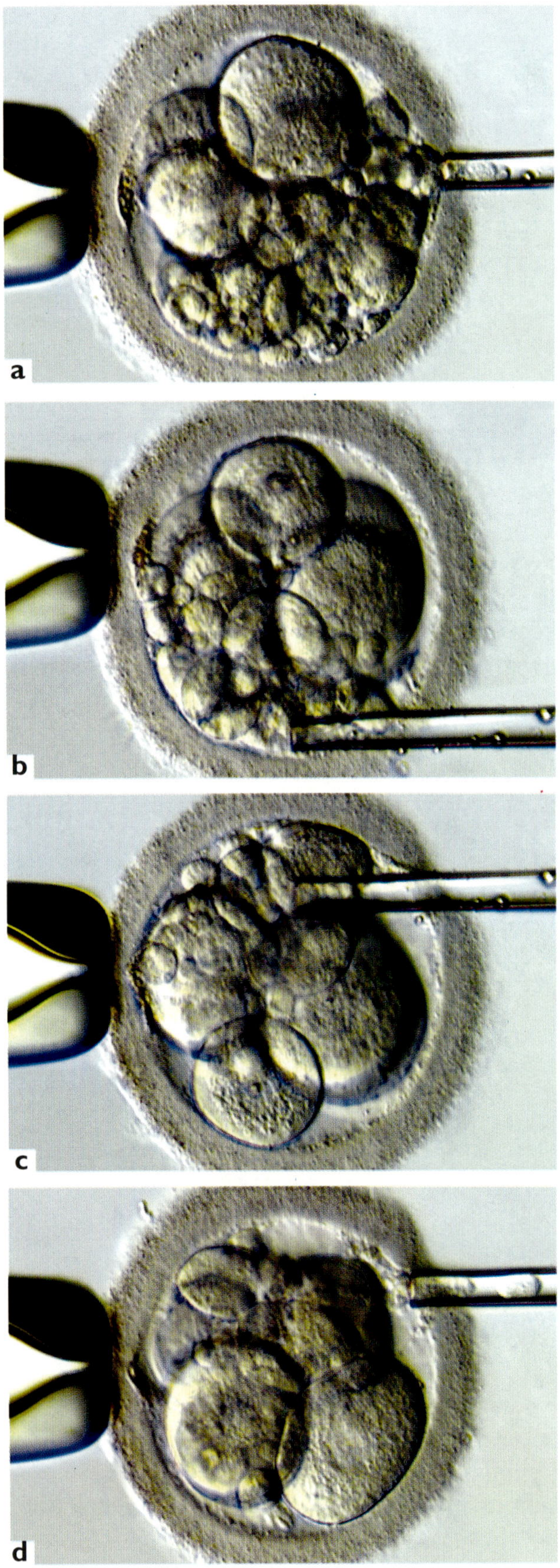

Figure 11.8 To facilitate visualization and removal of fragments, the preembryo can be rotated on the holding micropipette (a–d)

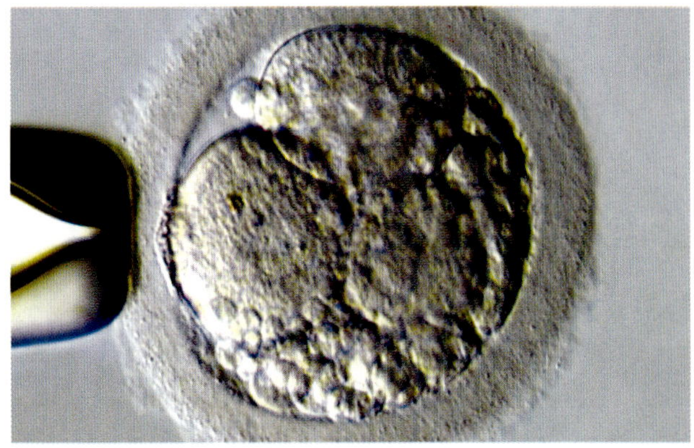

Figure 11.9 A poor-quality preembryo before AHA and fragment removal

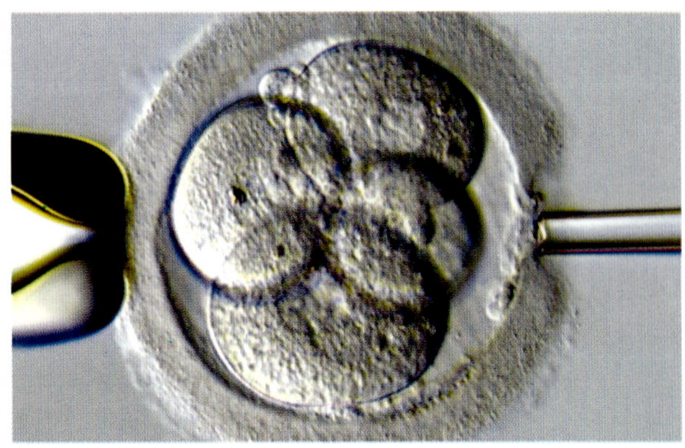

Figure 11.10 The same preembryo as in Figure 11.9 has been much improved in appearance after AHA and clearing of fragments

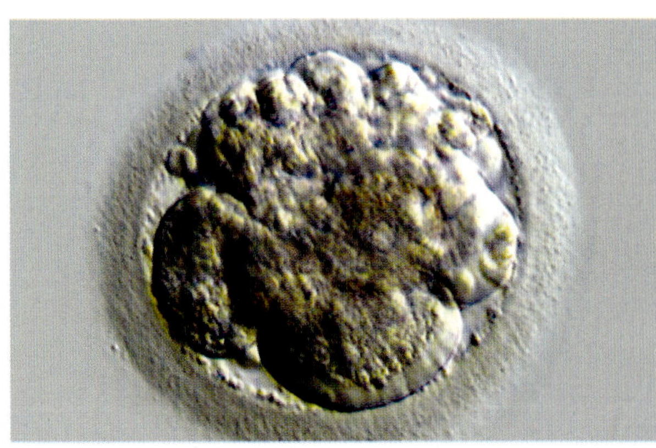

Figure 11.11 On day 2 and pre-AHA, a preembryo exhibits four blastomeres with clear cortical areas and > 30% fragmentation

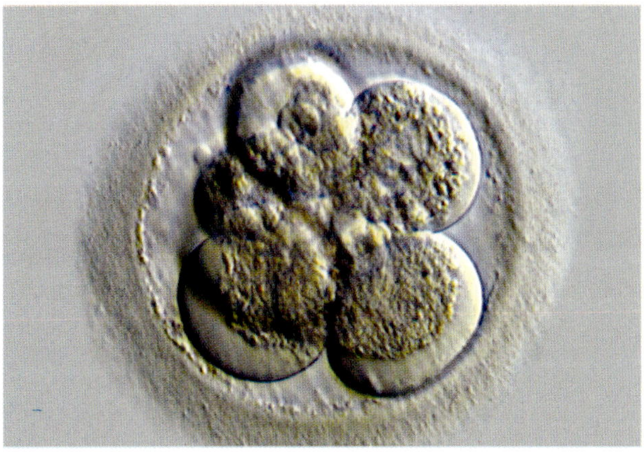

Figure 11.12 On day 3, the day after AHA was carried out, the same preembryo as in Figure 11.11 displays six or seven irregularly shaped blastomeres, still with clear cortical areas, but without further development of fragments. After intrauterine transfer together with another preembryo that was hatched on day 2 because of severe fragmentation, a clinical pregnancy was established, resulting in the birth of a normal child

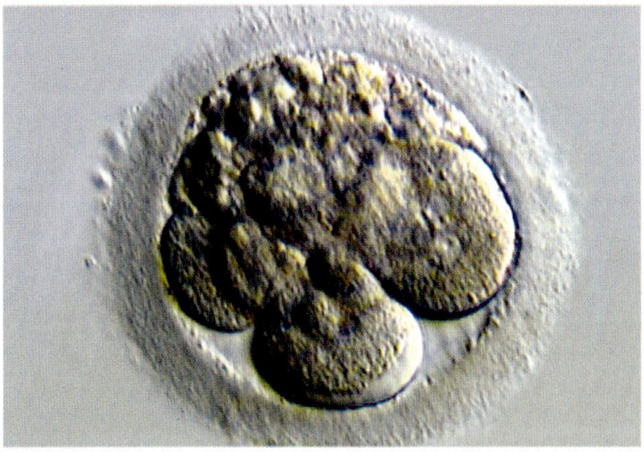

Figure 11.13 Control non-hatched preembryo from the same patient as in Figure 11.11. On day 2, the preembryo exhibits three blastomeres and significant fragmentation

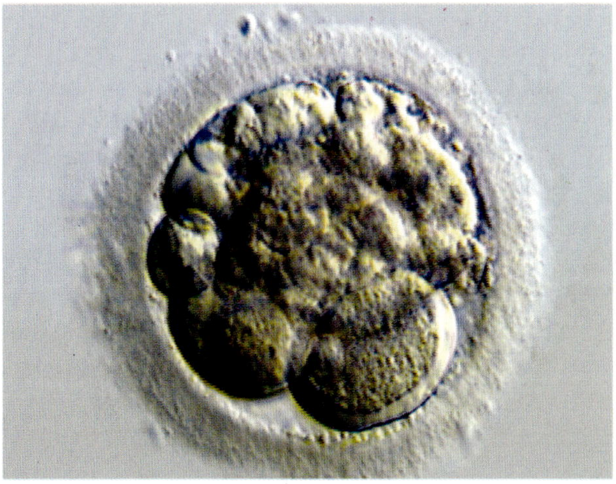

Figure 11.14 On day 3, the non-hatched preembryo exhibits only four blastomeres and increased fragmentation; this preembryo was not transferred

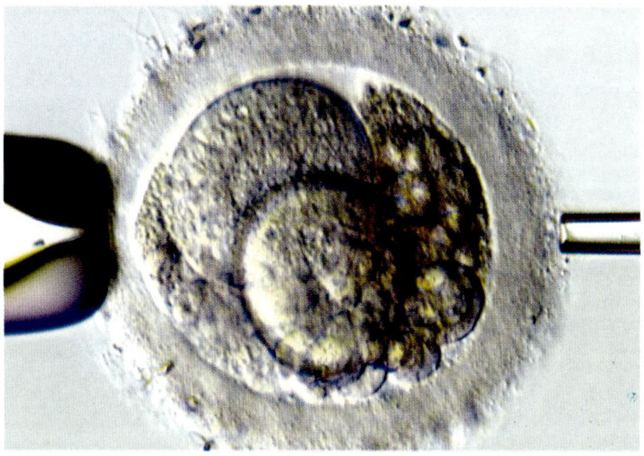

Figure 11.15 Preembryo frozen at the four-cell stage with two of four blastomeres surviving the thaw. The preembryo shows moderate fragmentation and a thick zona. It is oriented on the holding micropipette so that degenerative material and fragments are at a three-o'clock position

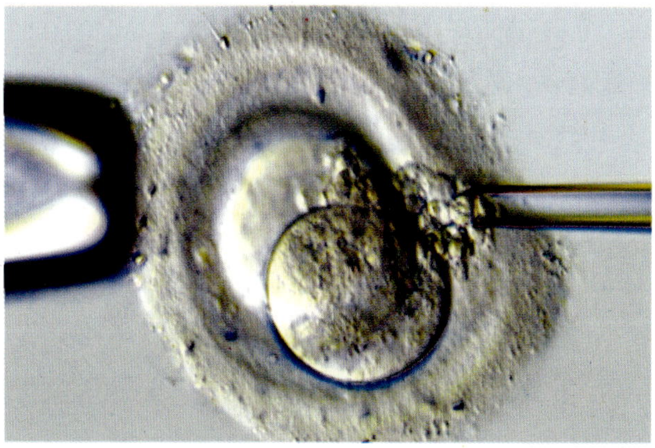

Figure 11.16 AHA is performed on the somewhat rigid, non-elastic zona. After thawing, degenerative material tends to be sticky so that fragment removal may be difficult

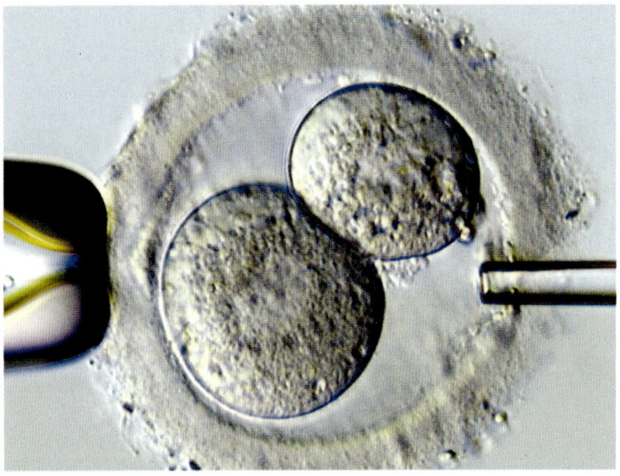

Figure 11.17 Cleaned preembryo after degenerative material and fragments have been removed

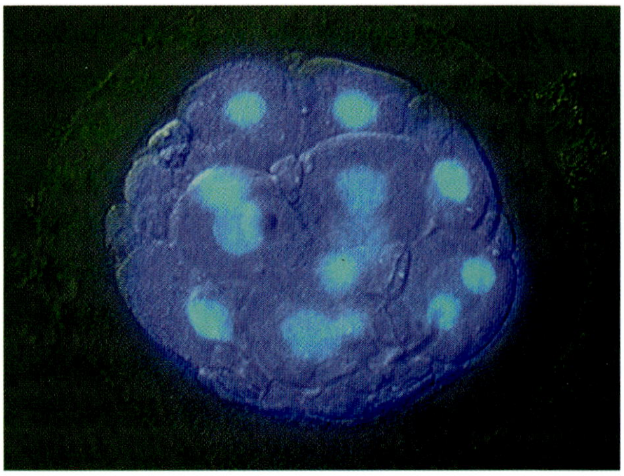

Figure 11.18 Arrested preembryo with 9 or 10 blastomeres and ~15% fragments, fixed and stained for DNA (DAPI staining; blue). This is a double exposure (DIC + DAPI). Some blastomeres show multinucleation. Note that the fragments at the ten-o'clock position do not contain DNA

Figure 12.1 Flowchart of procedures for preimplantation genetic diagnosis (PGD) in IVF according to time (D, day; W, week). Although some couples may be fertile and not in need of IVF, they may still be required to go through the IVF process to isolate gametes / preembryos for diagnosis. ICSI is necessary for polymerase chain reaction (PCR) analysis, regardless of semen quality, to eliminate the possibility of contamination from excess sperm DNA. Similarly, ICSI is preferred, though not absolutely necessary, for fluorescence in-situ hybridization (FISH). Freezing prezygotes after polar body biopsy and freezing biopsied preembryos may be feasible, but clinical success after cryopreservation of biopsied material remains to be evaluated. As PGD is still in a research stage, chorionic villus sampling (CVS) or amniocentesis is recommended to confirm results

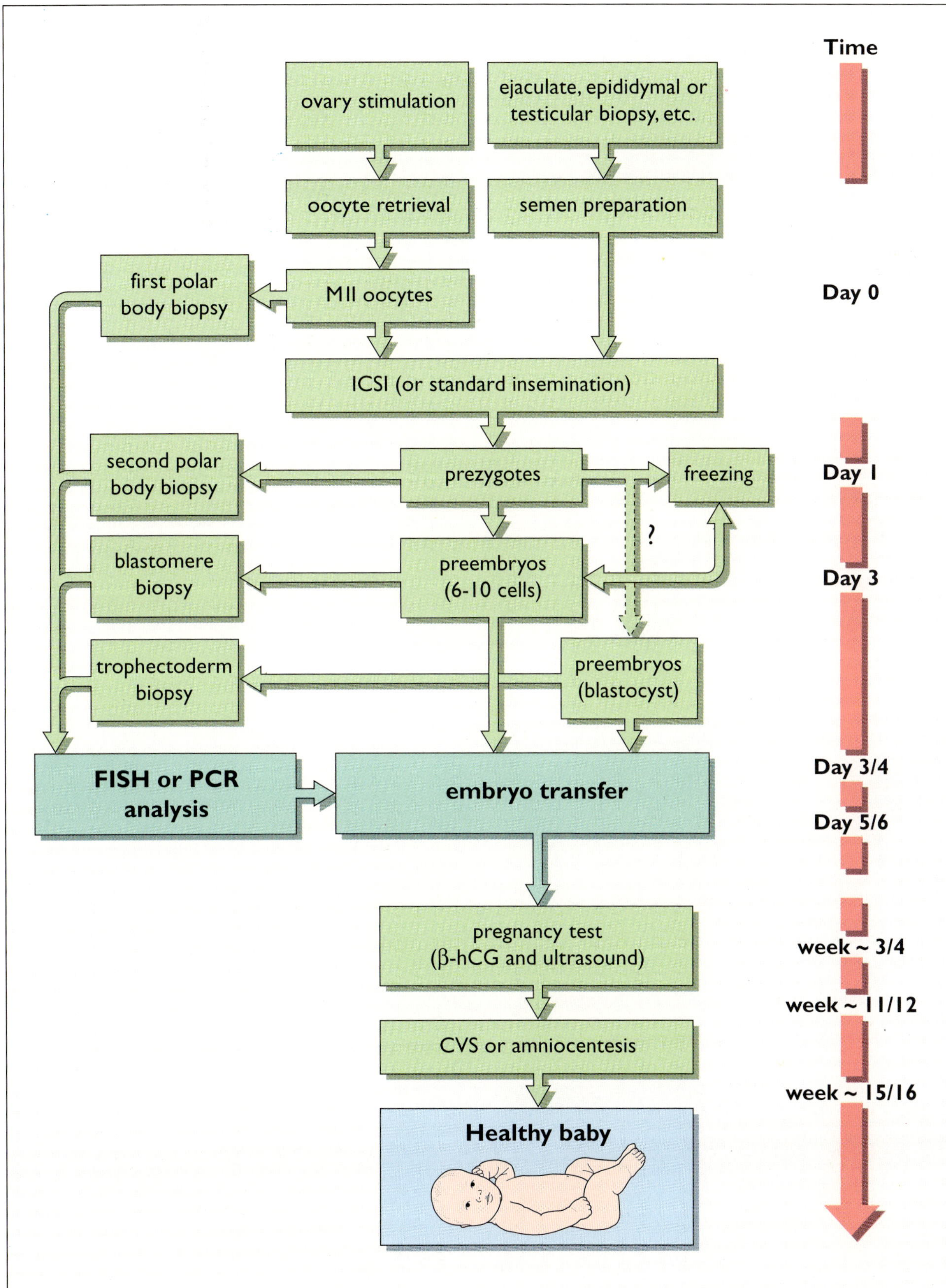
Time
ovary stimulation
ejaculate, epididymal or testicular biopsy, etc.
oocyte retrieval
semen preparation
first polar body biopsy
MII oocytes
Day 0
ICSI (or standard insemination)
second polar body biopsy
prezygotes
freezing
Day 1
?
blastomere biopsy
preembryos (6-10 cells)
Day 3
trophectoderm biopsy
preembryos (blastocyst)
FISH or PCR analysis
embryo transfer
Day 3/4
Day 5/6
pregnancy test (β-hCG and ultrasound)
week ~ 3/4
week ~ 11/12
CVS or amniocentesis
week ~ 15/16
Healthy baby

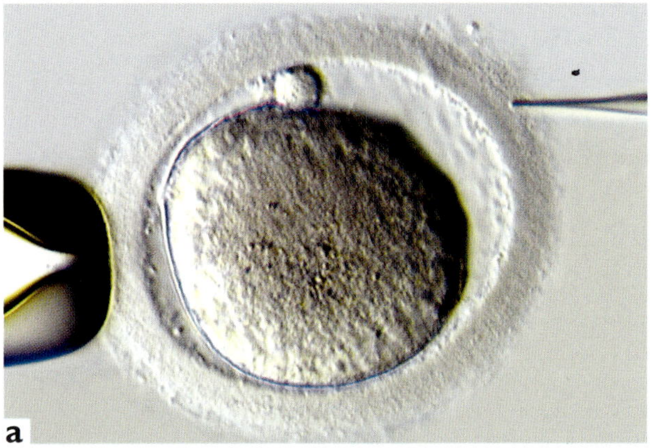

a

Figure 12.2 Among the approaches for polar body biopsy, a one-step technique utilizes a beveled needle to pierce the zona followed by negative pressure to suction out the polar body. Another method (a–d) uses a two-step approach. (a) First, the oocyte is held in place by a holding pipette with the polar body at a twelve-o'clock position. A sharp, thin, zona-dissection needle is used to penetrate the zona between one- and eleven-o'clock positions

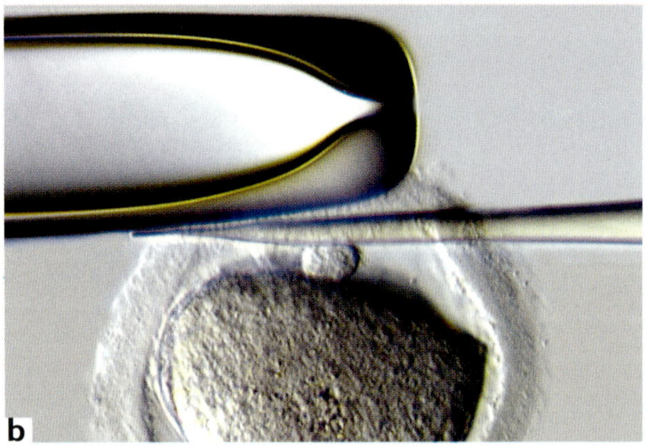

b

Figure 12.2 continued (b) The needle is pushed through the zona. The needle and oocyte are moved below the holding pipette, and a back-and-forth motion between the two glass microtools creates an opening in the zona which is approximately one-fifth the oocyte circumference. An opening may also be made by dissolving a portion of the zona with AT solution (as in AHA) or by using a laser[11]

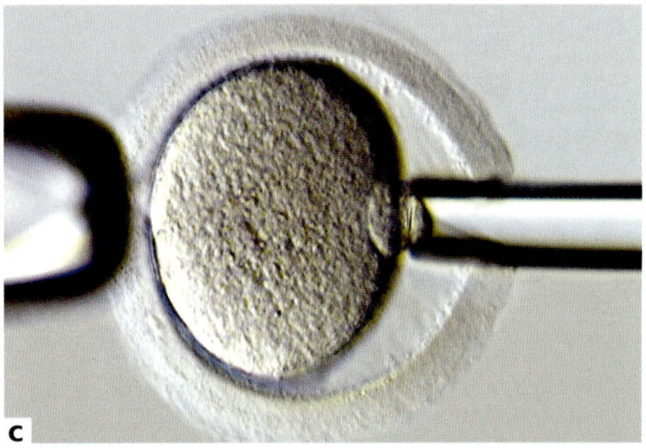

c

Figure 12.2 continued (c) After a slit or opening has been made, the oocyte is repositioned on the holding pipette with the opening and polar body facing three-o'clock. A smooth polished aspiration pipette (~20 μm internal diameter) is then used to gently suction out the polar body

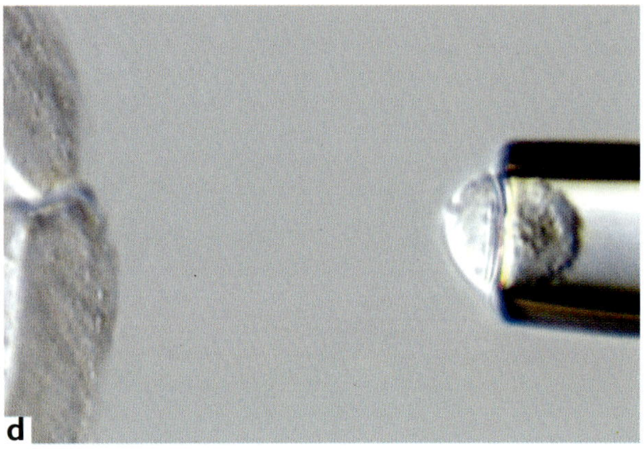

d

Figure 12.2 continued (d) Once removed, the polar body can be fixed for FISH chromosome analysis or used to exclude a single-gene defect by PCR

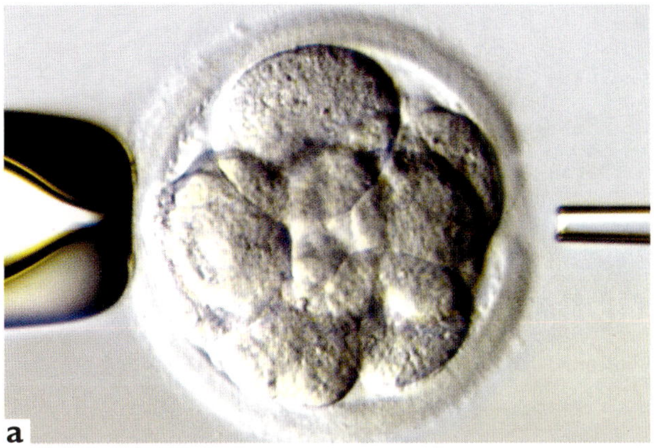

a

Figure 12.3 A common and reliable method for blastomere biopsy uses AT solution to open a hole in the zona (a–d). Ideally, the cell should lie clear of neighboring cells. (a) The cell to be biopsied is placed at a position between two- and four-o'clock. A slightly larger hole than for AHA is made (20–25 μm), using AT solution to allow easy passage of the biopsied cell. The size of the hole is particularly important when the preembryo has ≤6 blastomeres because of the larger blastomere diameters

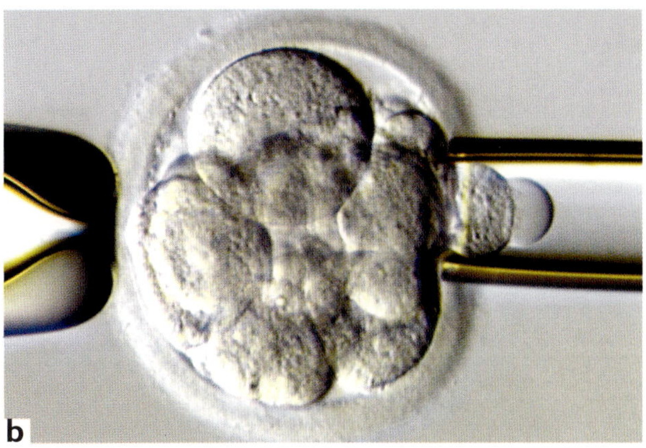

b

Figure 12.3 continued (b) After an appropriate hole has been made, the AT pipette is exchanged for a larger biopsy pipette. The well-polished tip of the biopsy pipette has an internal diameter of 45–55 μm and is preloaded with biopsy medium to avoid accidental oversuction of the blastomere. The pipette is slowly moved to the opening of the hole and the targeted cell; gentle suction is applied. Patience must be exercised when applying suction, especially if the preembryo has already begun compaction

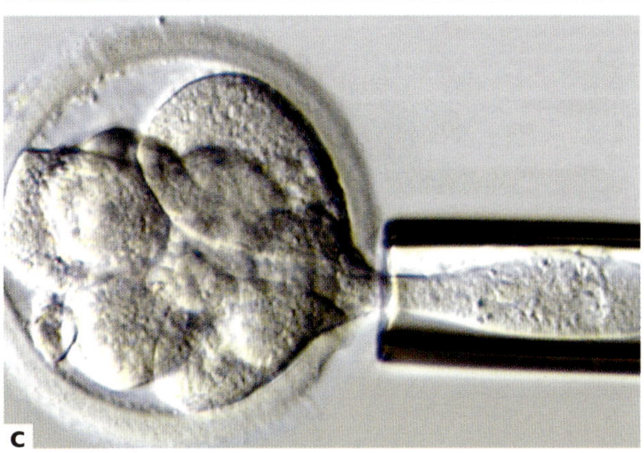

c

Figure 12.3 continued (c) Gently, the entire blastomere is pulled through the opening in the zona. After the blastomere has become detached from its neighboring cells and aspirated into the pipette, it is released nearby into the medium. A clear nucleus should be visible

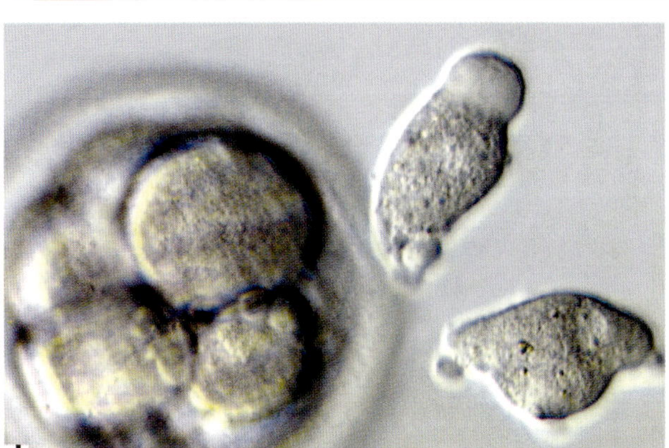

d

Figure 12.3 continued (d) Whenever possible, two blastomeres should be biopsied and analyzed independently to increase the accuracy of PGD

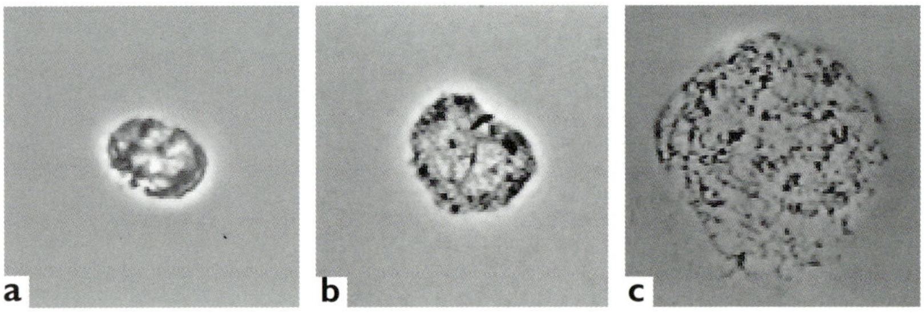

Figure 12.4 Phase-contrast microscopy (×200) showing blastomere fixation (a–c): One of two methods may be used: a classical air-drying method[17]; or a more recently developed spreading method using Tween-20 and HCl[18]. Ideally, an intact nucleus with little cytoplasm is obtained after appropriate fixation; in reality, various types of nuclei are observed by phase-contrast microscopy after fixation. In approximately one-third of fixed nuclei, a tightly condensed nucleus is seen (a); in another third, the nuclei are larger, but a clear boundary is observed (b); in the remaining third, chromosomal material may be dispersed, and no clear boundary is discernible (c)

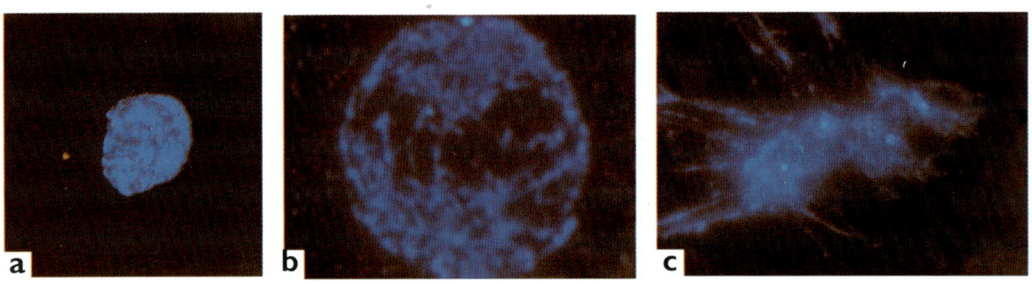

Figure 12.5 Blastomere fixation with DAPI staining (×400). As in Figure 12.4, three forms of nuclear morphology may be ascertained with DAPI staining used as a background for FISH analysis: (a) a tight and condensed nucleus; (b) a less condensed interphase nucleus; and (c) a very dispersed nucleus with no clear nuclear boundary

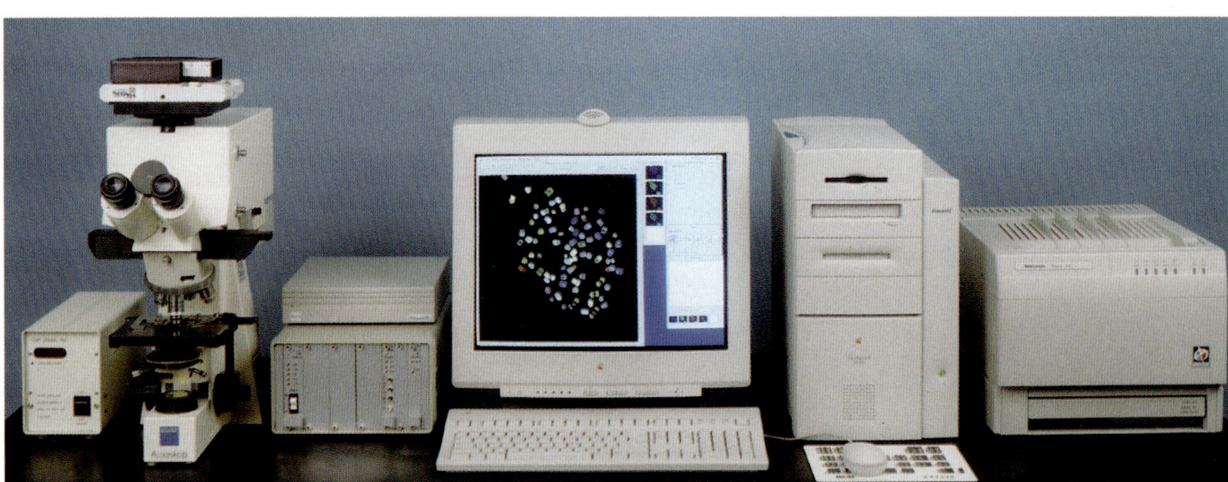

Figure 12.6 Imaging system for FISH–PGD. FISH results are analyzed under a fluorescent microscope using appropriate filters. Signals can be read directly and a diagnosis made. Recently, the development of new imaging systems has provided a much better means of not only analyzing FISH results, but also of creating imaging files that can be retrieved and studied at a later time. Computer software has been developed to assist in multicolor FISH analysis. (Courtesy of Vysis, Inc.)

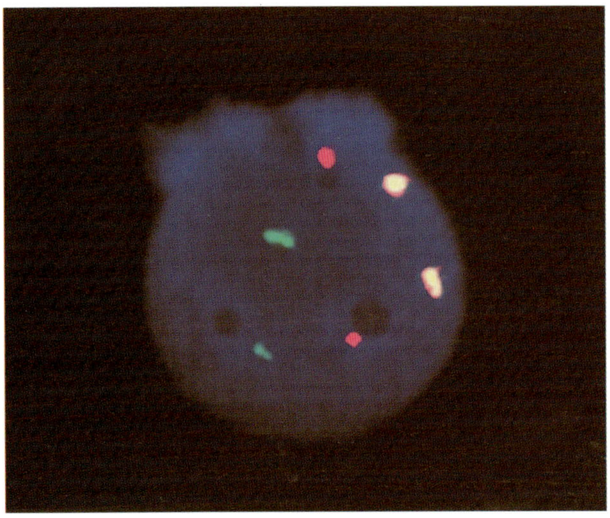

Figure 12.7 Normal XX cell with 2 × 16 and 2 × 18 chromosomes. The yellow X chromosomes are hybridized with a mixed probe (yellow color by 1 : 1 ratio of SpectrumOrange and SpectrumGreen probes (Vysis), and the two green chromosome 18s with the use of a chromosome 18-specific probe (SpectrumGreen; Vysis). The two red spots represent chromosome 16 (digoxigenin-labeled probe; Oncor). All three (X, 16, and 18) are specific for satellite DNA and, therefore, give strong and bright signals

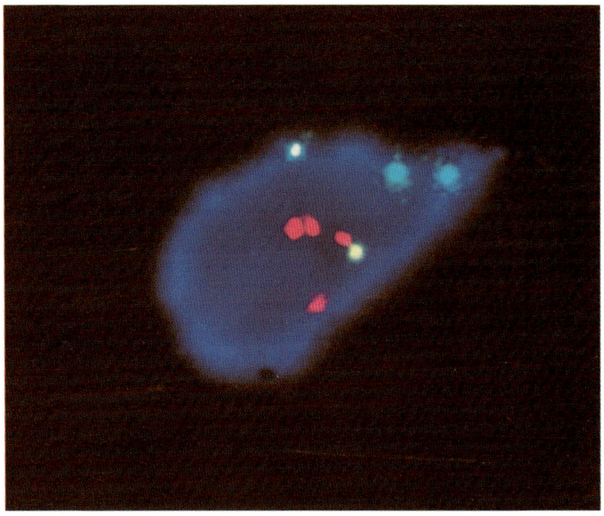

Figure 12.8 This XY cell with 2 × 18 and 4 × 13/21 chromosomes shows a normal finding of one yellow X chromosome (prepared as in Figure 12.7), one pale blue-green Y chromosome (SpectrumAqua; Vysis), two green chromosome 18s (as in Figure 12.7), and four red spots representing chromosomes 13 and 21 (13/21 probe; digoxigenin-labeled; Oncor). There is no distinction between chromosomes 13 and 21 as they share homology in the probe sequences

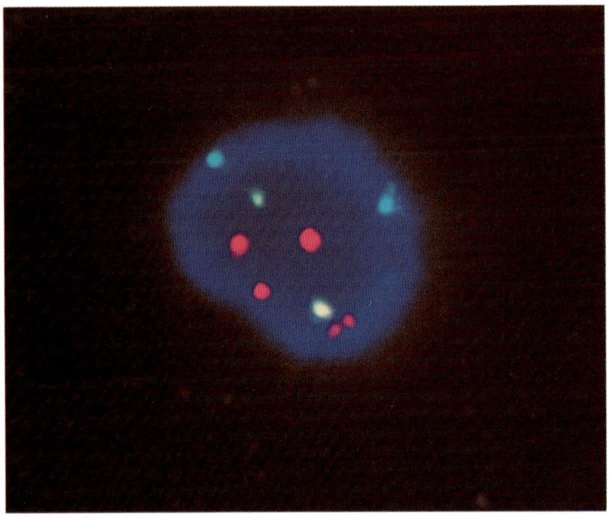

Figure 12.9 This XY cell with 2 × 18 and 5 × 13/21 chromosomes, viewed by the same probes as in Figures 12.7 and 12.8, shows an abnormal chromosome complement as indicated by five red spots. This represents a chromosome complement involving either trisomy 13 or trisomy 21

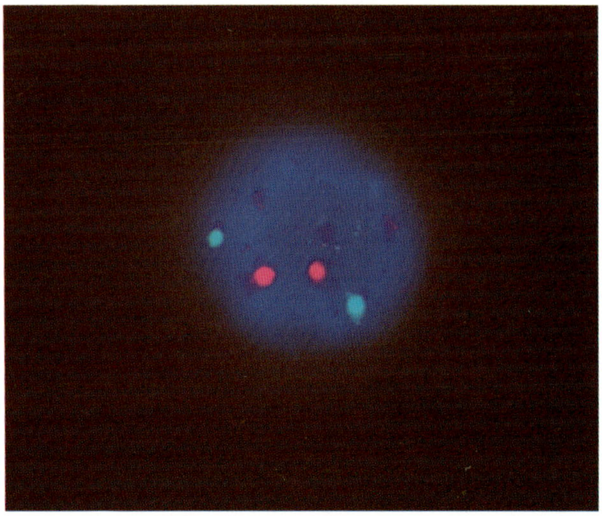

Figure 12.10 Normal 2 × 13, 2 × 21 chromosomes. To further distinguish chromosomes 13 and 21, locus-specific probes may be used. Shown here is a nucleus hybridized with specific probes for chromosomes 13 and 21 (LSI 13 SpectrumGreen and LSI 21 SpectrumOrange; Vysis)

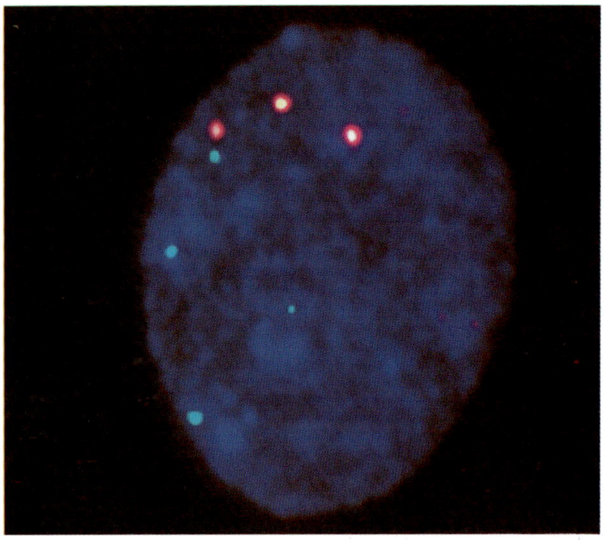

Figure 12.11 Triploid nucleus. When specific chromosome X and chromosome 18 probes are used, a nucleus with 3×X (yellow) and 3×18 (green) can be identified

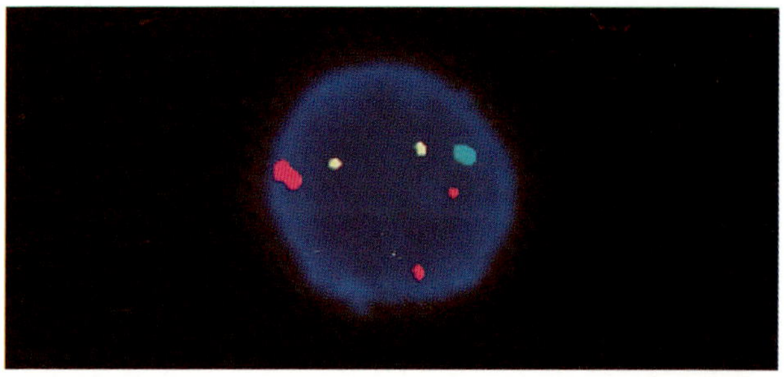

Figure 12.12 Overlapping signals. In some cases, signals are not clearly distinguishable. Using probes as in Figures 12.8 and 12.9, two clear X chromosomes are identified by two yellow dots. However, there are only three clearly separated red dots, one of which appears to be much larger than the other two, suggesting an overlapping signal. The green dot (chromosome 18) is less obviously overlapping as it appears to be only slightly larger than a normal signal. In such cases, a definitive diagnosis may not be possible for chromosome 18

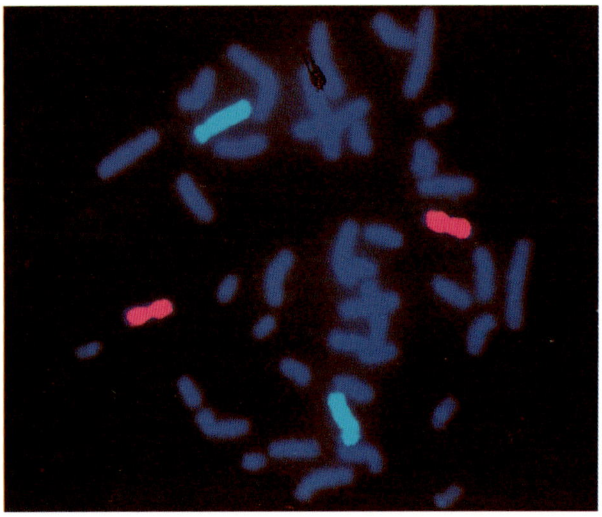

Figure 12.13 Chromosome painting probes for staining specific chromosomes have recently been proposed for use in the detection of chromosome translocations. In this example, a metaphase preparation from normal lymphocytes is hybridized with a whole chromosome painting probe (WCP 4, SpectrumGreen and WCP 11, SpectrumOrange; Vysis). The two normal chromosome 4s are painted green and the two normal chromosome 11s are orange

Figure 12.14 *(Facing page, upper left)* Painting probes can reveal a balanced translocation. This metaphase preparation from the lymphocytes of a patient with a reciprocal balanced translocation [46XX, t(4;11)(q21;q13)] was hybridized with two whole chromosome painting probes (reversed color combinations compared with Figure 12.13; WCP 4, SpectrumOrange and WCP 11, SpectrumGreen; Vysis). A normal chromosome 4 (orange) is located near the center of the metaphase plate, and a normal chromosome 11 (green) lies above it and slightly to the right. The chromosomes carrying the balanced translocation sit directly to the left and right of the large normal orange chromosome. A translocated segment of chromosome 4 is attached to chromosome 11 at a nine-o'clock position, and a small green segment from chromosome 11 is linked to chromosome 4 at a three-o'clock position. As demonstrated by the small nucleus to the lower right of the larger metaphase plate, painting probes are not useful for analyzing translocations at interphase of the cell cycle

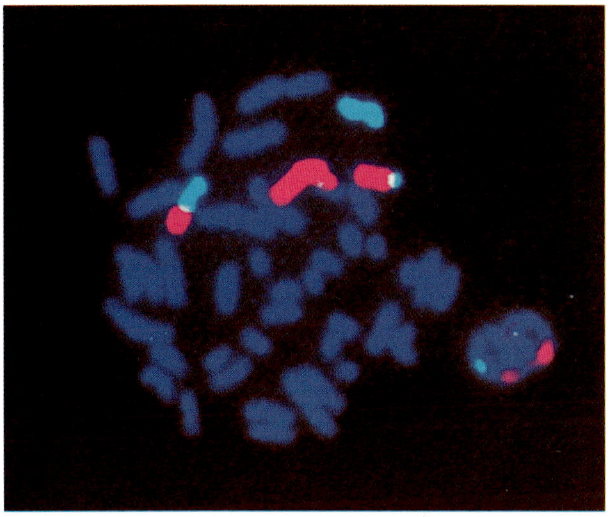

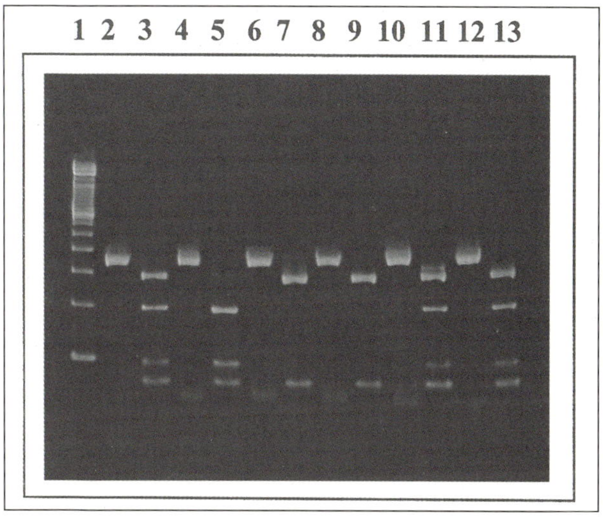

Figure 12.16 PCR–PGD for sickle cell anemia, another common genetic disorder for which methods are available to detect the specific mutation[20]. With this approach, also using a nested PCR technique, a 364-bp DNA fragment is amplified. There are two Dde I sites in a normal DNA fragment and three DNA fragments after DNA is digested with enzyme. Because the sickle cell mutation abolishes one Dde I site, only two fragments remain after enzymatic digestion of the amplified DNA of an affected individual. In a carrier who is heterozygous for the allele, both DNA digestion patterns are present. Lane 1, DNA size marker (100-bp ladder); lanes 2, 4, 6, 8, 10, 12, amplified DNA from five single blastomeres before enzyme digestion; lane 5, Dde I digested DNA from a normal blastomere (showing 201-, 90-, and 74-bp bands); lanes 3, 11, 13, Dde I digested DNA from three carrier blastomeres (showing 291-, 201-, 90-, and 74-bp bands); lanes 7, 9, Dde I digested DNA from two affected blastomeres (showing 291- and 74-bp bands)

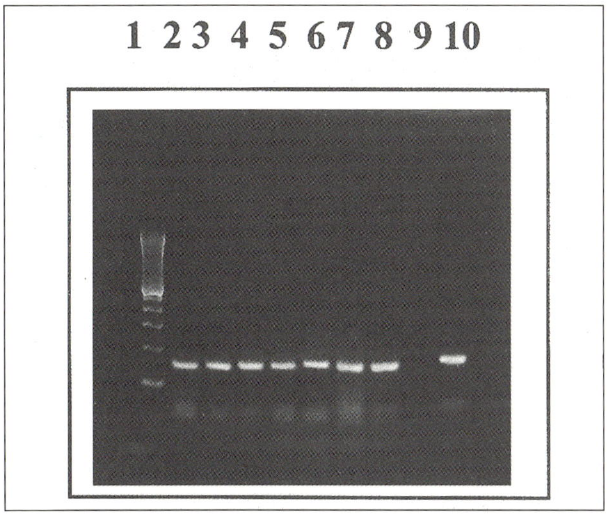

Figure 12.15 Successful PCR amplification of exon 10 of the CFTR (cystic fibrosis) gene from seven single blastomeres of an unaffected preembryo using a protocol described by Handyside and colleagues[19]. The most common mutation on the CFTR gene is located on exon 10 (ΔF508). By a nested PCR approach, a DNA fragment of 154 base pairs (bp) can be obtained from a normal individual. In an affected individual with a 3-bp nucleotide deletion, a 151-bp DNA fragment is amplified whereas a carrier may possess both 151- and 154-bp fragments. Lane 1, DNA size marker (100-bp ladder); lanes 2–8, PCR products from a single cell (nest PCR); lane 9, cell-wash medium (negative control); lane 10, genomic DNA as template (positive control)

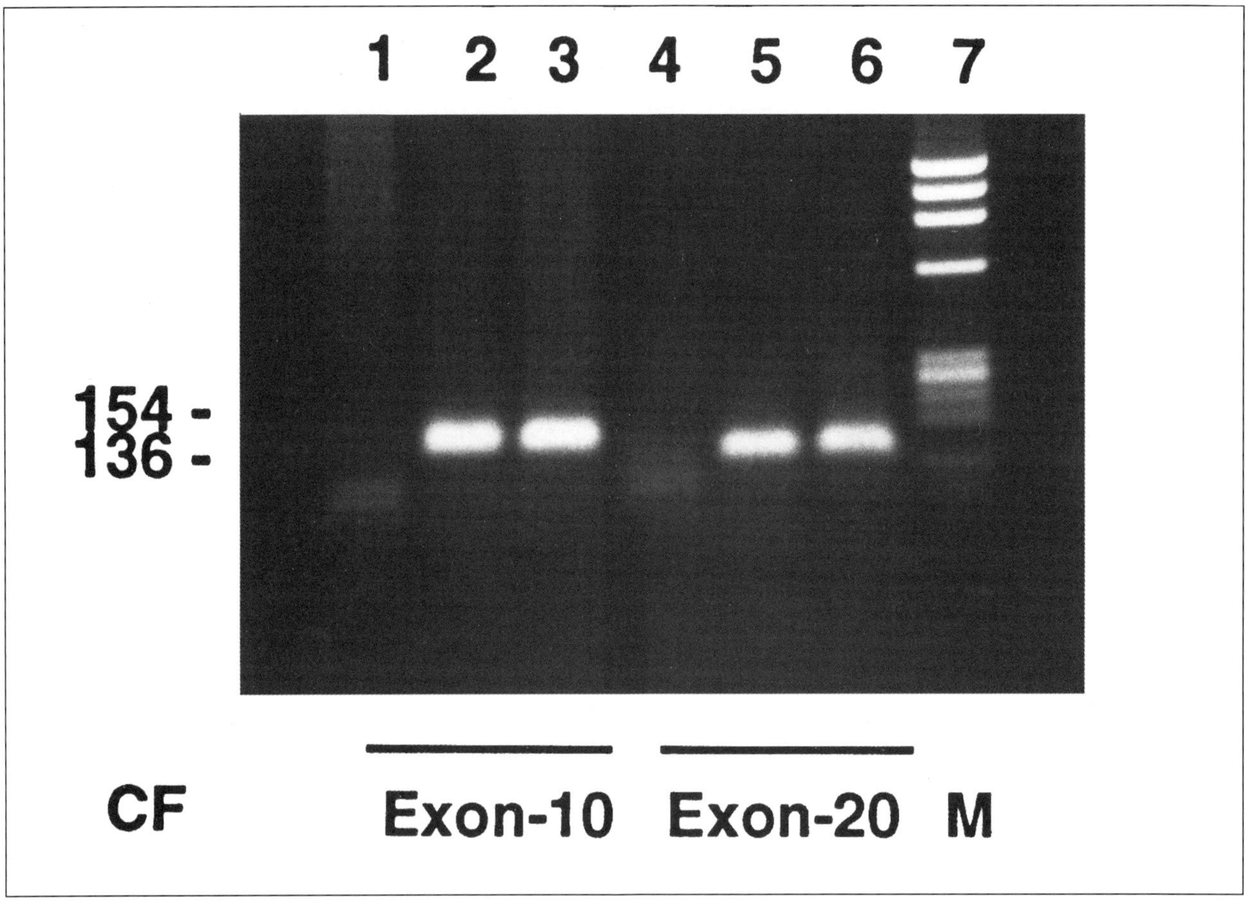

Figure 12.17 Multiplex PCR for cystic fibrosis exons 10 and 20. PCR is so powerful a tool that not only can a single mutation be detected, but two or more may also be analyzed. Thus, in cases where compound mutations are involved with one partner carrying one mutation and the other partner carrying another, multiplex PCR may be applied. If a partner has a ΔF508 mutation (located on the CFTR gene exon 10), and the other has a W1282X mutation (located on the CFTR gene exon 20), multiplex PCR may detect both loci in a single blastomere of their offspring.

Multiplex PCR is accomplished by adding both pairs of primers in the first round of PCR, after which aliquots (for example, 2–5 μl) are taken from the first PCR as templates for the second round of PCR. In this example, lanes 1 and 4 are negative controls, and lanes 2 and 3 are amplified DNA fragments from exon 10, using Handyside et al. protocol[19]. Lanes 5 and 6 are amplified DNA fragments (exon 20), using a protocol developed in our own laboratory (unpublished). Both DNA fragments for exons 10 and 20 are amplified from a single cell (lanes 2 and 5 are from blastomere 1, and lanes 3 and 6 from blastomere 2)

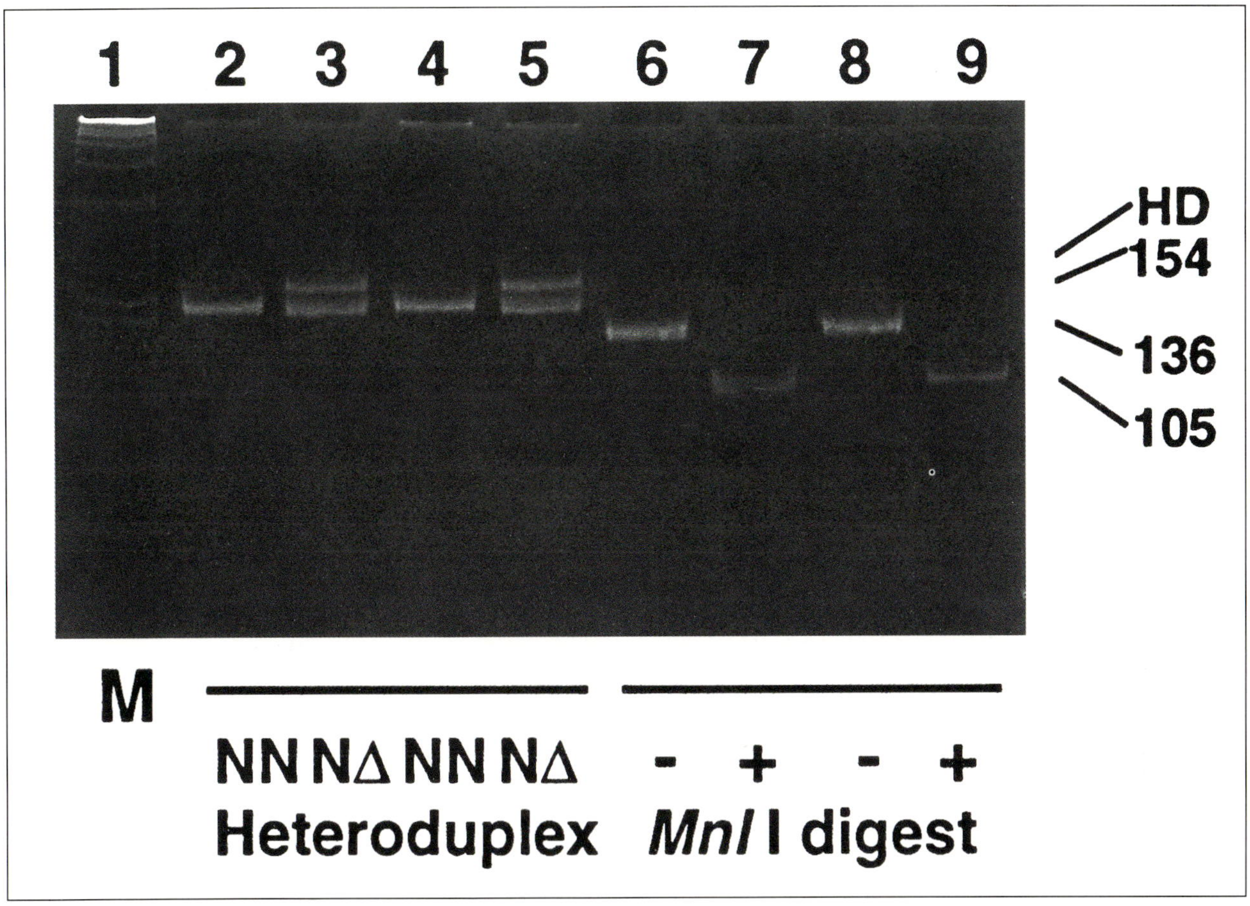

Figure 12.18 Heteroduplex formation and restriction enzyme analysis. A detailed procedure for heteroduplex formation has been described[19]. As in Figure 12.17, after multiplex PCR for CF exons 10 and 20, both products from blastomeres 1 and 2 are subjected to the two different mutation detection methods, and both results may be obtained from all individual cells (lanes 2 and 7 are from blastomere 1, and lanes 4 and 9 from blastomere 2)

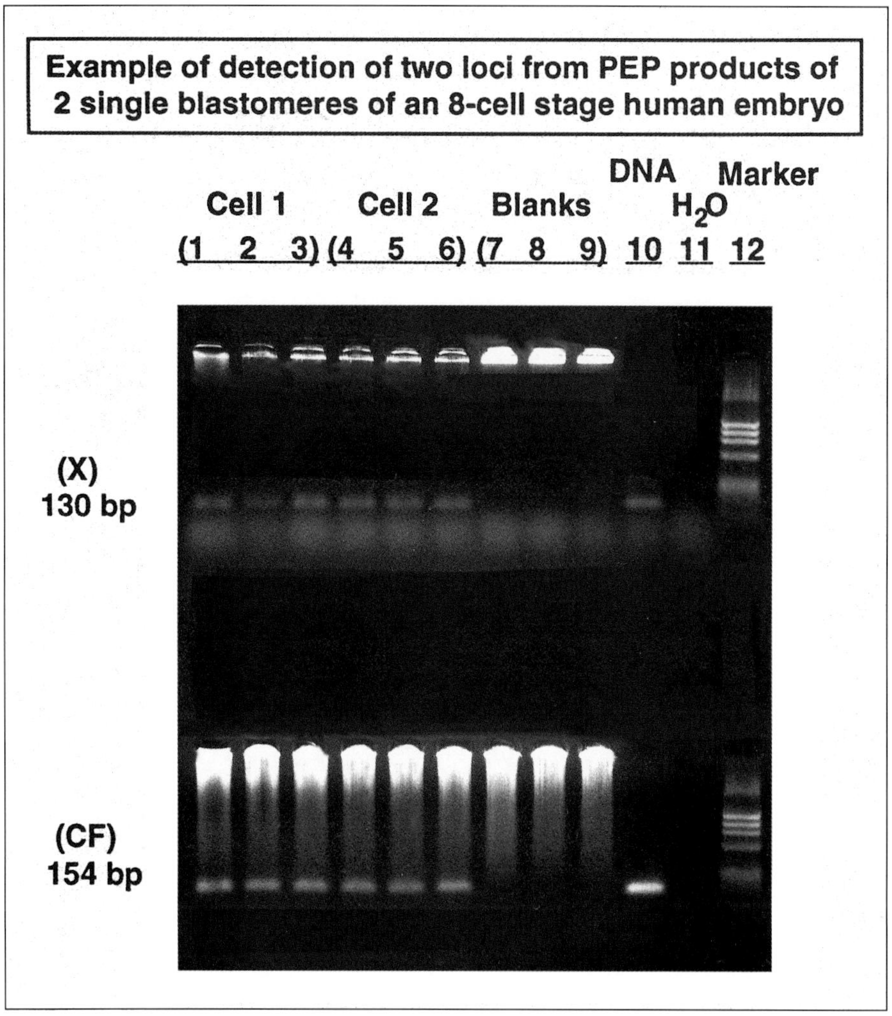

Figure 12.19 Whole genome amplification. Primer extension preamplification (PEP) was reported a few years ago by Zhang and colleagues[8]. Using this technique, whole genomic DNA from a single sperm was successfully amplified using 15-bp oligonucleotide random primers. Similarly, DNA from single blastomeres may be amplified. Aliquots of PEP products were tested with two specific sequences. Three aliquots from each PEP product were used as PCR templates. PCR-amplified products were analyzed by gel electrophoresis. Typically, a 130-bp fragment can be amplified from the human X chromosome (X)[21], and a 154-bp fragment can be amplified from exon 10 of the cystic fibrosis (CF) gene[19]. (Courtesy of Xu *et al.*[9], reproduced with permission)

Index

The page numbers in **bold** refer to figures.

P